Fundamentals of Nuclear Pharmacy
Fifth Edition

Gopal B. Saha

Fundamentals of
Nuclear Pharmacy

Fifth Edition

With 102 Figures

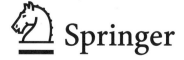 Springer

Gopal B. Saha, Ph.D.
Director of Nuclear Chemistry and Pharmacy
Department of Molecular and Functional Imaging
The Cleveland Clinic Foundation
Cleveland, OH 44195
USA

Library of Congress Cataloging-in-Publication Data
Saha, Gopal B.
    Fundamentals of nuclear pharmacy / Gopal B. Saha. — 5th ed.
      p.   cm.
    Includes bibliographical references and index.
    ISBN 0-387-40360-4 (alk. paper)
    1. Radiopharmaceuticals.   2. Nuclear medicine.   I. Title.
    RS431.R34S24   2003
    616.07'575—dc21   2003052971

ISBN-10: 0-387-40360-4   Printed on acid-free paper.
ISBN-13: 978-0387-40360-1

Printed in the United States of America.   (BS/EB)

9 8 7 6 5 4 3 2 (corrected second printing)

springeronline.com

*To those whose appreciation
has made this book successful*

Preface

The fifth edition of this book has been prompted by its great appreciation in the nuclear medicine community and a constant demand for upgrading with all the new developments in radiopharmaceutical chemistry and clinical nuclear medicine over the past 6 years. In the revision process, obsolete items have been replaced with new, up-to-date items.

The scope and contents of this edition are the same as those of the past editions. It serves as a textbook on nuclear chemistry and pharmacy for nuclear medicine residents and technologists as well as a reference book for many nuclear medicine physicians and radiologists.

The book has 16 chapters. At the end of each chapter, a set of questions and suggested reading materials related to the chapter are provided. As usual, Chapters 1 to 6 have only minor changes because the basic nature of the subject matter does not change over time. Some minor changes in Chapter 4 reflect the addition of newer equipment. Chapter 7 has been extensively revised by deleting clinically obsolete radiopharmaceuticals and adding new ones. A section on positron emission tomography (PET) radiopharmaceuticals has been added in this chapter. Chapters 8 to 10 do not have any major changes except updated information, a new absorbed dose list in Table 10.2, and a new section on effective doses in Chapter 10. Chapter 11 is thoroughly revised to include all new, up-to-date U.S. Food and Drug Administration and Nuclear Regulatory Commission regulations and guidelines. A section on European Regulations has been added to the chapter. No revisions have has been made in Chapter 12. Many changes have been made in Chapter 13 by removing obsolete imaging agents and adding new ones for different organs. Currently, molecular imaging has become the prime topic of interest in imaging modalities, and so a new chapter, Chapter 14, has been added to briefly discuss the subject. The former Chapter 14 has become Chapter 15 with the addition of a new therapeutic radiopharmaceutical. Adverse reactions and iatrogenic alterations in the biodistribution of radiopharmaceuticals are presented in Chapter 16 without any change.

Assistance and support from the members of our department is greatly appreciated.

As with other editions of my two books, Mrs. Rita Konyves made an extraordinary effort to type and complete the manuscript of this book in a timely manner, and I am very thankful and grateful to her.

I am grateful to Robert Albano, senior medical editor, and others at Springer-Verlag New York, Inc., for all their support in publishing my books.

Cleveland, Ohio   Gopal B. Saha

Contents

1
The Atom

According to Bohr's atomic theory, an atom is composed of a nucleus at the center and one or more electrons rotating around the nucleus along different energy orbits. The nucleus is primarily composed of protons and neutrons, collectively called nucleons. For an atom of a given element, the number of electrons moving around the nucleus equals the number of protons, balancing the electrical charge of the nucleus. The size of an atom is of the order of 10^{-8} cm (1 angstrom, Å) and that of a nucleus is of the order of 10^{-13} cm (equal to a unit termed the fermi, F). The electron configuration of the atom determines the chemical properties of an element, whereas the nuclear structure characterizes the stability and radioactive decay of the nucleus of an atom.

Electronic Structure of the Atom

The Bohr atomic theory states that electrons in an atom rotate around the nucleus in discrete *energy orbits* or *shells*. These energy shells, referred to as the K shell, L shell, M shell, N shell, and so forth, are stationary and arranged in order of increasing energy. When there is a transition of an electron from an upper orbit to a lower orbit, the energy difference between the two orbits is released as the photon radiation. If the electron is raised from a lower orbit to an upper orbit, the energy difference between the two orbits is absorbed and must be supplied for the transition to occur.

According to the quantum theory, each shell is designated by a quantum number n, called the *principal quantum number*, and denoted by integers, for example, 1 for the K shell, 2 for the L shell, 3 for the M shell, 4 for the N shell, and 5 for the O shell (Table 1.1). Each energy shell is subdivided into *subshells* or *orbitals*, which are designated as s, p, d, f, and so forth. For a principal quantum number n, there are n orbitals in the main shell. These orbitals are assigned *azimuthal quantum numbers*, l, which designate the electron's angular momentum and can assume numerical values of $l = 0, 1, 2, \ldots, n - 1$. Thus for the s orbital $l = 0$, the p orbital $l = 1$, the d orbital $l = 2$, and so forth. According to the above description, the K shell

1

TABLE 1.1. Electron configuration in different energy shells.

Principal shell	Principal quantum number (n)	Orbital (l)	No. of electrons $= 2(2l+1)$ in each orbital	$2n^2$
K	1	$s(0)$	2	2
L	2	$s(0)$	2	
		$p(1)$	6	8
M	3	$s(0)$	2	
		$p(1)$	6	
		$d(2)$	10	18
N	4	$s(0)$	2	
		$p(1)$	6	
		$d(2)$	10	
		$f(3)$	14	32
O	5	$s(0)$	2	
		$p(1)$	6	
		$d(2)$	10	
		$f(3)$	14	
		$g(4)$	18	50

has one orbital, designated as $1s$; the L shell has two orbitals, designated as $2s$ and $2p$, and so forth. The orientation of the electron's magnetic moment in a magnetic field is described by the *magnetic quantum number, m*. The values of m can be $m = -l, -(l-1), \ldots, \ldots, (l-1), l$. Another quantum number, the *spin quantum number*, $s(s = -1/2$ or $+1/2)$, is assigned to each electron in order to specify its rotation about its own axis. Each orbital can accommodate a maximum of $2(2l+1)$ electrons and the total number of electrons in a given shell is $2n^2$. Thus, the K shell can contain only two electrons, the next L shell eight electrons, the M shell 18 electrons, the N shell 32 electrons, and the O shell 50 electrons. In atoms, the orbitals are

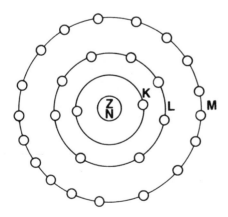

FIGURE 1.1. Schematic electron configuration of K, L, and M shells in a nickel atom.

filled in order of increasing energy; that is, the lowest energy orbital is filled in first.

The electron configuration in different orbitals and shells is illustrated in Table 1.1 and, for example, the structure of $_{28}$Ni is shown in Figure 1.1. Examples of the electron configurations of some elements are given below:

$_{11}$Na $1s^2 2s^2 2p^6 3s^1$

$_{18}$Ar $1s^2 2s^2 2p^6 3s^2 3p^6$

$_{26}$Fe $1s^2 2s^2 2p^6 3s^2 3p^6 3d^6 4s^2$

$_{43}$Tc $1s^2 2s^2 2p^6 3s^2 3p^6 3d^{10} 4s^2 4p^6 4d^6 5s^1$

$_{49}$In $1s^2 2s^2 2p^6 3s^2 3p^6 3d^{10} 4s^2 4p^6 4d^{10} 5s^2 5p^1$

Chemical Bonds

The electronic structure of the atom of an element determines to a large degree the chemical properties of the element. The periodic table has been devised to arrange the groups of elements of similar chemical properties in order of increasing atomic number. In the periodic table (Fig. 1.2) nine groups are presented vertically and seven periods are shown horizontally.

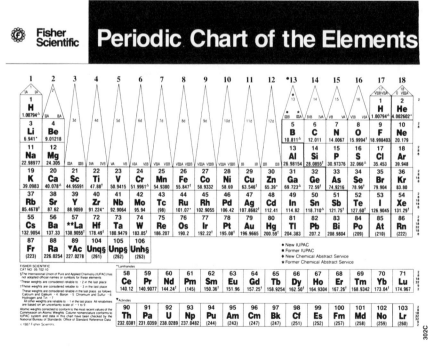

FIGURE 1.2. Periodic table of the elements. (Courtesy of Fisher Scientific Company, Pittsburgh, Pennsylvania.)

Each group contains elements of similar chemical properties, whereas the periods consist of elements having the same number of electron shells but dissimilar chemical properties. As can be seen in Figure 1.2, group VIIB consists of manganese, technetium, and rhenium, whose chemical properties are very similar. Period 2 contains lithium, beryllium, boron, carbon, nitrogen, oxygen, fluorine, and neon, all of which have the K shell and L shell in common, but are widely different in their chemical behavior.

The *valence* of an element is the tendency of the atom to lose or gain electrons in order to achieve a stable electron configuration. It is primarily determined by the number of electrons present in the outermost shell, referred to as the *valence shell*. In the most stable and chemically inert elements, such as neon, argon, krypton, and xenon, the valence shell has the electron configuration ns^2np^6. Helium, although a noble gas, has the configuration $1s^2$. The electrons in the valence shell are called the *valence electrons*. To achieve the stable electron configurations ns^2np^6, electrons can be added to or given up from the valence shell through chemical bond formation between the atoms of appropriate elements. All chemical bond formation is governed by the *octet rule*, which states that the electronic structure of each atom in a chemical bond assumes ns^2np^6 containing eight electrons, with the exception of hydrogen and lithium atoms, which essentially assume the structure $1s^2$. The energy involved in chemical bond formation is of the order of a few electron volts (eV). An electron volt is the energy acquired by an electron accelerated through a potential difference of 1 volt. There are three main types of chemical bonds, described below.

Electrovalent or Ionic Bond

An electrovalent or ionic bond is formed by the complete transfer of an electron from the valence shell of one atom to that of another atom. In ionic bonds two oppositely charged ions are held together in the compound by coulombic forces. The compound NaCl is formed as follows:

$$Na^+ + Cl^- \rightarrow NaCl$$

The sodium atom has the structure $1s^22s^22p^63s^1$, which can spare an electron to achieve the stable structure of neon, $1s^22s^22p^6$. On the other hand, the chlorine atom has the structure $1s^22s^22p^63s^23p^5$, which is short one electron in achieving the electronic structure of argon, $1s^22s^22p^63s^23p^6$. Thus, in the formation of NaCl, the sodium atom loses one electron to become Na^+ and the chlorine atom receives the electron to become Cl^-. Both ions are then held by an electrovalent bond. Because of their ionic properties, compounds with electrovalent bonds conduct electricity in the solid state as well as in solution.

Covalent Bond

In covalent bonds, each of the two atoms participating in bond formation contributes one electron to the bond. Both electrons are shared equally by each atom and, unlike electrovalent bonds, do not belong exclusively to one atom alone. The shared electrons are localized in the region between the two atoms and hence the molecules are nonionic. The following molecules are examples of covalent bonds:

H_2 H × H
HCl   H × Cl
$BeCl_2$ Cl × Be × Cl

Here the symbols × and · represent electrons from separate partners in the bond. Because the compounds with covalent bonds are nonionic, they are poor conductors of electricity.

Coordinate Covalent Bond

In a coordinate covalent bond, the pair of electrons required for bond formation is donated by only one atom to another that can accommodate two electrons in octet formation. These bonds are also called semipolar bonds, because only a partial positive charge is generated on the donor atom and a partial negative charge on the acceptor atom. The following molecules are examples of coordinate covalent bonds:

$$NH_4^+ \quad \left[\begin{array}{c} H \\ \times \\ H \times N \times H \\ \ddot{H} \end{array} \right]^+$$

$$H_3O^+ \quad \left[\begin{array}{c} H \times \ddot{O} \times H \\ \ddot{H} \end{array} \right]^+$$

In these examples, nitrogen and oxygen atoms have donated their lone pair of electrons to a hydrogen ion.

Some donor atoms with a lone pair of electrons are $\dot{N}:$, $\ddot{O}:$ $\ddot{S}:$, and so forth, and these atoms can form coordinate covalent bonds with various metal ions to form metal complexes.

Complex Formation

Metal complexes are produced by coordinate covalent bonds that are formed by the electrons donated by the chemical species having a lone pair of electrons. These complexes can be cationic, anionic, or neutral, examples of which are $[Co(NH_3)_6]^{3+}$, $[Fe(CN)_6]^{3-}$, and $[Ni(CO)_4]$, respectively.

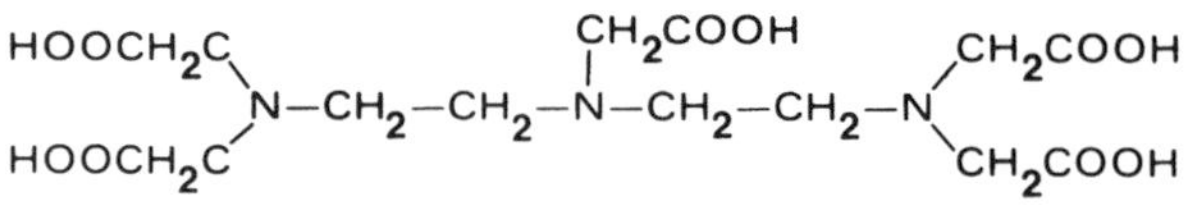

HOOCH$_2$C
        \
          N—CH$_2$—CH$_2$—N—CH$_2$—CH$_2$—N
        / | \
HOOCH$_2$C   CH$_2$COOH   CH$_2$COOH   CH$_2$COOH

Diethylenetriaminepentaacetic Acid   (DTPA; MW = 393)

FIGURE 1.3. Molecular structure of DTPA.

The chemical species such as NH$_3$,—CN, —SH, —COO, —NH$_2$, and CO are called *ligands*, which may be neutral or ionic in structure. The common characteristic of the ligands is that they all possess an unshared pair of electrons that can be donated to a metal ion to form a complex. These ligands are firmly attached to the metal ion, and the number of ligands in a complex is called the *coordination number* of the complex. For example, Co in $[Co(NH_3)_6]^{3+}$ has the coordination number 6.

A single ligand molecule can possess more than one donor atom and can donate more than one pair of electrons in the complex, provided spatial configuration permits. In such cases, more than one coordinate covalent bond is formed in the complex, and the mechanism of bond formation is called *chelation* (from Greek, meaning "clawlike configuration"). Such ligands are called *chelating agents*. Ethylenediaminetetraacetic acid (EDTA) and diethylenetriaminepentaacetic acid (DTPA) are typical examples of chelating agents; the structure of the latter is shown in Figure 1.3. Donor atoms are nitrogen in the amino groups and oxygen in carboxyl groups. Depending on the number of electron pair donating groups in the molecule, the ligands are named unidentate, bidentate, tridentate, and so on.

The stability of a metal complex is influenced by the sizes of the metal ion and the ligand, and the dipole moment of the ligand molecule. The smaller the size of the metal ion and the ligand, the more stable the coordinate covalent bond. Ligands with larger dipole moments form more stable complexes. The stability of a complex is also increased by chelation and the number of electron donor atoms in the chelating agent.

Various ^{99m}Tc-radiopharmaceuticals, such as ^{99m}Tc-DTPA and ^{99m}Tc-gluceptate, are complexes formed by coordinate covalent bonds between ^{99m}Tc and the chelating compounds. The coordination number of technetium in these complexes varies between 4 and 9.

Structure of the Nucleus

The nucleus of an atom is composed of protons and neutrons, collectively called *nucleons*. The characteristics of nucleons and electrons are summarized in Table 1.2. The number of protons in a nucleus is called the *atomic number* of the atom, denoted by Z. The number of neutrons is denoted by

TABLE 1.2. Characteristics of electrons and nucleons.

Particle	Charge	Mass (amu)[a]	Mass (kg)	Mass (MeV)[b]
Electron	-1	0.000549	0.9108×10^{-30}	0.511
Proton	$+1$	1.00728	1.6721×10^{-27}	938.78
Neutron	0	1.00867	1.6744×10^{-27}	939.07

[a] amu = 1 atomic mass unit = 1.66×10^{-27} kg = one twelfth of the mass of ^{12}C.
[b] 1 atomic mass unit = 931 MeV.

N. The total number of nucleons in a nucleus is referred to as the *mass number*, denoted by A. Thus, A is equal to $Z + N$. An elemental atom X having a mass number A, atomic number Z, and neutron number N is represented by $^A_Z X_N$. For example, the stable aluminum nucleus has 13 protons (Z) and 14 neutrons (N), and therefore its mass number is 27. Thus it is designated as $^{27}_{13}$Al$_{14}$. Since all the aluminum atoms have the same atomic number, and the neutron number can be calculated as $A - Z$, both the atomic number 13 and the neutron number 14 are omitted. Thus, the aluminum nucleus is normally designated as ^{27}Al. Alternatively, it is written as Al-27.

Different models have been postulated for the arrangement of the nucleons in a nucleus to explain various experimental observations. According to the Bohr liquid drop model, the nucleus is assumed to be spherical and composed of closely packed nucleons, and particle emission by the nucleus resembles evaporation of molecules from a liquid drop. This theory explains various phenomena, such as nuclear density, binding energy, energetics of particle emission by radioactive nuclei, and fission of heavy nuclei.

In the shell model, nucleons are arranged in discrete energy shells similar to the electron shells of the atom in the Bohr atomic theory. Nuclei containing 2, 8, 20, 50, 82, or 126 protons or neutrons are very stable, and these nucleon numbers are called *magic numbers*.

Nuclei are less stable if they contain an odd number of protons or neutrons, whereas nuclei with even numbers of protons and neutrons are more stable. The ratio of the number of neutrons to the number of protons (N/Z) is also an approximate index of the stability of a nuclide. This ratio equals 1 in the stable nuclei with a low atomic number, such as $^{12}_6$C, $^{16}_8$O, and $^{14}_7$N, and the ratio increases with the increasing atomic number of the nucleus. For example, it is 1.40 for $^{127}_{53}$I and 1.54 for $^{208}_{82}$Pb. Nuclei with N/Z different from the stable nuclei are unstable and decay by β-particle emission or electron capture. The shell model explains various nuclear characteristics such as the angular momentum, magnetic moment, and parity of the nucleus.

According to the classical electrostatic theory, a nucleus should not hold as a single entity because of the electrostatic repulsive forces among the protons in the nucleus. However, its stable existence has been explained by the postulation of a binding force, referred to as the *nuclear force*, which is much stronger than the electrostatic force and binds equally protons and neutrons in the nucleus. The nuclear force exists only in the nucleus and has no influence outside the nucleus. The short range of the nuclear force results in the very small size ($\sim 10^{-13}$ cm) and very high density ($\sim 10^{14}$ g/cm^3) of the nucleus.

The mass M of a nucleus is always less than the combined masses of the nucleons A in the nucleus. This difference in mass ($M - A$) is termed the *mass defect*, which has been used as energy in binding all the nucleons in the nucleus. This energy is the *binding energy* of the nucleus and needs to be supplied to separate all nucleons completely from each other. The binding energy of an individual nucleon has a definite value depending on the shell it occupies; it is approximately equal to the total binding energy divided by the number of nucleons. This energy is about 6 to 9 MeV and has to be supplied to remove a single nucleon from the nucleus.

Nomenclature

Several nomenclatures are important and need to be mentioned here. An exact nuclear composition including the mass number A, atomic number Z, and arrangement of nucleons in the nucleus identifies a distinct species, called the *nuclide*. If a nuclide is unstable or radioactive, it decays by spontaneous fission, or α-particle, β-particle, or γ-ray emission and the nuclide is termed a *radionuclide*. Nuclides of the same atomic number are called *isotopes* and exhibit the same chemical properties. Examples of oxygen isotopes are $^{15}_{8}O$, $^{16}_{8}O$, $^{17}_{8}O$, and $^{18}_{8}O$. Nuclides having the same number of neutrons but different atomic numbers are called *isotones*. Examples are $^{59}_{26}Fe$, $^{60}_{27}Co$, $^{62}_{29}Cu$, each having 33 neutrons. *Isobars* are nuclides with the same number of nucleons, that is, the same mass number, but a different number of protons and neutrons. For example, $^{67}_{29}Cu$, $^{67}_{30}Zn$, $^{67}_{31}Ga$, and $^{67}_{32}Ge$ are isobars having the same mass number 67. Nuclides having the same number of protons and neutrons but differing in energy states and spins are called *isomers*. ^{99}Tc and ^{99m}Tc are isomers of the same nuclide.

The nuclides, both stable and radioactive, are arranged in the form of a chart, referred to as the *chart of the nuclides*, a section of which is presented in Figure 1.4. Each nuclide is represented by a square containing various information such as the half-life, type and energy of radiations, and so forth, of the radionuclide and the neutron capture cross-section of the stable nuclides (see Chapter 4). The nuclides are arranged in increasing neutron number horizontally and in increasing proton number vertically. Each horizontal bar contains all isotopes of the same element; for example, all silicon isotopes are grouped in the horizontal block designated by the proton number 14. All isotones are grouped vertically; for example, $^{26}_{14}Si$, $^{25}_{13}Al$, and $^{24}_{12}Mg$ are isotones with 12 neutrons and are positioned in the vertical column identified by the neutron number 12. The diagonal nuclides in the chart are isobars, for example, $^{27}_{14}Si$, $^{27}_{13}Al$, and $^{27}_{12}Mg$. The radionuclides $^{24}_{13}Al$ and $^{26}_{13}Al$ each have an isomer.

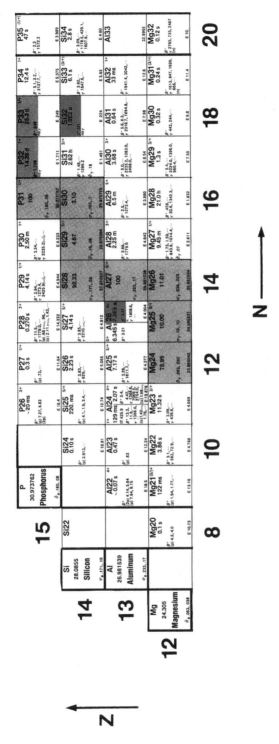

FIGURE 1.4. A section of the chart of the nuclides. (Courtesy of Knolls Atomic Power Laboratory, Schenectady, New York, operated by the General Electric Company for the United States Department of Energy Naval Reactor Branch.)

Questions

1. Describe the basic concept and significance of the Bohr atomic theory.
2. Write the electron configuration of $_6C$, $_{17}Cl$, $_{54}Xe$, $_{37}Rb$, $_{43}Tc$, and $_{49}In$.
3. What is the octet rule? Why is it necessary that the electron configuration of the atoms be ns^2np^6 in a chemical bond?
4. The compounds with electrovalent bonds dissociate mostly into ions in water, whereas those with covalent bonds rarely do so. Explain.
5. What are ligands and chelating agents? Define coordination number and explain complex formation.
6. Group the following nuclides into isotopes, isobars, isotones, and isomers: $^{13}_{6}C$, $^{12}_{6}C$, $^{14}_{6}C$, $^{14}_{5}B$, $^{17}_{8}N$, $^{17}_{8}O$, $^{19}_{10}Ne$, $^{113}_{49}In$, $^{113m}_{49}In$, $^{57}_{27}Co$, $^{57}_{26}Fe$, $^{57}_{28}Ni$.
7. Define mass defect and magic number. What does the mass defect account for?
8. Explain why the nuclear force differs from the electrostatic force in the nucleus of an atom.
9. Write the following nuclides in order of increasing stability: $^{88}_{39}Y$, $^{88}_{38}Sr$, $^{87}_{39}Y$.
10. What are the sizes of an atom and a nucleus? What is responsible for this size difference? What is the difference in magnitude between the chemical and nuclear binding energies?
11. The mass of $^{67}_{31}Ga$ is 66.9858. (a) Calculate the mass defect in MeV. (b) Calculate the average binding energy in MeV of each nucleon in $^{67}_{31}Ga$.

Suggested Reading

Cherry, SR, Sorensen JA, Phelps ME. *Physics in Nuclear Medicine*. 3rd ed. Philadelphia: Saunders; 2003.

Friedlander G, Kennedy JW, Miller JM. *Nuclear and Radiochemistry*. 3rd ed. New York: Wiley; 1981.

2
Radioactive Decay

Decay of Radionuclides

Some 3000 nuclides have been discovered thus far, and most are unstable. Unstable nuclei decay by spontaneous fission, α-particle, β-particle, or γ-ray emission, or electron capture in order to achieve stability. The stability of a nuclide is governed by the structural arrangement and binding energy of the nucleons in the nucleus. One criterion of stability is the neutron-to-proton ratio (N/Z) of the stable nuclides; the radionuclides decay to achieve the N/Z of the nearest possible stable nuclide. Radioactive decay by particle emission or electron capture changes the atomic number of the radionuclide, whereas decay by γ-ray emission does not.

Radionuclides may decay by any one or a combination of six processes: spontaneous fission, α decay, β^- decay, β^+ decay, electron capture, and isomeric transition. In radioactive decay, particle emission or electron capture may be followed by isomeric transition. In all decay processes, the energy, mass, and charge of radionuclides must be conserved. Each of these decay processes is briefly described below.

Spontaneous Fission

Fission is a process in which a heavy nucleus breaks down into two fragments typically in the ratio of 60:40. This process is accompanied by the emission of two or three neutrons with a mean energy of 1.5 MeV and a release of 200 MeV energy, which appears mostly as heat.

Fission in heavy nuclei can occur spontaneously or by bombardment with energetic particles. The probability of spontaneous fission is low and increases with mass number of the heavy nuclei. The half-life for spontaneous fission is 2×10^{17} years for ^{235}U and only 55 days for ^{254}Cf. It should be noted that spontaneous fission is an alternative to α decay or γ emission.

Alpha (α) Decay

Usually heavy nuclei such as radon, uranium, neptunium, and so forth decay by α-particle emission. The α particle is a helium ion containing two protons and two neutrons bound together in the nucleus. In α decay, the atomic number of the parent nuclide is therefore reduced by 2 and the mass number by 4. An example of α decay is

$$^{235}_{92}U \rightarrow ^{231}_{90}Th + ^{4}_{2}He^{2+}$$

An α transition may be followed by β^- emission or γ-ray emission or both. The α particles are monoenergetic, and their range in matter is very short (on the order of 10^{-6} cm) and is approximately 0.03 mm in body tissue.

Beta (β⁻) Decay

When a nucleus is "neutron rich" (i.e., has a higher N/Z ratio compared to the stable nucleus), it decays by β^--particle emission along with an antineutrino. An *antineutrino* ($\bar{\nu}$) is an entity almost without mass and charge and is primarily needed to conserve energy in the decay. In β^- decay, a neutron (n) essentially decays into a proton (p) and a β^- particle; for example,

$$n \rightarrow p + \beta^- + \bar{\nu}$$

The β^- particle is emitted with variable energy from zero up to the decay energy. The *decay or transition energy* is the difference in energy between the parent and daughter nuclides. An antineutrino carries away the difference between the β^- particle energy and the decay energy. The β^- decay may be followed by γ-ray emission, if the daughter nuclide is in an excited state and the number of γ rays emitted depends on the excitation energy. After β^- decay, the atomic number of the daughter nuclide is one more than that of the parent nuclide; however, the mass number remains the same for both nuclides.

Some examples of β^- decay are

$$^{131}_{53}I \rightarrow ^{131}_{54}Xe + \beta^- + \bar{\nu}$$

$$^{59}_{26}Fe \rightarrow ^{59}_{27}Co + \beta^- + \bar{\nu}$$

$$^{99}_{42}Mo \rightarrow ^{99m}_{43}Tc + \beta^- + \bar{\nu}$$

$$^{60}_{27}Co \rightarrow ^{60}_{28}Ni + \beta^- + \bar{\nu}$$

The radioactive decay of nuclides is represented schematically by decay schemes, and examples of the decay schemes of ^{131}I and ^{99}Mo are given in Figures 2.1 and 2.2, respectively.

The β^- particles emitted by radionuclides can produce what is called *bremsstrahlung* by interaction with surrounding medium. Electrons passing through matter are decelerated in the Coulomb field of atomic nuclei, and as a result, the loss in electron energy appears as continuous x rays. These

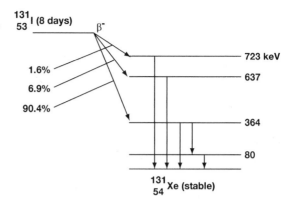

FIGURE 2.1. Decay scheme of ^{131}I. Eighty one percent of the total ^{131}I disintegrations decay by 364-keV γ-ray emission. The half-life of ^{131}I is shown in parentheses.

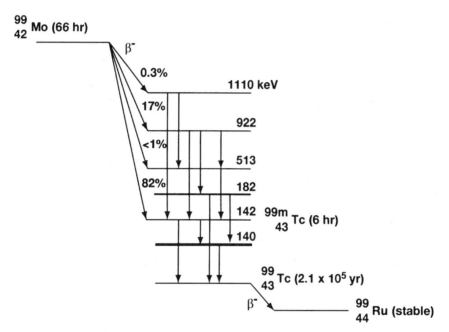

FIGURE 2.2. Decay scheme of ^{99}Mo. There is a 2-keV isomeric transition from the 142-keV level to the 140-keV level, which occurs by internal conversion. Approximately 87% of the total ^{99}Mo ultimately decays to ^{99m}Tc and the remaining 13% decays to ^{99}Tc. (The energy levels are not shown in scale.)

x rays are called bremsstrahlung (German for "braking" or "slowing down" radiation) and are used in radiographic procedures. The probability of producing bremsstrahlung increases with increasing electron energy and increasing atomic number of the medium. In tungsten, for example, a 10-MeV electron loses about 50% of its energy by bremsstrahlung, whereas a 100-MeV electron loses more than 90% of its energy by this process.

Positron or β^+ Decay

Nuclei that are "neutron deficient" or "proton rich" (i.e., have an N/Z ratio less than that of the stable nuclei) can decay by β^+-particle emission accompanied by the emission of a neutrino (v), which is an opposite entity of the antineutrino. After β^+-particle emission, the daughter nuclide has an atomic number that is 1 less than that of the parent. The range of positrons is short in matter. At the end of the path of β^+ particles, positrons combine with electrons and are thus annihilated, each event giving rise to two photons of 511 keV that are emitted in opposite directions. These photons are referred to as *annihilation radiations*.

In β^+ decay, a proton transforms into a neutron by emitting a β^+ particle and a neutrino; for example,

$$p \rightarrow n + \beta^+ + v$$

Since a β^+ particle can be emitted with energy between zero and decay energy, the neutrino carries away the difference between decay energy and β^+ energy. We know that a neutron is equivalent to one proton plus an electron. Therefore, in β^+ decay, a mass equivalent of two electrons are created by the conversion of a proton to a neutron, i.e., 1.02 MeV is needed to create these two particles. So positron emission takes place only when the energy difference between the parent and daughter nuclides is equal to or greater than 1.02 MeV. Some examples of β^+ decay are:

$$^{64}_{29}\text{Cu} \rightarrow {}^{64}_{28}\text{Ni} + \beta^+ + v$$

$$^{18}_{9}\text{F} \rightarrow {}^{18}_{8}\text{O} + \beta^+ + v$$

$$^{15}_{8}\text{O} \rightarrow {}^{15}_{7}\text{N} + \beta^+ + v$$

$$^{52}_{26}\text{Fe} \rightarrow {}^{52}_{25}\text{Mn} + \beta^+ + v$$

The decay scheme of ^{18}F is presented in Figure 2.3.

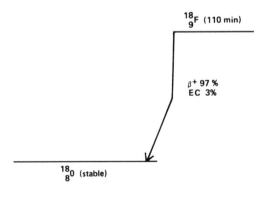

FIGURE 2.3. Decay scheme of ^{18}F. The positrons are annihilated in medium to give rise to two 511-keV γ rays emitted in opposite directions.

Electron Capture (EC)

When a nucleus has a smaller N/Z ratio compared to the stable nucleus, as an alternative to β^+ decay, it may also decay by the so-called electron capture process, in which an electron is captured from the extranuclear electron shells, thus transforming a proton into a neutron and emitting a neutrino. For this process to occur, the energy difference between the parent and daughter nuclides is usually, but not necessarily, less than 1.02 MeV. Nuclides having an energy difference greater than 1.02 MeV may also decay by electron capture. The atomic number of the parent is reduced by 1 in this process. Some examples of electron capture decay are:

$$^{67}_{31}\text{Ga} + e^- \rightarrow {}^{67}_{30}\text{Zn} + v$$

$$^{111}_{49}\text{In} + e^- \rightarrow {}^{111}_{48}\text{Cd} + v$$

$$^{57}_{27}\text{Co} + e^- \rightarrow {}^{57}_{26}\text{Fe} + v$$

Usually the K-shell electrons are captured because of their proximity to the nucleus; the process is then called K capture. Thus in L capture, an L shell electron is captured, and so on. The vacancy created in the K shell after electron capture is filled by the transition of electrons from an upper level (probably the L shell and possibly the M or N shell). The difference in energies of the electron shells will appear as an x ray that is characteristic of the daughter nucleus. These x-rays are termed characteristic K x-rays, L x-rays and so on belonging to the daughter nuclide. The probability of electron capture increases with increasing atomic number, because electron shells in these nuclei are closer to the nucleus. The decay scheme of ^{111}In is given in Figure 2.4.

Isomeric Transition (IT)

A nucleus can remain in several excited energy states above the ground state that are defined by quantum mechanics. All these excited states are referred to as *isomeric states* and decay to the ground state, with a lifetime of frac-

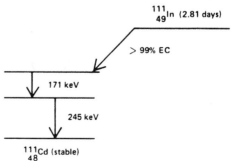

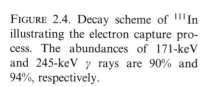

FIGURE 2.4. Decay scheme of ^{111}In illustrating the electron capture process. The abundances of 171-keV and 245-keV γ rays are 90% and 94%, respectively.

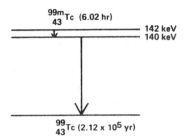

FIGURE 2.5. Decay scheme of ^{99m}Tc illustrating isomeric transition. Ten percent of the decay follows internal conversion.

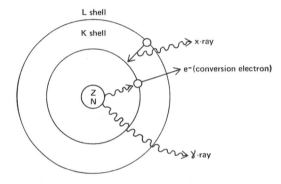

FIGURE 2.6. Internal conversion process. Nuclear excitation energy is transferred to a K shell electron, which is then emitted and the vacancy is filled by the transition of an electron from the L shell. The energy difference between the L shell and the K shell appears as the characteristic K x ray.

tions of picoseconds to many years. The decay of an upper excited state to a lower excited state is called the isomeric transition. In β^-, β^+, or electron capture decay, the parent nucleus may reach any of these isomeric states of the daughter nucleus in lieu of the ground state, and therefore these decay processes are often accompanied by isomeric transition. In isomeric transition, the energy difference between the energy states may appear as γ rays. When isomeric states are long lived, they are referred to as *metastable states* and can be detected by appropriate instruments. The metastable state is denoted by "m," as in ^{99m}Tc. The decay scheme of ^{99m}Tc is given in Figure 2.5.

There is a probability that instead of emitting a γ-ray photon, the excited nucleus may transfer its excitation energy to an electron in the extranuclear electron shell of its own atom, particularly the K shell, which is then ejected, provided the excitation energy is greater than the binding energy of the K shell electron (Fig. 2.6). The ejected electron is referred to as the *conversion electron* and will have the kinetic energy equal to $E_\gamma - E_B$, where E_γ is the excitation energy and E_B is the binding energy of the ejected electron. This process is an alternative to γ-ray emission and is termed *internal conversion*. The ratio of the conversion electrons (N_e) to the observed γ rays (N_γ) is referred to as the conversion coefficient, given by $\alpha = N_e/N_\gamma$. The larger the conversion coefficient, the smaller the number of observed γ rays. The probability of internal conversion is higher when the transition energy is low.

When an electron is ejected from, for example, the K shell by internal conversion, an upper shell electron will fall into the vacancy of the K shell, and the difference in energy between the two shells will appear as a K x ray that is characteristic of the daughter nuclide. The corresponding conversion coefficient is designated α_K. Similarly, it is also probable that instead of K shell electrons, $L, M, \ldots$ shell electrons are ejected, followed by the emission of $L, M, \ldots$ x rays in this process. The corresponding conversion coefficients then will be $\alpha_L, \alpha_M, \ldots$. The total conversion coefficient is given by the sum of all possible conversion coefficients; that is, $\alpha_T = \alpha_K + \alpha_L + \cdots$.

As an alternative to characteristic x-ray emission in either electron capture or internal conversion process, the transition energy between the two shells can be transferred to an orbital electron, which is then emitted from the atom, if energetically permitted. The process is referred to as the *Auger process*. The electron emitted is called an Auger electron and is similar to a conversion electron in internal conversion. The vacancy in the shell due to an Auger process is filled by an electron transition from the upper shells, followed by emission of characteristic x rays or Auger electrons as in internal conversion. Whether a particular vacancy in a given shell will result in the emission of a characteristic x ray or an Auger electron is a matter of probability. The fraction of vacancies in a given shell that are filled with accompanying x-ray emission and no Auger electron, is referred to as the *fluorescence yield*. The fluorescence yield increases with the increasing atomic number of the atom. The transition energy (i.e., the characteristic x-ray energy) between the two shells is always less than the binding energy of an electron in the lower shell, and therefore cannot eject it. For example, the K characteristic x-ray energy is always less than the binding energy of the K-shell electron, so the latter cannot undergo the Auger process and cannot be emitted as an Auger electron.

Radioactive Decay Equations

General Equation

As already mentioned, radionuclides are unstable and decay by particle emission, electron capture, or γ-ray emission. The decay of radionuclides is a random process, that is, one cannot tell which atom from a group of atoms will decay at a specific time. Therefore, one can only talk about the average number of radionuclides disintegrating during a period of time. This gives the disintegration rate of that particular radionuclide.

The number of disintegrations per unit time (disintegration rate), $-dN/dt$, of a radionuclide at any time is proportional to the total number of radioactive atoms present at that time. Mathematically,

$$-dN/dt = \lambda N \tag{2.1}$$

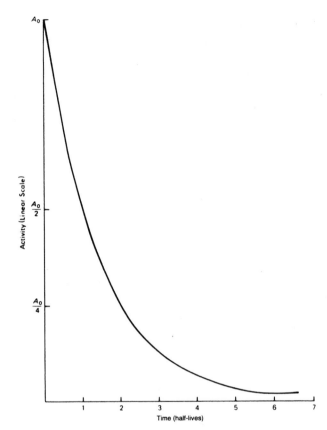

FIGURE 2.7. Plot of radioactivity versus time on a linear graph. The time is plotted in units of half-life. The graph shows an exponential decay of radioactivity with time.

where N is the number of radioactive atoms and λ is a *decay constant* that is defined as the probability of disintegration per unit time for the radioactive atom. The disintegration rate, $-dN/dt$, is termed the radioactivity or simply the activity of a radionuclide and denoted by A. It should be clearly understood from the above equation that the same amount of radioactivity means the same disintegration rate for any radionuclide, but the total number of atoms present and the decay constant may be different for different radionuclides. From the above statements, the following equation can be written:

$$A = \lambda N \tag{2.2}$$

From a knowledge of the decay constant and radioactivity of a radionuclide, one can calculate the total number of atoms or the total mass of the radionuclide present (using Avogadro's number, 1 gram · atom (g · atom) = 6.02×10^{23} atoms).

Equation (2.1) is a differential equation and can be solved by proper integration. The solution of this equation leads to

$$N_t = N_0 e^{-\lambda t} \tag{2.3}$$

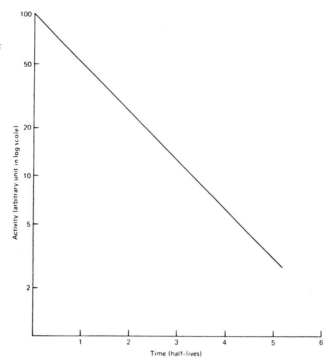

FIGURE 2.8. Plot of the data in Fig. 2.7 on a semilogarithmic graph showing a straight-line relationship.

where N_0 and N_t are the number of radioactive atoms present at $t = 0$ and time t, respectively. Equation (2.3) represents the exponential decay of any radionuclide. In terms of radioactivity Eq. (2.3) may be written

$$A_t = A_0 e^{-\lambda t} \qquad (2.4)$$

The graphical representations of the above equation are given in Figures 2.7 and 2.8 on linear and semilogarithmic plots, respectively.

Half-Life and Mean Life

Every radionuclide is characterized by a *half-life*, which is defined as the time required to reduce its initial activity to one half. It is usually denoted by $t_{1/2}$ and is unique for a given radionuclide. The decay constant λ of a radionuclide is related to half-life by

$$\lambda = 0.693/t_{1/2} \qquad (2.5)$$

To determine the half-life of a radionuclide, its radioactivity is measured at different time intervals and plotted on semilogarithmic paper, resulting in a straight line as in Figure 2.8. The slope of the straight line is λ, and the half-life is determined by Eq. (2.5). It can also be simply read from the graph as the time difference between the two values of activities where one value is one-half of the other. For a very long-lived radionuclide, it is determined by Eq. (2.2) from the knowledge of its activity and the number of atoms present.

From the definition of half-life, it is understood that A_0 is reduced to $A_0/2$ in one half-life of decay, to $A_0/4$, that is, $A_0/2^2$ in two half-lives, to $A_0/8$, that is, $A_0/2^3$ in three half-lives, and so forth. In n half-lives of decay, it is reduced to $A_0/2^n$. Thus the radioactivity A_t at time t can be calculated from the initial radioactivity A_0 by

$$A_t = \frac{A_0}{2^n} = \frac{A_0}{2^{(t/t_{1/2})}} \tag{2.6}$$

Here the number of half-lives n is equal to $(t/t_{1/2})$, where t is the time of decay and $t_{1/2}$ is the half-life of the radionuclide. As an example, suppose a radioactive sample with a half-life of 10 days contains 250 mCi radioactivity. The radioactivity of the sample after 23 days would be $250/2^{(23/10)} = 250/2^{2.3} = 250/4.92 = 50.8$ mCi.

Another relevant quantity of a radionuclide is its *mean life*, which is the average life of a group of the radioactive atoms. It is denoted by τ and related to decay constant λ and half-life $t_{1/2}$ as follows:

$$\tau = 1/\lambda \tag{2.7}$$

$$\tau = t_{1/2}/0.693 = 1.44t_{1/2} \tag{2.8}$$

In one mean life, the activity of a radionuclide is reduced to 37% of its initial value.

Units of Radioactivity

Radioactivity is expressed in units called *curies*. Historically, it was initially defined as the disintegration rate of 1 g radium, which was considered to be 3.7×10^{10} disintegrations per second. Later the disintegration rate of 1 g radium was found to be slightly different from this value, but the original definition of curie was still retained:

$$1 \text{ curie (Ci)} = 3.7 \times 10^{10} \text{ disintegrations per second (dps)}$$

$$= 2.22 \times 10^{12} \text{ disintegrations per minute (dpm)}$$

$$1 \text{ millicurie (mCi)} = 3.7 \times 10^7 \text{ dps}$$

$$= 2.22 \times 10^9 \text{ dpm}$$

$$1 \text{ microcurie } (\mu\text{Ci}) = 3.7 \times 10^4 \text{ dps}$$

$$= 2.22 \times 10^6 \text{ dpm}$$

The System Internationale (SI) unit for radioactivity is *becquerel* (Bq), which is defined as one disintegration per second. Thus

$$1 \text{ becquerel (Bq)} = 1 \text{ dps} = 2.7 \times 10^{-11} \text{ Ci}$$

$$1 \text{ kilobecquerel (kBq)} = 10^3 \text{ dps} = 2.7 \times 10^{-8} \text{ Ci}$$

$$1 \text{ megabecquerel (MBq)} = 10^6 \text{ dps} = 2.7 \times 10^{-5} \text{ Ci}$$

$$1 \text{ gigabecquerel (GBq)} = 10^9 \text{ dps} = 2.7 \times 10^{-2} \text{ Ci}$$

$$1 \text{ terabecquerel (TBq)} = 10^{12} \text{ dps} = 27 \text{ Ci}$$

Similarly,

$$1 \text{ Ci} = 3.7 \times 10^{10} \text{ Bq} = 37 \text{ GBq}$$

$$1 \text{ mCi} = 3.7 \times 10^7 \text{ Bq} = 37 \text{ MBq}$$

$$1 \text{ } \mu\text{Ci} = 3.7 \times 10^4 \text{ Bq} = 37 \text{ kBq}$$

Calculations

Two examples of calculations related to radioactivity are presented below.

Problem 2.1
Calculate the total number of atoms and total mass of ^{131}I present in 5 mCi (185 MBq) ^{131}I ($t_{1/2} = 8$ days).

Answer

$$\lambda \text{ for } {}^{131}\text{I} = \frac{0.693}{8 \times 24 \times 60 \times 60} = 1.0 \times 10^{-6} \text{ sec}^{-1}$$

$$A = 5 \times 3.7 \times 10^7 = 1.85 \times 10^8 \text{ dps}$$

Using Eq. (2.2),

$$N = \frac{A}{\lambda} = \frac{1.85 \times 10^8}{1 \times 10^{-6}} = 1.85 \times 10^{14} \text{ atoms}$$

Since 1 g · atom ^{131}I $= 131$ g ^{131}I $= 6.02 \times 10^{23}$ atoms of ^{131}I (Avogadro's number),

$$\text{Mass of } {}^{131}\text{I in 5 mCi (185 MBq)} = \frac{1.85 \times 10^{14} \times 131}{6.02 \times 10^{23}}$$

$$= 40.3 \times 10^{-9} \text{ g}$$

$$= 40.3 \text{ ng}$$

Therefore, 5 mCi ^{131}I contains 1.85×10^{14} atoms and 40.3 ng ^{131}I.

Problem 2.2
At 11:00 A.M., the ^{99m}Tc radioactivity was measured as 9 mCi (333 MBq) on a certain day. What was the activity at 8:00 A.M. and 4:00 P.M. on the same day ($t_{1/2}$ for ^{99m}Tc = 6 hr)?

Answer

Time from 8:00 A.M. to 11:00 A.M. is 3 hr;

$$A_t = 9 \text{ mCi (333 MBq)}$$

$$A_0 = ?$$

Using Eq. (2.4),

$$9 = A_0 e^{-0.1155 \times 3}$$

$$A_0 = 9 \times e^{0.3465}$$

$$= 12.7 \text{ mCi (470 MBq) at 8:00 A.M.}$$

Time from 11:00 A.M. to 4:00 P.M. is 5 hr;

$$A_0 = 9 \text{ mCi}$$

$$A_t = ?$$

Using Eq. (2.4),

$$A_t = 9 \times e^{-0.1155 \times 5}$$

$$= 9 \times e^{-0.5775}$$

$$= 5.05 \text{ mCi (187 MBq) at 4:00 P.M.}$$

Successive Decay Equations

General Equation

In the above section, we have derived equations for the activity of any radionuclide that is decaying. Here we shall derive equations for the activity of a radionuclide that is growing from another radionuclide and at the same time, is itself decaying.

If a parent radionuclide p decays to a daughter radionuclide d, which in turn decays, then the rate of growth of radionuclide d becomes

$$\frac{dN_d}{dt} = \lambda_p N_p - \lambda_d N_d \qquad (2.9)$$

$\lambda_p N_p$ is the growth rate of the daughter from the parent, and $\lambda_d N_d$ is the decay rate of the daughter. By integration, Eq. (2.9) becomes

$$(A_d)_t = \lambda_d N_d = \frac{\lambda_d (A_p)_0}{\lambda_d - \lambda_p} (e^{-\lambda_p t} - e^{-\lambda_d t}) \qquad (2.10)$$

Equation (2.10) gives the net activity of radionuclide d at time t due to the growth from the decay of radionuclide p. If there is an initial activity $(A_d)_0$ of radionuclide d, then the term $(A_d)_0 e^{-\lambda_d t}$ has to be added to Eq. (2.10). Thus,

$$(A_d)_t = \lambda_d N_d = \frac{\lambda_d (A_p)_0}{\lambda_d - \lambda_p} (e^{-\lambda_p t} - e^{-\lambda_d t}) + (A_d)_0 e^{-\lambda_d t} \qquad (2.11)$$

Transient Equilibrium

If $\lambda_d > \lambda_p$, that is, $(t_{1/2})_d < (t_{1/2})_p$, then $e^{-\lambda_d t}$ in Eq. (2.11) is negligible compared to $e^{-\lambda_p t}$ when t is sufficiently long. Eq. (2.11) then becomes

$$(A_d)_t = \frac{\lambda_d (A_p)_0}{\lambda_d - \lambda_p} e^{-\lambda_p t} = \frac{\lambda_d (A_p)_t}{\lambda_d - \lambda_p} \qquad (2.12)$$

This relationship is called the *transient equilibrium*. This equilibrium holds true when $(t_{1/2})_p$ and $(t_{1/2})_d$ differ by a factor of about 10 to 50. It can be seen from Eq. (2.12) that the daughter activity is always greater than the parent activity. Initially, the daughter activity grows owing to the decay of the parent radionuclide, reaches a maximum followed by an equilibrium, and then decays with a half-life of the parent. The time to reach maximum activity is given by

$$t_{max} = \frac{1.44 \times (t_{1/2})_p \times (t_{1/2})_d \times \ln[(t_{1/2})_p/(t_{1/2})_d]}{[(t_{1/2})_p - (t_{1/2})_d]} \qquad (2.13)$$

A typical example of transient equilibrium is ^{99}Mo ($t_{1/2} = 66$ hr) decaying to ^{99m}Tc ($t_{1/2} = 6.0$ hr) represented in Fig. 2.9. Because overall 87% of ^{99}Mo decays to ^{99m}Tc, the ^{99m}Tc activity is lower than the ^{99}Mo activity in the time activity plot (Fig. 2.9). The ^{99m}Tc activity reaches a maximum in about 23 hr, i.e., about 4 half-lives of ^{99m}Tc, followed by the equilibrium.

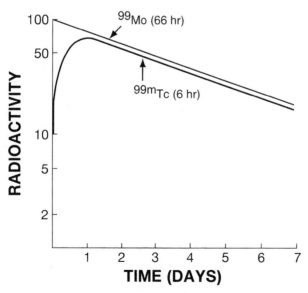

FIGURE 2.9. Plot of logarithm of ^{99}Mo and ^{99m}Tc activities versus time showing transient equilibrium. The activity of the daughter ^{99m}Tc is less than that of the parent ^{99}Mo, because only 87% of ^{99}Mo decays to ^{99m}Tc radionuclide. If 100% of the parent were to decay to the daughter, then the daughter activity would be higher than the parent activity after reaching equilibrium, as recognized from Eq. (2.12).

Problem 2.3
Yttrium-87 ($t_{1/2} = 80$ hr) decays to ^{87m}Sr ($t_{1/2} = 2.83$ hr). The activity of a pure sample of ^{87}Y is calibrated at noon on Wednesday and measured to be 300 mCi (11.1 GBq). Calculate the activity of ^{87m}Sr at 6:00 P.M. on Wednesday and at 6:00 P.M. on Thursday.

Answer
In Eq. (2.10), we have

$$\lambda_p = \frac{0.693}{80} = 0.0087 \text{ hr}^{-1}$$

$$\lambda_d = \frac{0.693}{2.83} = 0.2449 \text{ hr}^{-1}$$

$$\frac{\lambda_d}{\lambda_d - \lambda_p} = \frac{0.2449}{0.2449 - 0.0087} = 1.0368$$

$$(A_p)_0 = 300 \text{ mCi}$$

$$t = 6 \text{ hr (from noon to 6 P.M. Wednesday)}$$

$$e^{-\lambda_p t} = e^{-0.0087 \times 6} = 0.9491$$

$$e^{-\lambda_d t} = e^{-0.2449 \times 6} = 0.2301$$

$$(A_d)_t = ?$$

Using the above values in Eq. (2.10), the activity of ^{87m}Sr at 6:00 P.M. on Wednesday can be calculated as

$$(A_d)_t = 1.0368 \times 300 \times (0.9491 - 0.2301) = 223.6 \text{ mCi (8.27 GBq)}$$

For the activity of ^{87m}Sr at 6:00 P.M. on Thursday, we assume a transient equilibrium between ^{87}Y and ^{87m}Sr because the half-lives of the parent and daughter nuclides differ by a factor of 28, and more than 10 half-lives (i.e., 30 hr) of the daughter nuclide have elapsed between noon Wednesday and 6:00 P.M. on Thursday. Using Eq. (2.12), we have

$$t = 30 \text{ hr}$$

$$(A_p)_t = 300 \times e^{-0.0087 \times 30} = 231.1 \text{ mCi}$$

$$(A_d)_t = 1.0368 \times 231.1 = 239.6 \text{ mCi}$$

Therefore, the activity of ^{87m}Sr at 6:00 P.M. on Thursday is 239.6 mCi (8.87 GBq).

Secular Equilibrium

When $\lambda_d \gg \lambda_p$, that is, the parent half-life is much longer than that of the daughter nuclide, in Eq. (2.12) we can neglect λ_p compared to λ_d. Then Eq. (2.12) reduces to

$$(A_d)_t = (A_p)_t \tag{2.14}$$

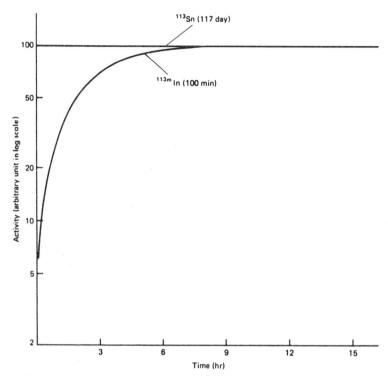

FIGURE 2.10. Plot of logarithm of ^{113}Sn and ^{113m}In activities illustrating secular equilibrium. In secular equilibrium, activities of the parent ^{113}Sn and the daughter ^{113m}In become the same and both decay with the same $t_{1/2}$ of ^{113}Sn.

Equation (2.14) is called the *secular equilibrium* and is valid when the half-lives of the parent and the daughter differ by more than a factor of 100. In secular equilibrium, the parent and daughter radioactivities are equal and both decay with the half-life of the parent nuclide. A typical example of secular equilibrium is ^{137}Cs ($t_{1/2} = 30$ years) decaying to ^{137m}Ba ($t_{1/2} = 2.6$ min). A graphical representation of secular equilibrium between ^{113}Sn ($t_{1/2} = 117$ days) and ^{113m}In ($t_{1/2} = 100$ min) is shown in Figure 2.10.

Problem 2.4
Germanium-68 has a half-life of 280 days and decays to ^{68}Ga, whose half-life is 68 min. The activity of a pure sample of ^{68}Ge is calibrated to be 450 mCi (16.7 GBq) at noon on Tuesday. Calculate the activity of ^{68}Ga at midnight on Tuesday and at 5:00 P.M. on Wednesday.

Answer
The time from Tuesday noon to midnight Tuesday is 12 hr and the time from Tuesday noon until 5:00 P.M. Wednesday is 29 hr. Since the half-lives of ^{68}Ge and

^{68}Ga differ by a factor of about 5800, a secular equilibrium is established between the two nuclides within 12 hr ($\sim$11 half-lives of ^{68}Ga) and 29 hr. The decay of ^{68}Ge in a 29-hr period is negligible, and therefore the activity of ^{68}Ge at both midnight Tuesday and 5:00 P.M. on Wednesday would be approximately 450 mCi (16.7 GBq). Then, according to Eq. (2.14), the activity of ^{68}Ga at these times would also be 450 mCi (16.7 GBq).

Statistics of Counting

Although it is beyond the scope of this book to discuss the details of statistics related to radioactive disintegration, it would be appropriate to describe briefly the salient points of statistics as applied to the measurement of radioactivity. Since nuclear pharmacists and technologists are routinely involved in radioactive counting, the following discussion of statistics will be helpful in determining how long a radioactive sample should be counted and how many counts should be accumulated for better precision and accuracy.

Error, Accuracy, and Precision

In the measurement of any quantity, an *error* or a deviation from the true value of the quantity is likely to occur. There are two types of errors—systematic and random. Systematic errors arise from malfunctioning equipment and inappropriate experimental conditions and can be corrected by rectifying the situation. Random errors arise from random fluctuations in the experimental conditions, for example, high-voltage fluctuations or fluctuations in the quantity to be measured, such as the radioactive decay.

The *accuracy* of a measurement indicates how closely it agrees with the "true" value. The *precision* of a series of measurements describes the reproducibility of the measurement and indicates the deviation from the "average" value. Remember that the average value may be far from the true value of the measurement. The closer the measurement is to the average value, the higher the precision, whereas the closer the measurement is to the true value, the more accurate the measurement. Precision can be improved by eliminating the random errors, whereas both the random and systematic errors must be eliminated for better accuracy.

Standard Deviation

The standard deviation for a group of measurements indicates the precision of the measurements. Radioactive disintegration follows the Poisson distribution law, and from this one can show that if a radioactive sample gives an average count of $\bar{n}$, then its standard deviation σ is given by

$$\sigma = \sqrt{\bar{n}} \tag{2.15}$$

The mean is then expressed as

$$\bar{n} \pm \sigma$$

The standard deviations in radioactive measurements indicate the statistical fluctuation of radioactive disintegration. If a single count, n, of a radioactive sample is quite large, then n can be estimated as close to $\bar{n}$ and substitute for it in Eq. (2.15) (i.e., $\sigma = \sqrt{n}$). For example, the standard deviation of the measurement of a radioactive sample giving 10,000 counts will be 100.

If we make a series of measurements repeatedly on a radioactive sample giving a mean count $\bar{n}$, then 68% of all measurements would fall within 1 standard deviation on either side of the mean, that is, in the range of $\bar{n} - \sigma$ to $\bar{n} + \sigma$. This is called the "68% confidence level" for $\bar{n}$. Similarly, 95% of the measurements will fall within 2 standard deviations ($\bar{n} - 2\sigma$ to $\bar{n} + 2\sigma$), and 99% of the data within 3 standard deviations ($\bar{n} - 3\sigma$ to $\bar{n} + 3\sigma$). These are designated as the 95% and 99% confidence levels, respectively.

A more useful quantity in the statistical analysis of the counting data is the percent standard deviation, which is given by

$$\% \, \sigma = \frac{\sigma}{n} \times 100 = \frac{100\sqrt{n}}{n} = \frac{100}{\sqrt{n}} \tag{2.16}$$

Equation (2.16) indicates that as n increases, the $\% \, \sigma$ decreases, and hence the precision of the measurement increases. Thus, the precision of a count of a radioactive sample can be increased by accumulating a large number of counts. For a count of 10,000, $\% \, \sigma$ is 1%, whereas for 1,000,000, $\% \, \sigma$ is 0.1%.

Problem 2.5
How many counts should be collected in a sample in order to have a 1% error at 95% confidence level?

Answer
95% confidence level is 2σ, i.e., $2\sqrt{n}$

$$1\% \text{ error} = \frac{2\sigma \times 100}{n} = \frac{2\sqrt{n} \times 100}{n}$$

$$\text{Therefore, } 1 = \frac{200}{\sqrt{n}}$$

$$\sqrt{n} = 200$$

$$n = 40,000 \text{ counts}$$

Standard Deviation of Count Rates

The standard deviation of a count rate is

$$\sigma_c = \sigma / t$$

where σ is the standard deviation of the total count n obtained in time t. Since n is equal to the count rate c times the time of counting t,

$$\sigma_c = \sqrt{n}/t = \sqrt{ct}/t = \sqrt{c/t} \qquad (2.17)$$

Problem 2.6
A radioactive sample is counted for 8 min and gives 3200 counts. Calculate the count rate and standard deviation for the sample.

Answer

$$\text{Count rate } c = 3200/8 = 400 \text{ counts per minute (cpm)}$$

$$\text{Standard deviation } \sigma_c = \sqrt{c/t} = \sqrt{400/8} \simeq 7$$

Therefore, the average count rate is 400 ± 7 cpm.

Propagation of Errors

Situations may arise in which two quantities, x and y, with their respective standard deviations, σ_x and σ_y, are either added, subtracted, multiplied, or divided. The standard deviations of results of these arithmetic operations are expressed by the following equations:

$$\text{Addition} : \sigma_{x+y} = \sqrt{\sigma_x^2 + \sigma_y^2} \qquad (2.18)$$

$$\text{Subtraction} : \sigma_{x-y} = \sqrt{\sigma_x^2 + \sigma_y^2} \qquad (2.19)$$

$$\text{Multiplication} : \sigma_{(x\times y)} = (x \times y)\sqrt{(\sigma_x/x)^2 + (\sigma_y/y)^2} \qquad (2.20)$$

$$\text{Division} : \sigma_{(x/y)} = (x/y)\sqrt{(\sigma_x/x)^2 + (\sigma_y/y)^2} \qquad (2.21)$$

Problem 2.7
A radioactive sample gives an average count of 9390 ± 95 and the counting time for each count is 20 ± 1 min. Calculate the average count rate and its standard deviation.

Answer

$$\text{Count rate } c = \frac{9390}{20} = 470 \text{ cpm}$$

$$\text{Standard deviation } \sigma_c = (9390/20)\sqrt{(95/9390)^2 + (1/20)^2}$$

$$= 470\sqrt{0.0026}$$

$$= 470 \times 0.051$$

$$= 24$$

Thus, the average count rate is 470 ± 24 cpm.

Questions

1. Describe how the N/Z ratio of a radionuclide determines whether a radionuclide would decay by β^- or β^+ emission or electron capture.
2. Why is an antineutrino emitted in β^- decay?
3. What is the threshold for β^+ emission? If the decay energy between two radionuclides is 1.3 MeV, are both β^+ emission and electron capture possible?
4. Discuss bremsstrahlung and internal conversion. What are the common characteristics of electron capture and internal conversion?
5. An excited nucleus with 190 keV energy ejects a K-shell electron of an atom by internal conversion. What is the kinetic energy of the electron if the binding energy of the K-shell electron is 20 keV?
6. The internal conversion coefficient of a 0.169-MeV photon is 0.310. Calculate the abundance in percent of the photon emission.
7. Calculate (a) the disintegration rate per minute and (b) the activity in curies and becquerels present in 1 μg ^{111}In ($t_{1/2} = 2.8$ days).
8. Calculate the total number of atoms and total mass of ^{99m}Tc present in 15 mCi (555 MBq) ^{99m}Tc activity ($t_{1/2} = 6$ hr).
9. If the radioactivity of ^{197}Hg ($t_{1/2} = 65$ hr) is 100 mCi (3.7 GBq) on Wednesday noon, what is its activity (a) at 8 A.M. the Tuesday before and (b) at noon the Friday after?
10. State the specific conditions of transient equilibrium and secular equilibrium.
11. The half-lives of ^{99}Mo and ^{99m}Tc are 66 hr and 6 hr, respectively, and both are in transient equilibrium in a sample. If the ^{99}Mo activity is 75 mCi (2.8 GBq), what is the activity of ^{99m}Tc? (Assume 87% ^{99}Mo decay to ^{99m}Tc.)
12. How long will it take for a 10-mCi (370 MBq) sample of ^{32}P ($t_{1/2} = 14.3$ days) and a 100-mCi (3.7 GBq) sample of ^{67}Ga ($t_{1/2} = 3.2$ days) to possess the same activity?
13. What is the time interval during which ^{67}Ga ($t_{1/2} = 3.2$ days) decays to 37% of the original activity?
14. For the treatment of a thyroid patient, 100 mCi (3.7 GBq) ^{131}I is required. What amount of ^{131}I should be shipped if transportation takes 3 days?
15. How much time would it take for the decay of 8/9 of a sample of ^{68}Ge whose half-life is 280 days?
16. What is the half-life of a radionuclide if a sample of it gives 10,000 cpm and 2 hr later gives 3895 cpm?
17. Iodine-127 is the only stable isotope of iodine. What modes of decay would you expect for ^{125}I and ^{132}I?
18. If a radionuclide decays for a time interval equal to the mean life of the radionuclide, what fraction of the original activity has decayed?

19. Draw a graph of the following activity versus time and find the half-life of the radionuclide.

Time (hr)	cpm
4	8021
9	5991
15	4213
20	3153
26	2250
30	1789
38	1130

20. A radioactive sample gives 12,390 counts in 12 min. (a) What are the count rate and standard deviation of the sample? (b) If the sample contained a background count rate of 50 cpm obtained from a 2-min count, what would be the net count rate of the sample and its standard deviation?
21. How many counts of a radioactive sample are to be collected in order to have a 2% error at 95% confidence level?
22. How many standard deviations of a mean count of 82,944 is 576?
23. What is the minimum number of counts that would give 1 standard deviation confidence level and no more than a 3% error?

Suggested Reading

Cherry, SR, Sorensen JA, Phelps ME. *Physics in Nuclear Medicine*. 3rd ed. Philadelphia: Saunders; 2003.
Friedlander G, Kennedy JW, Miller JM. *Nuclear and Radiochemistry*. 3rd ed. New York: Wiley; 1981.

3
Instruments for Radiation Detection and Measurement

In nuclear medicine, it is necessary to ascertain the presence, type, intensity, and energy of radiations emitted by radionuclides, and these are accomplished by radiation-detecting instruments. The two commonly used devices are gas-filled detectors and scintillation detectors with associated electronics. These instruments are described below.

Gas-Filled Detectors

The operation of a gas-filled detector is based on the ionization of gas molecules by radiations, followed by collection of the ion pairs as current with the application of a voltage between two electrodes. The measured current is primarily proportional to the applied voltage and the amount of radiations. A schematic diagram of a gas-filled detector is shown in Figure 3.1.

The two most commonly used gas-filled detectors are ionization chambers and Geiger-Müller (GM) counters. The primary difference between the two devices lies in the operating voltage that is applied between the two electrodes. Ionization chambers are operated at 50 to 300 V, whereas the GM counters are operated at around 1000 V. Examples of ionization chambers are "Cutie-Pie" counters and dose calibrators, which are used for measuring high intensity radiation sources, such as output from x-ray machines (Cutie-Pie) and activity of radiopharmaceuticals (dose calibrators). The GM counters are used for detecting low level beta and gamma radiations.

Dose Calibrators

The dose calibrator is one of the most essential instruments in nuclear medicine for measuring the activity of radionuclides for formulating and dispensing radiopharmaceuticals. It is a cylindrically shaped, sealed chamber with a central well and is filled with argon and traces of halogen at high pressure. Its operating voltage is about 150 V. A typical dose calibrator is shown in Figure 3.2.

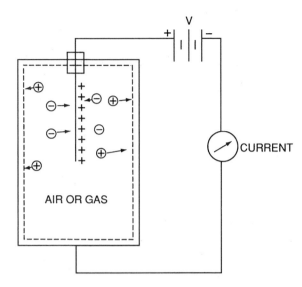

FIGURE 3.1. Schematic diagram of a gas-filled detector.

Because radiations of different types and energies produce different amounts of ionization (hence current), equal activities of different radionuclides generate different quantities of current. For example, current produced by 1 mCi (37 MBq) ^{99m}Tc is different from that by 1 mCi (37 MBq) ^{131}I. Isotope selectors are the feedback resistors to compensate for differences in ionization (current) produced by different radionuclides so the equal activities produce the same reading. In most dose calibrators, the isotope selectors for commonly used radionuclides are push-button types, whereas those for other radionuclides are set by a continuous dial. The settings of isotope selectors are basically the calibration factors for different radionuclides, which are determined by measuring the current produced by one millicurie of each radionuclide. The unknown activity of a radionuclide is then measured by its current divided by the calibration factor for that radionuclide, which is displayed in the appropriate unit on the dose calibrator. An activity range selector is a variable resistor that adjusts the range of activity (μCi, mCi, Ci or MBq, GBq) for display.

For measurement of the activity of a radionuclide, one first sets the calibration factor for the radionuclide using the appropriate push button or dial setting. Then the sample in a syringe, vial, or any other appropriate container is placed inside the chamber well of the dose calibrator, whereupon the reading of activity is displayed on the digital meter of the dose calibrator. The quality control methods of the dose calibrators are discussed in Chapter 8.

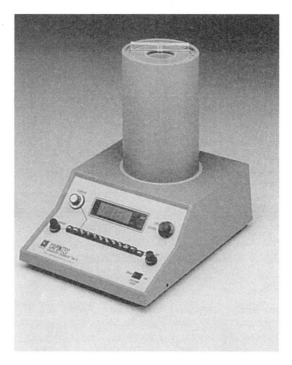

FIGURE 3.2. Isotope dose calibrator, Capintec model CRC-12. (Courtesy of Capintec, Inc.)

Geiger-Müller Counters

The GM counters are used for the measurement of exposure delivered by a radiation source and called *survey meters*. A typical GM survey meter is shown in Figure 3.3. The GM counter is one of the most sensitive detectors and can be constructed in different configurations. One end of the detector is made of a thin mica window that allows passage of beta particles and low energy gamma radiations that would otherwise be stopped by the metal cover provided for detection of gamma radiations. It is usually battery operated and operates as a ratemeter. The readings are given in micro-roentgen (μR) per hour, milliroentgen (mR) per hour, roentgen (R) per hour, or counts per minute (cpm). The GM counters do not have any energy-discriminative capabilities. Some GM counters are equipped with audible alarms or flashing light alarms that are triggered by radiations above a preset intensity. The latter kind is called an *area monitor*.

The GM counters are primarily used for area survey for contamination with low-level activity. According to Nuclear Regulatory Commission (NRC) regulations, these survey meters must be calibrated annually with standard sources such as ^{226}Ra and ^{137}Cs.

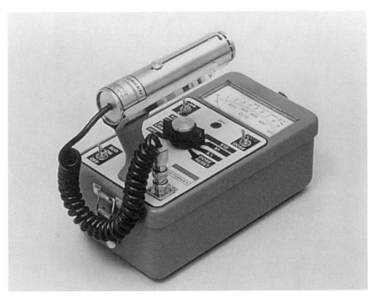

FIGURE 3.3. Geiger-Müller survey meter, Victoreen Model 290 Thyac IV (Courtesy of Victoreen, Inc.)

Scintillation Detecting Instruments

A variety of scintillation or γ-ray detecting equipment is currently used in nuclear medicine. The well counters, thyroid probes, and γ or scintillation cameras are most commonly used. All these instruments are γ-ray detecting devices and consist of a collimator (excluding well counter), sodium iodide detector, photomultiplier tube, preamplifier, pulse height analyzer, X, Y positioning circuit (only in scintillation cameras), and display or storage. Basically, γ rays from a source interact in the sodium iodide detector and light photons are emitted. The latter strike the photocathode of a photomultiplier (PM) tube and a pulse is generated at the end of the PM tube. The pulse is first amplified by a preamplifier and then by a linear amplifier. A pulse height analyzer sorts out the amplified pulses according to the desired energy of the γ ray and finally feeds the pulse into a scaler, magnetic tape, computer, cathode ray tube, or x-ray film.

Collimator

In all nuclear medicine equipment for imaging, a collimator is attached to the face of a sodium iodide detector to limit the field of view so that all radiations from outside the field of view are prevented from reaching the detector. Collimators are made of lead and have a number of holes of different shapes and sizes. In thyroid probes, they are single bore and cylindrical in shape. In scintillation cameras, collimators are classified as parallel hole, diverging, pinhole, and converging (see later), depending on the type of focusing.

When the number of holes in a collimator is increased, the sensitivity of the detector increases, but there is a comparable loss of septal thickness that results in septal penetration by relatively high energy γ rays and hence a loss in spatial resolution. One can increase the resolution[a] or the detail of the image by decreasing the size of the holes in a given collimator or increasing the length of the collimator. This results in a decrease in the sensitivity (i.e., γ-ray detection efficiency) of the camera.

Detector

For γ-ray detection, a sodium iodide crystal doped with a very small amount of thallium [NaI(Tl)] is most commonly used. Other detectors such as lithium-drifted germanium detector [Ge(Li)], bismuth germanate (BGO), barium fluoride (BaF$_2$), gadolinium oxyorthosilicate (GSO) and lutetium oxyorthosilicate (LSO) are also used for scintillation detection.

The choice of NaI(Tl) crystals for γ-ray detection is primarily due to their reasonable density (3.67 g/cm^3) and high atomic number of iodine ($Z = 53$) that result in efficient production of light photons (about 1 light photon per approximately 30 eV) upon interaction with γ rays in the presence of a trace amount of thallium (0.1–0.4 mole %). The light generated in the crystal is directed toward the PM tube by coating the outside surface of the crystal with reflector material such as magnesium oxide or by using light pipes between the crystal and the PM tube. Sodium iodide is hygroscopic and absorbed water causes color changes that distort light transmission to the PM tubes. Therefore, the crystals are hermetically sealed in aluminum containers. Room temperature should not be abruptly changed, because such changes in temperatures can cause cracks in the crystal. Also, mechanical stress must be avoided in handling them, because NaI crystals are very fragile.

The NaI(Tl) detectors of different sizes are used in different instruments. In well-type NaI(Tl) detectors, the crystals have a hole in the middle deep enough to cover the counting sample almost completely. In these crystals counting efficiency is very high and no collimator is needed. In thyroid probes and well counters, the smaller cylindrical but thicker (7.6 × 7.6 cm or 12.7 × 12.7 cm) NaI(Tl) crystals are used, whereas in scintillation cameras, the larger rectangular (33–59 cm) and thinner (0.64–1.9 cm) crystals are employed.

---

[a] Resolution is the minimum distance between two points in an image that can be detected by a detecting device.

Photomultiplier Tube

A PM tube consists of a light-sensitive photocathode at one end, a series (usually 10) of metallic electrodes called dynodes in the middle, and an anode at the other end—all enclosed in a vacuum glass tube. The PM tube is fixed on to the NaI(Tl) crystal with the photocathode facing the crystal with a special optical grease. The number of PM tubes in the thyroid probe and the well counter is one, whereas in scintillation cameras it varies from 19 to 94 which are attached on the back face of the NaI(Tl) crystal.

A high voltage of ~ 1000 V is applied from the photocathode to the anode of the PM tube in steps of ~ 100 V between dynodes. When a light photon from the NaI(Tl) crystal strikes the photocathode, photoelectrons are emitted, which are accelerated toward the immediate dynode by the voltage difference between the electrodes. The accelerated electrons strike the dynode and more secondary electrons are emitted, which are further accelerated. The process of multiplication of secondary electrons continues until the last dynode is reached, where a pulse of 10^5 to 10^8 electrons is produced. The pulse is then attracted to the anode and finally delivered to the preamplifier.

Preamplifier

The pulse from the PM tube is small in amplitude and must be amplified before further processing. It is initially amplified with a preamplifier that is placed close to the PM tube. A preamplifier is needed to adjust the voltage of the pulse shape and match the impedance levels between the detector and subsequent components so that the pulse is appropriately processed by the system.

Linear Amplifier

The output pulse from the preamplifier is further amplified and properly shaped by a linear amplifier. The amplified pulse is then delivered to a pulse height analyzer for analysis as to its voltage. The amplification of the pulse is defined by the amplifier gain given by the ratio of the amplitude of the outgoing pulse to that of the incoming pulse, and the gain can be adjusted in the range of 1 to 1000 by gain controls provided on the amplifier. The amplitudes of output pulses normally are of the order of 0 to 10 V.

Pulse Height Analyzer

Gamma rays of different energies can arise from a source, either from the same radionuclide or from different radionuclides, or due to scattering of γ-rays in the source. The pulses coming out of the amplifier may be different in amplitude due to differing γ-ray energies. The pulse height analyzer (PHA) is a device that selects for counting only those pulses falling within preselected voltage amplitude intervals or "channels" and rejects all others. This selection of pulses is made by control knobs, called the lower level and upper level, or the base and window, provided on the PHA. Proper choice of settings of these knobs determines the range of γ-ray energies that will be accepted for further processing such as recording, counting, and so on. In scintillation cameras, these two knobs are normally replaced by a peak voltage control and a percent window control. The peak voltage control relates to the desired γ-ray energy and the percent window control indicates the window width in percentage of the desired γ-ray energy, which is set symmetrically on each side of the peak voltage.

The above mode of counting is called *differential counting*, in which only pulses of preselected energy are counted. If γ rays of all energies or all γ rays of energies above a certain preselected energy need to be counted, the mode of counting is called *integral counting*, in which case only the lower level or base line is operative and the window mechanism is bypassed.

A pulse height analyzer normally selects only one range of pulses and is called a *single-channel analyzer* (SCA). A multichannel analyzer (MCA) is a device that can simultaneously sort out pulses of different energies into a number of channels. By using an MCA, one can obtain simultaneously a spectrum of γ rays of different energies arising from a source (Figure 3.4).

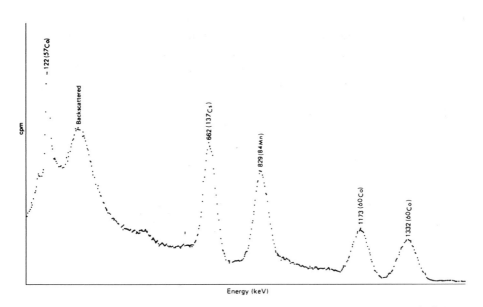

FIGURE 3.4. A γ-ray spectrum of different photon energies taken with a NaI(Tl) detector coupled to a multichannel analyzer.

Display or Storage

Information processed by the PHA can be displayed on a cathode ray tube (CRT) or an oscilloscope with a CRT. In a multichannel analyzer, a γ-ray spectrum can be displayed on the CRT. Pulses can also be counted for a predetermined number of counts or for a preset time by a scaler–timer device. A ratemeter can be used to display the pulses in terms of counts/min or counts/s. In the case of scintillation cameras, x-ray films and computers are employed to obtain images formed by the pulses. Pulses can be stored in a computer or on magnetic tape or disk for further processing later.

Scintillation Camera

A scintillation camera, also known as a gamma camera, basically operates on the same principles as described above. It consists of a collimator; detector; X, Y positioning circuit; PHA; and display or storage. Although PM tubes, preamplifiers, and linear amplifiers are also basic components of gamma cameras, their functions are the same as described above and, therefore, will not be discussed further here. A schematic electronics diagram of a scintillation camera is illustrated in Figure 3.5, and a typical scintillation camera is shown in Figure 3.6.

Collimator

As already mentioned, classification of collimators used in scintillation cameras depends primarily on the type of focusing, and also on the septal thickness of the holes. Depending on the type of focusing, collimators are classified as parallel hole, pinhole, converging, and diverging types; these are

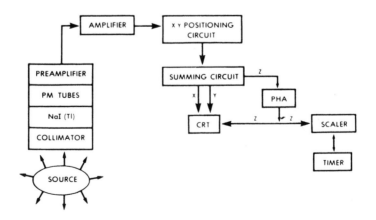

FIGURE 3.5. A schematic electronics diagram of a scintillation camera.

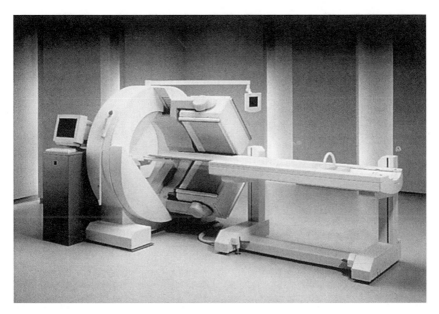

FIGURE 3.6. A scintillation camera. Siemens model E-CAM. (Image Courtesy of Siemens Medical Systems, Inc.)

COLLIMATOR DESIGNS

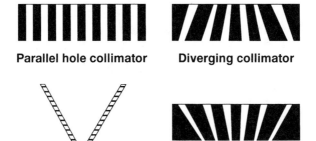

Parallel hole collimator   **Diverging collimator**

Pinhole collimator   **Converging collimator**

FIGURE 3.7. Several collimator designs.

illustrated in Figure 3.7. Pinhole collimators are used in imaging small organs such as thyroid glands. Converging collimators are employed when the target organ is smaller than the size of the detector, whereas diverging collimators are used in imaging organs such as lungs that are larger than the size of the detector. Parallel hole collimators are most commonly used in nuclear medicine procedures.

Parallel hole collimators are classified as high-resolution, all-purpose, and high-sensitivity types. Most manufacturers keep the size and number of holes the same for all these collimators, but only change the thickness. High-sensitivity collimators are made with smaller thickness than all-purpose collimators, whereas high-resolution collimators are made thickest of all. The deterioration in spatial resolution is related to the thickness of the collimator; thus, the high-sensitivity collimator shows the sharpest drop in spatial resolution, followed in order by the all-purpose and high-resolution collimators. For all parallel hole collimators, the spatial resolution is best at the collimator face and deteriorates with increasing distance between the collimator and the object. It is therefore desirable to image patients in close proximity to the collimator face.

Detector

The NaI(Tl) crystals used as the detector in scintillation cameras are mostly rectangular in shape and have the dimension between 33×43 cm and 37×59 cm with thickness varying between 0.64 cm and 1.9 cm. The most common thickness is 0.95 cm. The 0.64-cm thick detectors are usually used in portable cameras for nuclear cardiac studies.

Increasing the thickness of a crystal increases the probability of complete absorption of γ rays and hence the sensitivity of the detector. However, there is a probability of multiple interactions of a γ ray in a thick crystal and the X, Y coordinates of the point of γ-ray interaction can be obscured (see later). This results in poor resolution of the image of the organ. For this reason, thin NaI(Tl) crystals are used in scintillation cameras, but this decreases the sensitivity of the camera since many γ rays escape from the detector without interaction and only a few γ rays interact in the detector.

X, Y Positioning Circuit

When a γ ray interacts in the crystal, its exact location is determined by the X, Y positioning circuit in conjunction with an array of PM tubes. Many PM tubes (19–94) are mounted on the NaI(Tl) crystal in scintillation cameras. After γ-ray interaction in the crystal, a maximum amount of light will be received by the PM tube nearest to the point of interaction, whereas other PM tubes will receive an amount of light directly proportional to the solid angle subtended by the PM tube at the point of interaction. The X, Y positioning circuit sums up the output of different PM tubes and produces X and Y pulses in direct proportion to the X, Y coordinates of the point of interaction of γ rays and thus gives an image of the distribution of activity in a source. The pulses are stored in a computer, for further processing.

The larger the number of PM tubes, the better the depiction on the image of the X, Y coordinates of the point of γ-ray interaction, that is, better resolution of the image. Also, the higher the energy of γ rays, the better the resolution, because they produce more light in the crystal. However, it should be remembered that very high energy γ rays can penetrate the collimator septa and thus blur the image. Low energy γ rays (< 80 keV) are largely scattered in the source and the crystal and give poor resolution.

Pulse Height Analyzer

It is a circuit that sums up the output of all PM tubes to produce a pulse known as the Z pulse that represents the energy of a γ ray. The SCA analyzes the amplitude of the Z pulses and selects only those of desired energy by the use of appropriate peak energy and percent window settings. In many scintillation cameras, the energy selection is made automatically by pushbutton type isotope selectors designated for different radionuclides such as ^{131}I, ^{99m}Tc, and so on. In some scintillation cameras, two or three SCAs are used to select simultaneously two or three γ rays of different energies, particularly while imaging with ^{67}Ga and ^{111}In that possess two or three predominant γ rays. For most studies, a 20% window, centered on the photopeak, is used.

It should be pointed out that X, Y pulses are accepted only if the Z pulse is within the energy range selected by the PHA. If the Z pulses are outside this range, then X, Y pulses are discarded.

The above discussion is given for understanding the base principle of image formation with the pulses produced by interaction of radiation with the detectors. However, current gamma cameras use a digital technique in which each pulse is processed and analyzed by the PM tube nearest to the site of interaction of the radiation in the detector. Analog signals are digitized and stored in the computer. This technique provides accurate localization of the signal and improves the spatial resolution. These cameras are called digital cameras.

Display and Storage

Currently, most cameras employ digital computers in acquiring, storing, and processing of image data. Some cameras have built-in computers and use a single console for both the camera and the computer, while others have stand-alone computers that are custom-designed for the specific camera. In institutions having several scintillation cameras, a single, large-capacity computer is interfaced with all cameras to acquire and process the data. Instant images can be seen on a computer monitor as the data are collected. This is essential for positioning the detector on the organ of interest. Data are collected for a preset time or counts. Software for different purposes is normally provided by the commercial vendors. However, software for specific needs can be developed by an experienced computer specialist, if available in the nuclear medicine department.

Data from patient studies are needed to be stored for archiving and later processing. This is accomplished by storing them in a computer with a large memory using picture archiving communication systems (PACS).

Digital computers operate only with binary numbers. The information from a scintillation camera is usually in analog form, and must be digitized for processing by the computer. A device in the computer, known as the analog-to-digital converter (ADC), converts the analog signals into binary digits. An ADC is characterized by a bit, a unit of division of a certain range of pulses. A given range of pulses is equally divided into two parts by a one-bit ($2^1 = 2$) ADC, into four parts by a two-bit ($2^2 = 4$) ADC, and so on.

For X and Y pulses, six- to eight-bit ADCs are used, thus dividing the range of X or Y pulses into $2^6(64)$, $2^7(128)$, or $2^8(256)$ equal divisions. The two-dimensional analog image formed by the X and Y pulses is divided into 64×64, 128×128, or 256×256 picture elements, which are called *pixels*. Each pixel corresponds to a specific area on the crystal and also to a specific memory location in the computer. Thus, the ADC determines the pixel location for a γ-ray interaction in the crystal and a count is stored in the corresponding memory location in the computer. With increasing numbers of γ-ray interactions over a period of time, more counts are accumulated in appropriate locations and finally a digitized image is stored. The information can be retrieved later by proper manipulation of the computer and the image displayed on a monitor or recorded on film.

Tomographic Imagers

A basic limitation of the scintillation cameras is that they depict images of three-dimensional activity distributions in two-dimensional displays. Images of structures in the third dimension, depth, are obscured by the underlying and overlying structures. One way to solve this problem is to obtain images at different angles around the patient such as anterior, posterior, lateral, and oblique projections. However, success of the technique is limited because of the complexity of structures surrounding the organ of interest. Currently, tomographic techniques are employed to delineate the depth of the object of imaging.

The common tomographic technique is computed tomography, which is based on rigorous mathematical algorithms, to reconstruct the images at distinct focal planes (slices). Illustrations of four tomographic slices of the heart are shown in Figure 3.8. In nuclear medicine, two types of computed tomography are employed based on the type of radionuclides used: single photon emission computed tomography (SPECT), which uses γ-emitting radionuclides such as ^{99m}Tc, ^{123}I, ^{67}Ga, ^{111}In, and so forth, and positron emission tomography (PET), which uses β^+-emitting radionuclides such as ^{11}C, ^{13}N, ^{15}O, ^{18}F, ^{68}Ga, ^{82}Rb, and so forth.

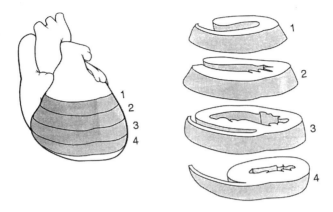

FIGURE 3.8. Four slices of the heart in the short axis (transverse).

Single Photon Emission Computed Tomography

The most common SPECT systems consist of a typical gamma camera with one to three NaI(Tl) detector heads mounted on a gantry, an on-line computer for acquisition and processing of data and a display system. The detector head rotates around the long axis of the patient at small angle increments (3°–10°) for 180° or 360° angular sampling. The data are stored in a 64 × 64 or 128 × 128 matrix in the computer for later reconstruction of the images of the planes (slices) of interest. Transverse, sagittal, and coronal images can be obtained from the collected data. Examples of SPECT images are shown in Chapter 13.

Positron Emission Tomography

The PET is based on the detection in coincidence of the two 511-keV photons emitted in opposite directions after annihilation of a positron from a positron emitter and an electron in the medium. Two photons are detected by two detectors in coincidence, and data collected over many angles around the body axis of the patient are used to reconstruct the image of the activity distribution in the slice of interest. Such coincidence counting obviates the need for a collimator to define the field of view. A schematic diagram of the PET system using four pairs of detectors is illustrated in Figure 3.9.

The detectors are primarily made of bismuth germanate (BGO), NaI(Tl), lutetium oxyorthosilicate (LSO), godolinium oxyorthosilicate (GSO), or barium fluoride (BaF$_2$), of which BGO is most commonly used in the PET systems.

The PET systems use multiple detectors distributed in two to eight circular, hexagonal, or octagonal circumferential rings around the patient. Each

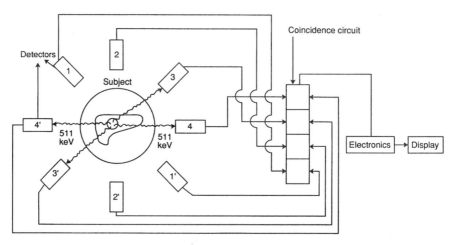

FIGURE 3.9. Schematic diagram of a PET system using four pairs of detectors.

detector is connected to the opposite detector by a coincidence circuit. Thus, all coincident counts from different slices over 360° angles around the patient are acquired simultaneously in a 64 × 64, 128 × 128, or higher matrix in a computer. The data are then processed to reconstruct the images depicting the activity distribution in each slice. Examples of PET images are illustrated in Chapter 13.

Another variety of camera is available, which is capable of counting in both PET and SPECT modes. These cameras have two detectors which rotate around the patient. In PET mode, data are acquired in coincidence and in SPECT mode, appropriate collimators are used. These cameras are called dual-head coincidence camera.

A new system, PET/CT, is currently available, which offers accurate matching of anatomic (CT) and functional (PET) images. Patients are imaged by both PET and CT in the same position of the patient, and images are then aligned to provide accurate diagnosis.

Questions

1. What are the differences between an ionization chamber and a Geiger-Müller counter?
2. What is the function of a push-button isotope selector on a dose calibrator?
3. Can you discriminate between 140-keV and 364-keV γ rays by a Geiger-Müller counter?
4. What type of instruments would you use for detection of (a) x-ray beam exposure, (b) spill of 1 mCi (37 MBq) ^{201}Tl, and (c) 10 mCi (370 MBq) ^{99m}Tc?

5. Describe how a scintillation camera works. Explain why the following are used in a scintillation camera: (a) a collimator, (b) many PM tubes, and (c) a thin NaI(Tl) crystal.
6. Define the resolution and sensitivity of a scintillation camera.
7. Describe how a digital computer works.
8. Describe the principles of tomographic imaging.
9. What is the difference between SPECT and PET?

Suggested Reading

Bushberg JT, Seibert JA, Leidholdt EM Jr, Boone JM. *The Essential Physics of Medical Imaging.* 2nd ed. Baltimore: Lippincott Williams & Wilkins; 2002.

Cherry SR, Sorensen JA, Phelps ME. *Physics in Nuclear Medicine.* 3rd ed. Philadelphia: Saunders; 2003.

Hendee WR, Ritenour ER. *Medical Imaging Physics.* 4th ed. Hoboken, NJ: Wiley; 2002.

Rollo FD, ed. *Nuclear Medicine Physics, Instrumentation and Agents.* St. Louis: Mosby; 1977.

4
Production of Radionuclides

In 1896, Becquerel discovered the natural radioactivity in potassium uranyl sulfate. Since then, Pierre and Marie Curie, E. Rutherford, and F. Soddy all made tremendous contributions to the discovery of many other radioactive elements. The work of all these scientists has shown that all elements found in nature with an atomic number greater than 83 (bismuth) are radioactive. Artificial radioactivity was first reported by I. Curie and F. Joliot in 1934. These scientists irradiated boron and aluminum targets with α particles from polonium and observed positrons emitted from the target even after the removal of the α-particle source. This discovery of induced or artificial radioactivity opened up a brand new field of tremendous importance. Around the same time, the discovery of the cyclotron, neutron, and deuteron by various scientists facilitated the production of many more artificial radioactivities. At present, more than 2700 radionuclides have been produced artificially in the cyclotron, the reactor, the neutron generator, and the linear accelerator.

Radionuclides used in nuclear medicine are mostly artificial ones. They are primarily produced in a cyclotron or a reactor. The type of radionuclide produced in a cyclotron or a reactor depends on the irradiating particle, its energy, and the target nuclei. Since they are expensive, these facilities are limited and supply radionuclides to remote facilities that do not possess such equipment. Very short-lived radionuclides are available only in the institutions that have the cyclotron or reactor facilities; they cannot be supplied to remote institutions or hospitals because they decay rapidly. For remote facilities, however, there is a secondary source of radionuclides, particularly short-lived ones, which is called a radionuclide generator discussed in detail in the next chapter.

Cyclotron-Produced Radionuclides

In a cyclotron, charged particles such as protons, deuterons, α particles, ^{3}He particles, and so forth are accelerated in circular paths in dees under vacuum by means of an electromagnetic field (Fig. 4.1). These accelerated particles

FIGURE 4.1. Schematics of a cyclotron. V, alternating voltage; S, ion source; A and B, dees with vacuum; D, deflector; W, window.

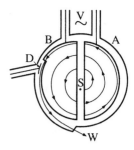

can possess a few kiloelectron volts (keV) to several billion electron volts (BeV) of energy depending on the design and type of the cyclotron. Since the charged particles move along the circular paths under the magnetic field with gradually increasing energy, the larger the radius of the particle trajectory, the higher the energy of the particle. In a given cyclotron, this relationship of energy to radius is definitely established. Heavy ions such as ^{16}O, ^{14}N, and ^{32}S have also been successfully accelerated in heavy-ion accelerators.

When targets of stable elements are irradiated by placing them in the external beam of the accelerated particles or in the internal beam at a given radius in a cyclotron, the accelerated particles irradiate the target nuclei and nuclear reactions take place. In a nuclear reaction, the incident particle may leave the nucleus after interaction, leaving some of its energy in it, or it may be completely absorbed by the nucleus, depending on the energy of the incident particle. In either case, a nucleus with excitation energy is formed and the excitation energy is disposed of by the emission of nucleons (i.e., protons and neutrons). Particle emission is followed by γ-ray emission when the former is no longer energetically feasible. Depending on the energy deposited by the incident particle, a number of nucleons are emitted randomly from the irradiated target nucleus, leading to the formation of different nuclides. As the energy of the irradiating particle is increased, more nucleons are emitted, and therefore a much greater variety of nuclides are produced.

Each nuclear reaction for the production of a nuclide has a definite threshold or Q energy, which is either absorbed or released in the reaction. This energy requirement arises from the difference between the masses of the target nucleus plus the irradiating particle and the masses of the product nuclide plus the emitted particles. In nuclear reactions requiring the absorption of energy, the irradiating particles must possess energy above the threshold energy; otherwise, the nuclear reaction would not take place. Furthermore, if the irradiating or emitted particles are charged, then an additional Coulomb energy due to the Coulomb barrier between the charged particle and the target nucleus or the emitting nucleus must be added to the Q value of the nuclear reaction.

An example of a simple cyclotron-produced radionuclide is ^{111}In, which is produced by irradiating ^{111}Cd with 12-MeV protons in a cyclotron. The nuclear reaction is written as follows:

$$^{111}Cd(p, n)\ ^{111}In$$

where ^{111}Cd is the target, the proton p is the irradiating particle, the neutron n is the emitted particle, and ^{111}In is the product radionuclide. In this case, a second nucleon may not be emitted because there may not be enough energy left after the emission of the first neutron. The excitation energy that is not sufficient to emit any more nucleons will be dissipated by γ-ray emission.

As another example, relatively high-energy nuclear reactions induced in ^{89}Y by irradiation with 40-MeV protons are listed below:

$$^{89}Y + p(40\,MeV) \rightarrow\ ^{89}Zr + n$$
$$\rightarrow\ ^{89}Y + p$$
$$\rightarrow\ ^{88}Zr + 2n$$
$$\rightarrow\ ^{88}Y + pn$$
$$\rightarrow\ ^{88}Sr + 2p$$
$$\rightarrow\ ^{87}Zr + 3n$$
$$\rightarrow\ ^{87}Y + p2n$$

Although all reactions mentioned in the above example are feasible, the most probable reactions are (p, 3n) and (p, p2n) reactions with 40-MeV protons.

As can be understood, radionuclides produced with atomic numbers different from those of the target isotopes theoretically should not contain any stable ("cold" or "carrier") isotope detectable by ordinary analytical methods, and such preparations are called *carrier-free*. In practice, however, it is impossible to have these preparations without the presence of any stable isotopes. Another term for these preparations is *no carrier added* (NCA), meaning that no stable isotope has been added purposely to the preparations.

The target material for irradiation must be pure and preferably mono-isotopic or at least enriched isotopic in order to avoid the production of extraneous radionuclides. The energy and type of the irradiating particle must be chosen so that contamination with undesirable radionuclides resulting from extraneous nuclear reactions can be avoided. Since various isotopes of different elements may be produced in a particular irradiating system, it is necessary to isolate isotopes of a single element; this can be accomplished by appropriate chemical methods such as solvent extraction, precipitation, ion exchange, and distillation. Cyclotron-produced radionuclides are usually neutron deficient and therefore decay by β^+ emisson or electron capture.

Methods of preparation of several useful cyclotron-produced radio-nuclides are described below.

Gallium-67

Gallium-67 can be produced by several nuclear reactions such as $^{66}Zn(d, n)$ ^{67}Ga (deuteron is denoted d), $^{68}Zn(p, 2n)$ ^{67}Ga, and $^{64}Zn(\alpha, p)$ ^{67}Ga. A pure natural zinc target or enriched zinc isotope in the form of oxide is irradiated with 20-MeV protons, 8-MeV deuterons, or 23-MeV α particles in a cyclo-tron at a certain beam current for a specified time. After irradiation the target is dissolved in $7N$ hydrochloric acid (HCl) and carrier-free ^{67}Ga is extracted with isopropyl ether. The organic phase is then evaporated to dryness in a water bath and the residue is taken up in dilute HCl for supply as gallium chloride. It may be complexed with citric acid to form gallium citrate, which is most commonly used in nuclear medicine.

Natural zinc targets can lead to impurities such as ^{66}Ga, which has a half-life of 9 hr, as compared to the 78-hr half-life of ^{67}Ga. The radio-contaminant ^{66}Ga can, however, be eliminated by allowing it to decay com-pletely before the chemical processing of ^{67}Ga. Enriched zinc isotope targets produce less radioactive impurities, but they are expensive to prepare.

Iodine-123

Iodine-123 is very useful in nuclear medicine because it has good radiation characteristics such as decay by electron capture, half-life of 13.2 hr and γ-ray emission of 159 keV. It is produced directly or indirectly in a cyclotron by several nuclear reactions. Direct nuclear reactions are those reactions whereby ^{123}I is produced directly and likely to be contaminated with other iodine radioisotopes such as ^{124}I and ^{125}I, depending on the type of target and the irradiating particle. Examples of such reactions are $^{121}Sb(\alpha, 2n)$, ^{123}I, $^{123}Te(p, n)$ ^{123}I, $^{122}Te(d, n)$ ^{123}I, and $^{124}Te(p, 2n)$ ^{123}I. Depending on the target composition and energy of the irradiating particles, other side reac-tions may produce various radioisotopes of iodine. In the direct methods, after irradiation the target is dissolved in mineral acid and iodine is collected by distillation into dilute sodium hydroxide (NaOH).

In the indirect method, the nuclear reaction is so chosen that ^{123}Xe is produced initially, which then decays with a half-life of 2.1 hr to produce ^{123}I. These reactions allow the production of ^{123}I free of other radioisotopes of iodine. Various reactions include $^{122}Te(\alpha, 3n)$ ^{123}Xe using 42- to 46-MeV α particles, $^{122}Te(^3He, 2n)$ ^{123}Xe using 20- to 30-MeV ^3He particles, $^{123}Te(^3He, 3n)$ ^{123}Xe using 25-MeV ^3He particles, and $^{127}I(p, 5n)$ ^{123}Xe using 60- to 70-MeV protons. In all cases except the last, the target con-sists of natural or enriched tellurium powder coated inside a water-cooled chamber that is irradiated with α or ^3He particles. During irradiation, helium gas is passed through the target, sweeping ^{123}Xe and some directly produced iodine isotopes. The gas mixture is initially passed through a trap maintained at $-79\,°C$ with solid carbon dioxide to remove iodine, and then through another trap maintained at $-196\,°C$ with liquid nitrogen to remove ^{123}Xe. Iodine can be removed simply by leaching the nitrogen trap. The major contaminant in these samples is $^{124}I(t_{1/2} = 4.2$ days). For the $^{127}I(p, 5n)\ ^{123}Xe$ reaction, the target is dissolved in aqueous potassium iodide, and ^{123}Xe is removed by helium gas bubbled through the solution and isolated by a liquid nitrogen trap. Such preparations contain ^{125}I as contaminant.

Another important method of producing pure ^{123}I is by the $^{124}Xe(p, 2n)$ ^{123}Cs reaction, in which case $^{123}Cs(t_{1/2} = 5.9\,min)$ decays to ^{123}Xe. The ^{124}Xe gas is contained under pressure in a chamber and the chamber is irradiated with protons. Sufficient time is allowed for ^{123}Cs to decay completely to ^{123}Xe, which is then processed as above to yield ^{123}I. Such preparations are ^{124}I-free.

Indium-111

Indium-111 is produced by the $^{111}Cd(p, n)\ ^{111}In$ and $^{109}Ag(\alpha, 2n)\ ^{111}In$ reactions. After irradiation with 15-MeV protons, the cadmium target is dissolved in mineral acid and the acidity is made $1N$ in HCl. The solution is passed through anion-exchange resin (Dowex-1). Indium-111 is removed by elution with $1N$ hydrochloric acid, leaving cadmium on the column. Similarly, the silver target is dissolved in mineral acid after irradiation with 30-MeV α particles, and ^{111}In is separated by the solvent extraction method.

Thallium-201

Thallium-201 is primarily produced by the $^{203}Tl(p,3n)\ ^{201}Pb$ reaction, whereby ^{201}Pb decays to ^{201}Tl with a half-life of 9.4 hr. Thallium-201 obtained in this way is pure and free of other contaminants. After irradiation with 35- to 45-MeV protons, the natural thallium target is dissolved in concentrated nitric acid and then evaporated to dryness. The residue is dissolved in 0.025M EDTA and passed through a Dowex resin column. Most of the thallium is adsorbed on the column, while ^{201}Pb passes through. The eluate is purified once more by passing through another Dowex resin column. The eluate containing ^{201}Pb is allowed to decay for 30–35 hr to produce ^{201}Tl and is then passed through a Dowex 1×8 column. $^{201}Tl^{3+}$ adheres to the column and ^{201}Pb passes through. $^{201}Tl^{3+}$ is eluted with hydrazine-sulfate solution, reducing Tl^{3+} to Tl^{1+}. The eluate is evaporated to dryness with HNO_3 and HCl and finally taken up with NaOH to give TlCl.

Short-Lived Radionuclides

Considerable interest has developed for the production of short-lived radionuclides and their clinical uses because of the availability of the positron emission tomography (PET) imaging systems. Among them are the key radionuclides such as ^{11}C, ^{13}N, ^{15}O, and ^{18}F, which decay by positron emission (hence annihilation radiations of 511 keV). These positron emitters are useful in imaging by PET. Because they have very short half-lives, a cyclotron or a medical cyclotron must be located on site in the laboratory. A medical cyclotron is a small version of a cyclotron and is used primarily for the production of radionuclides for medical applications; it provides low-energy charged particles of high intensity. In some medical cyclotrons, both deuterons and protons can be accelerated alternately.

Carbon-11

Carbon-11 has a half-life of 20.4 min and can be produced by ^{10}B(d, n) ^{11}C, ^{11}B(p, n) ^{11}C, and ^{14}N(p, α) ^{11}C reactions in the cyclotron. In the first two reactions, B_2O_3 is the target, and nitrogen gas in the third. Both ^{11}CO and ^{11}CO$_2$ are produced in boron targets, which are then flushed out by neutral gases. Either ^{11}CO is oxidized to have all the gas in ^{11}CO$_2$ form, or ^{11}CO$_2$ is reduced to have all the gas in ^{11}CO form. Both ^{11}CO and ^{11}CO$_2$ are commonly used as precursors in the preparation of various clinically useful compounds, such as ^{11}C-palmitate for myocardial perfusion imaging by PET.

The ^{14}N(p, α) ^{11}C reaction is carried out by bombardment of a mixture of $N_2 + H_2$ to give ^{11}C, with reacts with N_2 to give ^{11}CN, followed by radiolysis of ^{11}CN to give ^{14}CH$_4$ (95–100% radiochemical yield). Carbon-11-methane is allowed to react with NH_3 over platinum at 1000 °C to a give a 95% overall yield of H^{11}CN. Various biological molecules such as aliphatic amines, amino nitriles, and hydantoins have been labeled with ^{11}C using ^{11}CN as a precursor.

Nitrogen-13

Nitrogen-13 has a half-life of 10 min and is commonly used as NH_3. It is produced by the ^{12}C(d, n) ^{13}N reaction by bombarding Al_4C_3 or methane with 6- to 7- MeV deuterons, or by the ^{16}O(p, α) ^{13}N or ^{13}C(p, n) ^{13}N reaction. In the latter two reactions, a target of slurried mixture of ^{13}C powder and water is used for irradiation with 11- to 12-MeV protons. Nitrogen-13 is converted to NH_3 in aqueous medium. ^{13}NH$_3$ in the form of NH_4^+ ion is used primarily for myocardial perfusion imaging by PET. ^{13}NH$_3$ is also used to label glutamine and asparagine for assessment of viability of tissues.

Oxygen-15

Oxygen-15 has a half-life of 2 min and is produced by the ^{14}N(d, n) ^{15}O reaction by deuteron irradiation of gaseous nitrogen or by the ^{15}N(p, n) ^{15}O reaction by proton bombardment of enriched ^{15}N target. ^{15}O$_2$ is then passed over activated charcoal heated at 600 °C to convert it to C^{15}O and C^{15}O$_2$, which are then used for labeling hemoglobins and for clinical investigations of pulmonary and cardiac malfunctions. Oxygen-15-labeled water is prepared by mixing the N_2 target with H_2 gas and after irradiation, by passing the mixture over the palladium catalyst at 175 °C. ^{15}O-water is recovered in saline and is useful for cerebral and myocardial perfusion studies.

Fluorine-18

Fluorine-18 ($t_{1/2} = 110$ min) is commonly produced by the ^{18}O(p, n) ^{18}F reaction on a pressurized ^{18}O-water target. ^{18}F is recovered as F⁻ ion from water by passing the mixture through a column of quaternary ammonium resins, and ^{18}O-water can be reused as the target. Fluorine-18 is used primarily to label glucose to give ^{18}F-labeled fluorodeoxyglucose (FDG) for myocardial and cerebral metabolic studies. It is also used to label many potential ligands for a variety of tumors and recently approved by the U.S. Food and Drug Administration (FDA) for bone imaging.

Reactor-Produced Radionuclides

A variety of radionuclides are produced in nuclear reactors. A nuclear reactor is constructed with fuel rods made of fissile materials such as enriched ^{235}U and ^{239}Pu. These fuel nuclei undergo spontaneous fission with extremely low probability. Fission is defined as the breakup of a heavy nucleus into two fragments of approximately equal mass, accompanied by the emission of two to three neutrons with mean energies of about 1.5 MeV. In each fission, there is a concomitant energy release of 200 MeV that appears as heat and is usually removed by heat exchangers to produce electricity in the nuclear power plant.

Neutrons emitted in each fission can cause further fission of other fissionable nuclei in the fuel rod provided the right conditions exist. This obviously will initiate a chain reaction, ultimately leading to a possible meltdown situation in the reactor. This chain reaction must be controlled, which is accomplished by the proper size, shape, and mass of the fuel material and other complicated and ingenious engineering techniques. To control a self-sustained chain reaction, excess neutrons (more than one) are removed by positioning cadmium rods in the fuel core (cadmium has a high probability of absorbing a thermal neutron).

The fuel rods of fissile materials are interspersed in the reactor core with spaces in between. Neutrons emitted with a mean energy of 1.5 MeV from the surface of the fuel rod have a low probability of interaction with other nuclei and therefore do not serve any useful purpose. It has been found, however, that neutrons with thermal energy (0.025 eV) interact with many nuclei, efficiently producing various radionuclides. To make the high energy or so-called fast neutrons more useful, they are thermalized or slowed down by interaction with low molecular weight materials, such as water, heavy water, beryllium, and graphite, which are distributed in the spaces between the fuel rods. These materials are called *moderators*. The flux or intensity of the thermal neutrons so obtained ranges from 10^{11} to 10^{14} neutrons/ $(cm^2 \cdot sec)$ and they are important in the production of many radionuclides. When a target element is inserted in the reactor core, a thermal neutron will interact with the target nucleus with a definite probability to produce another nuclide. The probability of formation of a radionuclide by thermal neutrons varies from element to element.

In the reactor, two types of interaction with thermal neutrons are of considerable importance in the production of various useful radionuclides: fission of heavy elements and neutron capture or (n, γ) reaction. These two reactions are described below.

Fission or (n, f) Reaction

As already mentioned, fission is a breakup of a heavy nucleus into two fragments of approximately equal mass. When a target of heavy elements is inserted in the reactor core, heavy nuclei absorb thermal neutrons and undergo fission. Fissionable heavy elements are ^{235}U, ^{239}Pu, ^{237}Np, ^{233}U, ^{232}Th, and many others having atomic numbers greater than 90. Fission of heavy elements may also be induced in a cyclotron by irradiation with high-energy charged particles, but the fission probability depends on the type and energy of the irradiating particle. Nuclides produced by fission may range in atomic number from about 28 to nearly 65. These isotopes of different elements are separated by appropriate chemical procedures that involve precipitation, solvent extraction, ion exchange, chromatography, and distillation. These methods are described in detail in Chapter 8. The fission radionuclides are normally carrier-free or NCA, and therefore isotopes of high specific activity are available from fission. Since the chemical behavior of isotopes of many different elements is similar, contamination often becomes a serious problem in the isolation of a desired radionuclide; therefore, meticulous methods of purification are needed to remove the contaminants. The fission products are usually neutron rich and decay by β^- emission.

Many clinically useful radionuclides such as ^{131}I, ^{99}Mo, ^{133}Xe, and ^{137}Cs are produced by fission of ^{235}U. An example of thermal fission of ^{235}U is presented below, showing only a few representative radionuclides:

$$^{235}_{92}U + {}^1_0n \rightarrow {}^{236}_{92}U \rightarrow {}^{131}_{53}I + {}^{102}_{39}Y + 3{}^1_0n$$

$$\rightarrow {}^{99}_{42}Mo + {}^{135}_{50}Sn + 2{}^1_0n$$

$$\rightarrow {}^{117}_{46}Pd + {}^{117}_{46}Pd + 2{}^1_0n$$

$$\rightarrow {}^{133}_{54}Xe + {}^{101}_{38}Sr + 2{}^1_0n$$

$$\rightarrow\ {}^{137}_{55}Cs + {}^{97}_{37}Rb + 2{}^{1}_{0}n$$

$$\rightarrow\ {}^{155}_{62}Sm + {}^{78}_{30}Zn + 3{}^{1}_{0}n$$

$$\rightarrow\ {}^{156}_{62}Sm + {}^{77}_{30}Zn + 3{}^{1}_{0}n$$

It should be understood that many other nuclides besides those mentioned in the example are also produced.

Iodine-131

For chemical separation of ^{131}I from the irradiated ^{235}U target, the latter is dissolved in 18% NaOH by heating, and hydroxides of many metal ions are precipitated by cooling. The supernatant containing sodium iodide is acidified with sulfuric acid in a closed distillation system. Iodide is oxidized to iodine by the acid, and iodine is collected in a NaOH solution by distillation.

Molybdenum-99

For ^{99}Mo separation, the irradiated uranium target is dissolved in nitric acid and the solution is adsorbed on an alumina (Al_2O_3) column. The column is then washed with nitric acid to remove uranium and other fission product cations. Molybdenum is then eluted with ammonium hydroxide. It is further purified by adsorption of ammonium molybdate on Dowex-1 anion-exchange resin and washing of the column with concentrated HCl to remove other impurities. Ammonium molybdate is finally eluted with dilute HCl and ultimately used for the ^{99}Mo-^{99m}Tc generator. The ^{99}Mo radionuclide produced by fission is carrier-free or NCA and its most common contaminants are ^{131}I and ^{103}Ru.

Neutron Capture or (n, γ) Reaction

In neutron capture reaction, the target nucleus captures one thermal neutron and emits γ rays to produce an isotope of the same element. The radionuclide so produced is therefore not carrier-free and its specific activity (described later) is relatively low. This reaction takes place in almost all elements with varying probability. Since the target and the product nuclei belong to the same element, chemical separation is obviously unnecessary unless impurities develop due to decay of various radioisotopes or extraneous radionuclides produced by impurities in the target. In all these cases, chemical separation must be carried out.

Various useful radionuclides produced by this reaction are ^{131}Te (which produces ^{131}I by β^- decay with a half-life of 25 min), ^{99}Mo, ^{197}Hg, ^{59}Fe, ^{51}Cr, and many more. These radionuclides are often neutron rich and therefore decay by β^- emission. Some examples of neutron capture reactions are

$^{98}Mo(n, \gamma)$ ^{99}Mo, $^{196}Hg(n, \gamma)$ ^{197}Hg, and $^{50}Cr(n, \gamma)$ ^{51}Cr. Molybdenum-99 so produced is called the irradiated molybdenum as opposed to the fission molybdenum described earlier.

It should be pointed out that the neutron capture reaction is the basis of the neutron activation analysis of various trace metals. A sample containing trace metals is irradiated with thermal neutrons and the trace metal atom captures a neutron to produce a radionuclide that can be detected by radiation detectors. Neutron activation analysis has proved to be an important tool in detecting the presence of trace elements in forensic, industrial, and biological sciences.

Target and Its Processing

Various types of targets have been designed and used for both reactor and cyclotron irradiation. In the design of targets, primary consideration is given to heat deposition in the target by irradiation with neutrons in the reactor or charged particles in the cyclotron. In both cases, the temperature can rise to $1000\,°C$ and, if proper material is not used or a method of heat dissipation is not properly designed, the target is likely to be burned. For this reason, water cooling of the cyclotron probe to which the target is attached is commonly adopted. In the case of the reactor, the core cooling is sufficient to cool the target. Most often, the targets are designed in the form of a foil to maximize the heat dissipation.

The target element ideally should be monoisotopic or at least an enriched isotope to avoid extraneous nuclear reactions. The enrichment of a given isotope is made by an isotope separator and the degree of enrichment depends on the percent abundance of the isotope in the natural element. If the interfering nuclear reactions are minimal, then targets of natural abundance also can be used.

The common form of the target is metallic foil, for example, copper, aluminum, uranium, vanadium, and so on. Other forms of targets are oxides, carbonates, nitrates, and chlorides contained in an aluminum tubing which is then flattened. Aluminum tubing is used because of its high melting point. In some cases, compounds are deposited on the appropriate metallic foil by vacuum distillation or by electrodeposition and the products are then used as targets. A pneumatic tube is often used to carry the target to and from the inside of the reactor or the cyclotron. In special cases, such as in the production of ^{123}I, a chamber whose inside is coated with tellurium powder is used as the target (discussed earlier).

After irradiation, the target must be dissolved in an appropriate solvent, either an acid or an alkali. Various chemical methods, such as precipitation, ion exchange, solvent extraction, distillation, and gel chromatography, are employed to separate different isotopes from the target solution. These methods are described in detail in Chapter 8 (the chemical separation methods of all elemental radionuclides have been described in the Nuclear Science Series published by National Academy of Science–National Research Council of U.S.A.).

Equation for Production of Radionuclides

While irradiating a target for the production of a radionuclide, it is essential to know various parameters affecting its production, preferably in mathematical form, in order to estimate how much of it would be produced for a given set of parameters. These parameters are therefore discussed in some detail in a mathematical form.

The activity of a radionuclide produced by irradiation of a target material with charged particles in a cyclotron or with neutrons in a nuclear reactor is given by

$$A = IN\sigma(1 - e^{-\lambda t}) \tag{4.1}$$

where

A = activity in disintegrations per second of the radionuclide produced
I = intensity or flux of the irradiating particles [number of particles/ $(cm^2 \cdot sec)$]
N = number of target atoms
σ = formation cross-section (probability) of the radionuclide (cm^2); it is given in units of "barn," which is equal to $10^{-24} cm^2$
λ = decay constant given by $0.693/t_{1/2}(sec^{-1})$
t = duration of irradiation (sec)

Equation (4.1) indicates that the amount of radioactivity produced depends on the intensity and energy (related to the cross-section σ) of the incident particles, the amount of the target material, the half-life of the radionuclide produced, and the duration of irradiation. The term $(1 - e^{-\lambda t})$ is called the saturation factor and approaches unity when t is approximately five to six half-lives of the radionuclide in question. At that time, the yield of the product nuclide becomes maximum and its rates of production and decay become equal. For a period of irradiation of five to six half-lives, Eq. (4.1) becomes

$$A = IN\sigma \tag{4.2}$$

A graphic representation of Eqs. (4.1) and (4.2) is given in Figure 4.2.

The intensity of the irradiating particles is measured by various physical techniques, the description of which is beyond the scope of this book; however, the values are available from the operator of the cyclotron or the reactor. The cross-sections of various nuclides are determined by experimental methods using Eq. (4.1), and they have been compiled and published

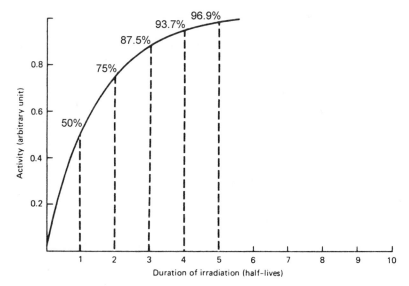

FIGURE 4.2. Production of radionuclides in a reactor or a cyclotron. The activity produced reaches a maximum (saturation) in five to six half-lives of the radionuclide.

by many investigators. The number of atoms N of the target is calculated from the weight W of the material irradiated, the atomic weight A_w and natural abundance K of the target atom, and Avogadro's number (6.02×10^{23}) as follows:

$$N = \frac{W \times K}{A_w} \times 6.02 \times 10^{23} \tag{4.3}$$

After irradiation, isotopes of different elements may be produced and therefore separated by the appropriate chemical methods. These radionuclides are identified and quantitated by the NaI(Tl) or Ge(Li) detectors coupled to a multichannel pulse height analyzer. They may also be assayed in an ionization chamber if the amount of radioactivity is high.

We shall now do two problems using Eq. (4.1) to calculate the radioactivity of the commonly used radionuclides produced by irradiation in a cyclotron or a nuclear reactor.

Problem 4.1
In a nuclear reactor, 10 g ^{235}U is irradiated with 2×10^{14} neutrons/(cm^2 · sec) for 10 days. Calculate the radioactivity of ^{99}Mo produced if its $t_{1/2}$ is 66 hr and formation cross-section by fission is 10^{-26} cm^2.

Answer

Number of g · atoms in 10 g ^{235}U $= 10/235$

Number of atoms of ^{235}U $= (10/235) \times 6.02 \times 10^{23} = 2.56 \times 10^{22}$

$$\lambda \text{ for } ^{99}\text{Mo} = \frac{0.693}{66 \times 60 \times 60} = 2.91 \times 10^{-6} \text{ sec}^{-1}$$

$$t = 10 \times 24 \times 60 \times 60 = 8.64 \times 10^5 \text{ sec}$$

Using Eq. (4.1),

$$A(\text{dps}) = 2 \times 10^{14} \times 2.56 \times 10^{22} \times 10^{-26} \times [1 - \exp(-2.91 \times 10^{-6} \times 8.64 \times 10^5)]$$

$$= 4.71 \times 10^{10} \text{ dps}(47.1 \text{ GBq})$$

Since 1 Ci $= 3.7 \times 10^{10}$ dps, the activity A of ^{99}Mo is calculated as

$$A = \frac{4.71 \times 10^{10}}{3.7 \times 10^{10}} = 1.27 \text{ Ci}$$

Problem 4.2

Calculate the radioactivity of ^{111}In produced by irradiation of 1 g ^{111}Cd with a proton beam current of 1 microampere (μA) per cm^2 in a cyclotron for a period of 10 hr. The half-life of ^{111}In is 2.8 days and its cross-section for formation by the (p, n) reaction is 1 barn.

Answer

Since 1 ampere is equal to 1 coulomb (C)/sec and 1 proton carries 1.6×10^{-19} C, the number of protons in 1 μA/cm^2 is

$$I = \frac{1 \times 10^{-6}}{1.6 \times 10^{-19}} = 6.25 \times 10^{12} \text{ protons}/(\text{cm}^2 \cdot \text{sec})$$

$$N = \frac{1}{111} \times 6.02 \times 10^{23} = 5.42 \times 10^{21} \text{ atoms } ^{111}\text{Cd}$$

$$\lambda = \frac{0.693}{2.8 \times 24 \times 60 \times 60} = 2.86 \times 10^{-6} \text{ sec}^{-1} \text{ for } ^{111}\text{In}$$

$$t = 10 \times 60 \times 60 = 3.60 \times 10^4 \text{ sec}$$

Using Eq. (4.1),

$$A(\text{dps}) = 6.25 \times 10^{12} \times 5.42 \times 10^{21} \times 10^{-24}$$

$$\times [1 - \exp(-2.86 \times 10^{-6} \times 3.6 \times 10^4)]$$

$$= 3.39 \times 10^{10} \times (1 - 0.9022)$$

$$= 3.32 \times 10^9 \text{ dps } (3.32 \text{ GBq})$$

$$A = \frac{3.32 \times 10^9}{3.7 \times 10^7} \text{ mCi}$$

$$= 89.7 \text{ mCi}$$

Using this example, activities of ^{67}Ga, ^{123}I, and other cyclotron-produced radionuclides can be calculated from the knowledge of all the relevant parameters.

In Table 4.1, the radiation characteristics and production methods of several useful radionuclides are presented.

Specific Activity

Specific activity is defined as the radioactivity per unit mass of a radionuclide or a labeled compound. For example, suppose that 100 mg ^{131}I-labeled albumin contains 150 mCi (5.55 GBq) ^{131}I radioactivity. Its specific activity would be 150/100, that is, 1.5 mCi/mg or 55.5 MBq/mg. Sometimes it is confused with concentration, which is defined as the radioactivity per unit volume of a sample. A 10-ml solution containing 45 mCi (1.67 GBq) radioactivity will have a concentration of 4.5 mCi/ml (167 MBq/ml). Specific activity is at times expressed in terms of the radioactivity per mole of a labeled compound, for example, mCi/mole (MBq/mole) or mCi/μmole (MBq/μmole) for ^{3}H-, ^{14}C-, and ^{35}S-labeled compounds.

The specific activity of a carrier-free radionuclide sample is related to the half-life of the radionuclide: the shorter the half-life, the higher the specific activity. For example, carrier-free ^{99m}Tc and ^{131}I have specific activities of 5.27×10^{6} mCi/mg (1.95×10^{5} GBq/mg) and 1.25×10^{5} mCi/mg (4.6×10^{3} GBq/mg), respectively. The derivation of these values should be understood from the following problem.

Problem 4.3
What is the specific activity of carrier-free ^{111}In($t_{1/2} = 67$ hr)?

Answer
In 1 mg ^{111}In, the number of atoms N of ^{111}In is

$$N = \frac{1 \times 10^{-3} \times 6.02 \times 10^{23}}{111}$$

The decay constant λ of ^{111}In is

$$\lambda = \frac{0.693}{67 \times 60 \times 60} \text{ sec}^{-1}$$

$$A = \lambda N$$

$$= \frac{0.693 \times 10^{-3} \times 6.02 \times 10^{23}}{67 \times 60 \times 60 \times 111} \text{ dps}$$

$$= 1.56 \times 10^{13} \text{ dps}$$

$$= 4.22 \times 10^{5} \text{ mCi}$$

TABLE 4.1. Characteristics of commonly used radionuclides.

Nuclide	Physical half-life	Mode of decay (%)	γ-ray energy[a] (MeV)	Abundance (%)	Common production method
^3_1H	12.3 yr	$\beta^-(100)$	—	—	$^6\text{Li}(n,\alpha)^3\text{H}$
$^{11}_6\text{C}$	20.4 min	$\beta^+(100)$	0.511 (annihilation)	200	$^{10}\text{B}(d,n)^{11}\text{C}$ $^{14}\text{N}(p,\alpha)^{11}\text{C}$
$^{13}_7\text{N}$	10 min	$\beta^+(100)$	0.511 (annihilation)	200	$^{12}\text{C}(d,n)^{13}\text{N}$ $^{16}\text{O}(p,\alpha)^{13}\text{N}$ $^{13}\text{C}(p,n)^{13}\text{N}$
$^{14}_6\text{C}$	5730 yr	$\beta^-(100)$	—	—	$^{14}\text{N}(n,p)^{14}\text{C}$
$^{15}_8\text{O}$	2 min	$\beta^+(100)$	0.511 (annihilation)	200	$^{14}\text{N}(d,n)^{15}\text{O}$ $^{15}\text{N}(p,n)^{15}\text{O}$
$^{18}_9\text{F}$	110 min	$\beta^+(97)$ EC(3)	0.511 (annihilation)	194	$^{18}\text{O}(p,n)^{18}\text{F}$
$^{32}_{15}\text{P}$	14.3 days	$\beta^-(100)$	—	—	$^{32}\text{S}(n,p)^{32}\text{P}$
$^{51}_{24}\text{Cr}$	27.7 days	EC(100)	0.320	9	$^{50}\text{Cr}(n,\gamma)^{51}\text{Cr}$
$^{52}_{26}\text{Fe}$	8.3 hr	$\beta^+(56)$ EC(44)	0.165 0.511 (annihilation)	100 112	$^{55}\text{Mn}(n,4n)^{52}\text{Fe}$ $^{50}\text{Cr}(\alpha,2n)^{52}\text{Fe}$
$^{57}_{27}\text{Co}$	271 days	EC(100)	0.014 0.122 0.136	9 86 11	$^{56}\text{Fe}(d,n)^{57}\text{Co}$
$^{58}_{27}\text{Co}$	71 days	$\beta^+(14.9)$ EC(85.1)	0.811	99.5	$^{55}\text{Mn}(\alpha,n)^{58}\text{Co}$
$^{59}_{26}\text{Fe}$	45 days	$\beta^-(100)$	1.099 1.292	56 43	$^{58}\text{Fe}(n,\gamma)^{59}\text{Fe}$
$^{60}_{27}\text{Co}$	5.2 yr	$\beta^-(100)$	1.173 1.332	100 100	$^{59}\text{Co}(n,\gamma)^{60}\text{Co}$
$^{62}_{28}\text{Zn}$	9.3 hr	$\beta^+(8)$ EC(92)	0.420 0.511 0.548 0.597	25 31 15 26	$^{63}\text{Cu}(p,2n)^{62}\text{Zn}$
$^{62}_{29}\text{Cu}$	9.7 min	$\beta^+(97)$ EC(3)	0.511 (annihilation)	194	$^{62}\text{Ni}(p,n)^{62}\text{Cu}$ or $^{62}\text{Zn}\xrightarrow[9.3\,\text{hr}]{\beta^+,\text{EC}}{}^{62}\text{Cu}$
$^{67}_{29}\text{Cu}$	2.6 days	$\beta^-(100)$	0.185 0.92	49 23	$^{67}\text{Zn}(n,p)^{67}\text{Cu}$
$^{67}_{31}\text{Ga}$	78.2 hr	EC(100)	0.093 0.184 0.300 0.393	40 20 17 5	$^{68}\text{Zn}(p,2n)^{67}\text{Ga}$
$^{68}_{31}\text{Ga}$	68 min	$\beta^+(89)$ EC(11)	0.511 (annihilation)	178	$^{68}\text{Zn}(p,n)^{68}\text{Ga}$
$^{82}_{37}\text{Rb}$	75 s	$\beta^+(95)$ EC(5)	0.511 (annihilation) 776	190 13	$^{82}\text{Sr}\xrightarrow[25.5\,\text{days}]{\text{EC}}{}^{82}\text{Rb}$
$^{82}_{38}\text{Sr}$	25.5 days	EC(100)	—	—	$^{85}\text{Rb}(p,4n)^{82}\text{Sr}$
$^{89}_{38}\text{Sr}$	50.6 days	$\beta^-(100)$	—	—	$^{88}\text{Sr}(n,\gamma)^{89}\text{Sr}$
$^{90}_{38}\text{Sr}$	28.5 yr	$\beta^-(100)$	—	—	$^{235}\text{U}(n,f)^{90}\text{Sr}$
$^{90}_{39}\text{Y}$	2.7 days	$\beta^-(100)$	—	—	$^{89}\text{Y}(n,\gamma)^{90}\text{Y}$
$^{99}_{42}\text{Mo}$	66 hr	$\beta^-(100)$	0.181 0.740 0.780	6 12 4	$^{98}\text{Mo}(n,\gamma)^{99}\text{Mo}$ $^{235}\text{U}(n,f)^{99}\text{Mo}$

TABLE 4.1 (*continued*)

Nuclide	Physical half-life	Mode of decay (%)	γ-ray energy[a] (MeV)	Abundance (%)	Common production method
$^{99m}_{43}$Tc	6.0 hr	IT(100)	0.140	90	^{99}Mo $\xrightarrow[\text{66 hr}]{\beta^-}$ ^{99m}Tc
$^{111}_{49}$In	2.8 days	EC(100)	0.171	90	^{111}Cd(p, n)^{111}In
			0.245	94	
$^{113m}_{49}$In	100 min	IT(100)	0.392	64	^{112}Sn(n, γ)^{113}Sn
					^{113}Sn $\xrightarrow[\text{117 days}]{\text{EC}}$ ^{113m}In
$^{123}_{53}$I	13.2 hr	EC(100)	0.159	83	^{121}Sb(α, 2n)^{123}I
$^{124}_{53}$I	4.2 days	β^+ (23)	0.511	46	^{124}Te(p, n)^{124}I
		EC(77)	(annihilation)		
$^{125}_{53}$I	60 days	EC(100)	0.035	7	^{124}Xe(n, γ)^{125}Xe
			x ray(0.027–0.032)	140	^{125}Xe $\xrightarrow[\text{17 hr}]{\text{EC}}$ ^{125}I
$^{131}_{53}$I	8.0 days	β^-(100)	0.284	6	^{130}Te(n, γ)^{131}Te
			0.364	81	^{235}U(n, f)^{131}Te
			0.637	7	^{131}Te $\xrightarrow[\text{25 min}]{\beta^-}$ ^{131}I
					^{235}U(n, f)^{131}I
$^{133}_{54}$Xe	5.3 days	β^-(100)	0.081	37	^{235}U(n, f)^{133}Xe
$^{137}_{55}$Cs	30.0 yr	β^-(100)	0.662	85	^{235}U(n, f)^{137}Cs
$^{153}_{62}$Sm	1.9 days	β^-(100)	70	5	^{152}Sm(n, γ)^{153}Sm
			103	28	
$^{186}_{75}$Re	3.8 days	β^-(92)	137	9	^{185}Re(n, γ)^{186}Re
		EC(8)			
$^{201}_{81}$Tl	73 hr	EC(100)	0.167	9.4	^{203}Tl(p, 3n)^{201}Pb
			x ray(0.069–0.083)	93	^{201}Pb $\xrightarrow[\text{9.3 hr}]{\text{EC}}$ ^{201}Tl

Data from Browne E, Finestone RB. *Table of Radioactive Isotopes.* New York: Wiley; 1986.
[a] γ rays with abundance less than 4% and those having energy less than 20 keV have not been cited.
NOTE: IT, isomeric transition; EC, electron capture; f, fission; d, deuteron; n, neutron; p, proton; α, alpha particle.

Therefore, the specific activity of ^{111}In is 4.22×10^5 mCi/mg or 1.56×10^4 GBq/mg.

The specific activity of a carrier-free or NCA radionuclide can be calculated by the following formula.

$$\text{Specific activity (mCi/mg)} = \frac{3.13 \times 10^9}{A \times t_{1/2}} \qquad (4.4)$$

where

A is the mass number of the radionuclide
$t_{1/2}$ is the half-life in hours of the radionuclide

The specific activity of a radiopharmaceutical is an important information for a particular nuclear medicine test and is often provided on the label posted on the vial. Low specific activity is of little value in some labeling procedures because the cold atoms compete with radioactive atoms for the binding sites of the reacting molecules and thus lower the labeling yield. Similarly in nuclear medicine studies cold atoms in low-specificity sample compromises the uptake of the tracer in the tissue of interest in vivo. On the other hand, high specific activity can cause radiolysis in the solution of a compound, resulting in the breakdown of the compound into undesirable impurities. Proteins are denatured by high specific activities.

Questions

1. Describe the different methods of production of radionuclides and discuss the merits and disadvantages of each method.
2. If ^{127}I is irradiated with protons in a cyclotron and three neutrons are emitted from the nucleus, what is the product of the nuclear reaction? Write the nuclear reaction.
3. In fission, how many neutrons are emitted and what is their average energy? What is the average energy released in fission?
4. Why are cadmium rods and graphite used in the reactor?
5. Outline the procedure for separating ^{131}I and ^{99}Mo from the fission products of ^{235}U.
6. (a) Calculate the activity in millicuries of ^{123}I produced by the $^{121}Sb\,(\alpha, 2n)\,^{123}I$ reaction, when 200 mg natural antimony (natural abundance of ^{121}Sb is 57.3%) is irradiated for 2 hr with an α-particle beam of 25-MeV energy and an intensity of 10^{14} particles/ $(cm^2 \cdot sec)$. The cross-section for formation of $^{123}I\,(t_{1/2} = 13.2\,hr)$ is 28 mbarns.
   (b) What is the number of ^{123}I atoms produced after irradiation?
   (c) What is the activity of ^{123}I 6 hr after irradiation?
7. Calculate the specific activities of carrier-free or NCA ^{131}I, ^{99m}Tc, ^{32}P, and $^{67}Ga\,(t_{1/2} = 8\,days, 6\,hr, 14.3\,days,\ and\ 78\,hr,\ respectively)$.
8. Why is the specific activity of radionuclides higher in fission than in the (n, γ) reaction?
9. Is the specific activity higher for radionuclides having a longer half-life?
10. Calculate the duration of irradiation necessary to produce 600 mCi (22.2 GBq) of ^{99}Mo by irradiating 4 g of ^{235}U in the nuclear reactor whose thermal neutron flux is 2×10^{14} neutrons/$cm^2 \cdot sec$. (Assume the formation cross-section of ^{99}Mo is 20 mbarns and the half-life of ^{99}Mo is 66 hr.)

Suggested Reading

Friedlander G, Kennedy JW, Miller JM. *Nuclear and Radiochemistry*. 3rd ed. New York: Wiley; 1981.

Gelbard AS, Hara T, Tilbury RS, Laughlin JS. Recent aspects of cyclotron production of medically useful radionuclides. In: *Radiopharmaceuticals and Labelled Compounds*. Vienna: IAEA; 1973:239.

Poggenburg JK. The nuclear reactor and its products. *Semin Nucl Med*. 1974; 4:229.

Saha GB. Miscellaneous radiotracers for imaging. In: Rayudu GVS, ed. *Radiotracers for Medical Applications*. Boca Raton, Fla: CRC Press; 1983; II:119.

Saha GB, MacIntyre WJ, Go RT. Cyclotrons and positron emission tomography for clinical imaging. *Semin Nucl Med* 1992; 22:150.

Silvester DJ. Accelerator production of medically useful radionuclides. In: *Radiopharmaceuticals and Labelled Compounds*. Vienna: IAEA; 1973; I:197.

Silvester DJ, Waters SL. Radionuclide production. In Sodd VJ, Allen DR, Hoogland DR, Ice RD, eds. *Radiopharmaceuticals II*. New York: Society of Nuclear Medicine; 1979:727.

5
Radionuclide Generators

Principles of a Generator

The use of short-lived radionuclides has grown considerably, because larger dosages of these radionuclides can be administered to the patient with only minimal radiation dose and produce excellent image quality. This increasing appreciation of short-lived radionuclides has led to the development of radionuclide generators that serve as convenient sources of their production. A generator is constructed on the principle of the decay-growth relationship between a long-lived parent radionuclide and its short-lived daughter radionuclide. The chemical property of the daughter nuclide must be distinctly different from that of the parent nuclide so that the former can be readily separated. In a generator, basically a long-lived parent nuclide is allowed to decay to its short-lived daughter nuclide and the latter is then chemically separated. The importance of radionuclide generators lies in the fact that they are easily transportable and serve as sources of short-lived radionuclides in institutions far from the site of a cyclotron or reactor facility.

A radionuclide generator consists of a glass or plastic column fitted at the bottom with a fritted disk. The column is filled with adsorbent material such as cation- or anion-exchange resin, alumina, and zirconia, on which the parent nuclide is adsorbed. The daughter radionuclide grows as a result of the decay of the parent until either a transient or a secular equilibrium is reached within several half-lives of the daughter, after which the daughter appears to decay with the same half-life as the parent. Because there are differences in chemical properties, the daughter activity is eluted in a carrier-free state with an appropriate solvent, leaving the parent on the column. After elution, the daughter activity starts to grow again in the column until an equilibrium is reached in the manner mentioned above; the elution of activity can be made repeatedly. A schematic of a typical generator is presented in Figure 5.1. The vial containing the eluant is first inverted onto needle A, and another evacuated vial is inverted onto the other needle B. The vacuum in the vial on needle B draws the eluant through the column and elutes the daughter nuclide, leaving the parent nuclide on the column.

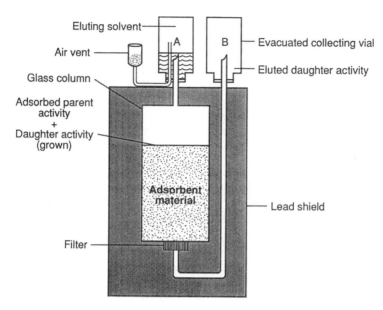

FIGURE 5.1. Typical generator system. The daughter activity grown by the decay of the parent is separated chemically from the parent. The eluent in vial A is drawn through the column and the daughter nuclide is collected in vial B under vacuum.

A radionuclide generator must be sterile and pyrogen-free. The generator system may be sterilized either by autoclaving the entire column or by preparing it from sterile materials under aseptic conditions. Often, bacteriostatic agents are added to the generator column to maintain sterility or a membrane filter unit is attached to the end of the column. Elution or "milking" of the generator is carried out under aseptic conditions.

An ideal radionuclide generator should be simple, convenient, rapid to use, and give a high yield of the daughter nuclide repeatedly and reproducibly. It should be properly shielded to minimize radiation exposure, and sturdy and compact for shipping. The generator eluate should be free from the parent radionuclide and the adsorbent material. Other extraneous radioactive contaminants should be absent in the eluate. The daughter nuclide should decay to a stable or very long-lived nuclide so that the radiation dose to the patient is minimal. Even though the parent activity may be eluted in an extremely small quantity (10^{-5}–10^{-6} times the daughter activity), the radiation dose to the patient may become appreciable if it has a long effective half-life (see Chapter 6).

The first commercial radionuclide generator was the ^{132}Te($t_{1/2} = 78$ hr)–^{132}I ($t_{1/2} = 2.3$ hr) system developed at the Brookhaven National Laboratory in the early 1960s. Since then, a number of other generator systems have been developed and tried for routine use in nuclear medicine. Only a few of these generators are of importance in nuclear medicine; they are the

TABLE 5.1. Several generator systems useful in nuclear medicine.

Parent	Parent $t_{1/2}$	Nuclear reaction	Daughter	Daughter $t_{1/2}$	Mode of daughter decay	Principal photon energy (keV) (% abundance)	Column	Eluant
^{99}Mo	66 hr	Fission ^{98}Mo(n,γ)	^{99m}Tc	6 hr	IT[a]	140 (90)	Al$_2$O$_3$	0.9% NaCl
^{113}Sn	115 days	^{112}Sn(n,γ)	^{113m}In	99.5 min	IT	392 (64)	ZrO$_2$	0.05 N HCl
^{87}Y	80 hr	^{88}Sr(p,2n)	^{87m}Sr	2.8 hr	IT	388 (82)	Dowex 1 $\times$ 8	0.15 M NaHCO$_3$
^{68}Ge	271 days	^{69}Ga(p,2n)	^{68}Ga	68 min	β^+	511 (178)	Al$_2$O$_3$ SnO$_2$	0.005 M EDTA 1 N HCl
^{62}Zn	9.3 hr	^{63}Cu(p,2n)	^{62}Cu	9.7 min	β^+	511 (194)	Dowex 1 $\times$ 8	2 N HCl
^{137}Cs	30 yr	Fission	^{137m}Ba	2.6 min	IT	662 (85)	Ammonium molybdophosphate	0.1 N HCl + 0.1 N NH$_4$Cl
^{81}Rb	4.6 hr	^{79}Br(α,2n)	^{81m}Kr	13 sec	IT	190 (67)	BioRad AG 50	Water or air
^{82}Sr	25.5 days	^{85}Rb(p,4n)	^{82}Rb	75 sec	β^+	511 (190)	SnO$_2$	0.9% NaCl
^{191}Os	15.4 days	^{190}Os(n,γ)	^{191m}Ir	4.9 sec	IT	129 (26)	BioRad AG1	4% NaCl
^{195}Hg	41.5 hr	^{197}Au(p,3n)	^{195m}Au	30.6 sec	IT	262 (68)	Silica gel coated with ZnS	Sodium thiosulfate solution

Data from Browne E, Firestone RB. *Table of Radioactive Isotopes*. 1st ed. New York: Wiley; 1986.

[a] IT, isomeric transition.

^{99}Mo–^{99m}Tc, ^{113}Sn–^{113m}In, ^{82}Sr–^{82}Rb, and ^{68}Ge–^{68}Ga systems. Several generator systems, including those above, are presented in Table 5.1 along with their properties.

Important Radionuclide Generators

^{99}Mo–^{99m}Tc Generator

The ^{99}Mo radionuclide has a half-life of 66 hr and decays by β^- emission; 87% of its decay goes ultimately to the metastable state ^{99m}Tc and the remaining 13% to the ground state ^{99}Tc. It has photon transitions of 740 keV and 780 keV. The radionuclide ^{99m}Tc has a half-life of 6 hr and decays to ^{99}Tc by isomeric transition of 140 keV. Approximately 10% of these transitions are via internal conversion. The ground state ^{99}Tc has a half-life of 2.1×10^5 years and decays to stable ^{99}Ru by β^- emission.

Because the half-lives of ^{99}Mo and ^{99m}Tc differ by a factor of about 11, these two radionuclides lend themselves to the construction of a useful generator. The extreme usefulness of this generator is due to the excellent radiation characteristics of ^{99m}Tc, namely its 6-hr half-life, very little electron emission, and a high yield of 140-keV γ rays (90%), which are nearly ideal for the current generation of imaging devices in nuclear medicine.

Construction

Liquid Column Generator

The ^{99}Mo–^{99m}Tc generator was first introduced at the Brookhaven National Laboratory. Before this generator was developed, the ^{99m}Tc radioactivity used to be extracted with methyl ethyl ketone (MEK) from a 20% NaOH solution (pH $\sim$ 10–12) of ^{99}Mo. After extraction, the organic phase was evaporated and the ^{99m}TcO$_4^-$ dissolved in isotonic saline for clinical use. This method of solvent extraction has been employed to construct the liquid-liquid extractor type of generator for the ^{99}Mo–^{99m}Tc system. The basic principle involves placing the 20% NaOH solution of ^{99}Mo in a glass column and then letting MEK flow through the column from the bottom. MEK will extract ^{99m}TcO$_4^-$ leaving ^{99}Mo in the aqueous solution. Repeated elutions of the column can be made after or before the transient equilibrium between ^{99}Mo and ^{99m}Tc is reached. The advantage of this generator is that the cost of ^{99m}Tc is low. But the disadvantage is that it needs a lot of manipulation in the overall method. It is rarely used in nuclear medicine.

Solid Column Generator

The solvent extraction technique has been replaced by the solid column generator for obtaining ^{99m}Tc. The ^{99}Mo–^{99m}Tc or "Moly" generator is constructed with alumina (Al$_2$O$_3$) loaded in a plastic or glass column. The amount of alumina used is of the order of 5 to 10 g, depending on the total activity of ^{99}Mo. The ^{99}Mo radioactivity is adsorbed on alumina in the chemical form MoO$_4^{2-}$ (molybdate) and in various amounts. The column is thoroughly washed with 0.9% NaCl solution to remove any undesirable activity. Currently, all generators are made with fission-produced ^{99}Mo.

The generator columns are shielded with lead for radiation protection. Some commercial firms use depleted uranium in lieu of lead for shielding high ^{99}Mo activity generators (8.3–16.6 Ci or 307–614 GBq) because ^{238}U has higher Z and therefore attenuates γ rays more efficiently (depleted uranium is natural uranium from which ^{235}U has been removed, leaving only ^{238}U).

After adsorption of ^{99}Mo on alumina, ^{99m}Tc grows by the decay of ^{99}Mo according to Eq. (2.10) until its maximum activity is reached after approximately four half-lives of ^{99m}Tc. At equilibrium and thereafter, the ^{99m}Tc radioactivity follows the half-life of ^{99}Mo. The typical decay–growth relationship between ^{99}Mo and ^{99m}Tc is illustrated in Figure 5.2 for a 100-mCi (3.7-GBq) generator.

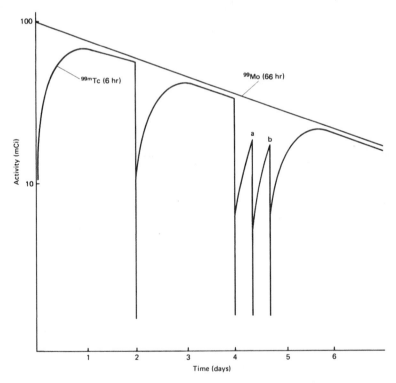

FIGURE 5.2. Typical decay-growth relationship of ^{99}Mo and ^{99m}Tc activities in a Moly generator. On day 2, ^{99m}Tc activity is eluted with saline and then starts growing after elution. The yield of ^{99m}Tc is approximately 80% to 90%. It takes approximately 24 hr to reach maximum activity of ^{99m}Tc after elution. Positions a and b indicate elutions of ^{99m}Tc activity at 8 hr and 17 hr after elution on day 4.

The ^{99m}Tc radionuclide is eluted as sodium pertechnetate ($Na^{99m}TcO_4$) with a 0.9% NaCl solution (saline without any additivies). After elution, the ^{99m}Tc radioactivity starts to grow again. Elution may be carried out, if needed, even before equilibrium is reached (*a* and *b* in Figure 5.2). The amount of ^{99m}Tc activity obtained in this case will depend on the time elapsed between the previous and present elutions.

The ^{99}Mo–^{99m}Tc generators are available from several commercial suppliers. In some commercial generators, isotonic saline is provided in a bottle that is placed inside the generator housing, and aliquots of saline are used up to elute ^{99m}Tc-pertechnetate ($^{99m}TcO_4^-$) using evacuated vials. Evacuated vials of different volumes are often supplied for elution in order to have approximately the same daily concentrations of ^{99m}Tc activity. Larger volume vials are used in the beginning of the week, and smaller volume vials are used in the latter part of the week. In other generators, vials with definite volumes of saline for each elution are provided. A commercial generator supplied by Mallinckrodt Medical, Inc. is shown in Figure 5.3.

There are two types of Moly generators, wet column generators and dry column generators, supplied by different commercial firms. The difference between the two types is that in a dry column generator after routine elution the leftover saline in the column is drawn out by using an evacuated vial without adding any more saline. The suggestion for a dry column generator came from the fact that radiation can cause radiolysis of water in a wet generator resulting in the formation of hydrogen peroxide (H_2O_2) and

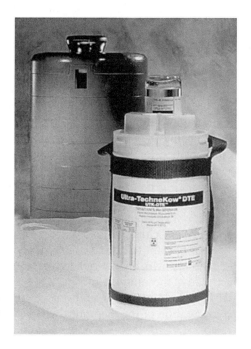

FIGURE 5.3. A ^{99}Mo–^{99m}Tc generator (Ultra-Technekow DTE). (Courtesy of Mallinckrodt Medical, Inc.)

perhydroxyl free radical ($HO_2^{\cdot}$). These species are oxidants and, if present in the ^{99m}Tc eluate, can interfere with the technetium chemistry outlined in Chapter 6. The radiolysis of water is likely to be greater in the high activity generator. Also, in wet column generators, saline in the tubing may possibly freeze in extremely cold weather, thus preventing elution until thawed.

Yield of ^{99m}Tc

It is often necessary to calculate the theoretical yield of ^{99m}Tc one would obtain after elution from a generator at a given time. The yields at various times can be calculated from Eq. (2.10) as follows (the mass numbers of ^{99m}Tc and ^{99}Mo have been omitted in equations in order to avoid complications in representing different symbols):

$$\lambda_{Mo} = 0.693/66 = 0.0105\,\text{hr}^{-1}$$

$$\lambda_{Tc} = 0.693/6 = 0.1155\,\text{hr}^{-1}$$

Then Eq. (2.10) becomes

$$A_{Tc} = 1.1(A_{Mo})_0(e^{-0.0105t} - e^{-0.1155t}) \tag{5.1}$$

where t is the time in hours elapsed after the previous elution. If there is any activity of ^{99m}Tc left from the previous elution, that should also be added. Thus,

$$A_{Tc} = 1.1(A_{Mo})_0(e^{-0.0105t} - e^{-0.1155t}) + (A_{Tc})_0\,e^{-0.1155t} \tag{5.2}$$

Since 87% of all ^{99}Mo nuclides ultimately decay to ^{99m}Tc, this factor should be included in the above equation by multiplying A_{Mo} by 0.87. Taking this factor into consideration, Eq. (5.2) reduces to

$$A_{Tc} = 0.957(A_{Mo})_0(e^{-0.0105t} - e^{-0.1155t}) + (A_{Tc})_0 e^{-0.1155t} \tag{5.3}$$

From Eq. (5.3), one can calculate the theoretical yield of ^{99m}Tc from a Moly generator at a given time. For practical reasons, it is not possible to obtain a complete yield of ^{99m}Tc from a generator as predicted by Eq. (5.3). The yield may be reduced by a column defect, such as channeling in the adsorbent bed, or by autoradiolysis due to high radioactivity whereby the chemical form of ^{99m}Tc changes. The practical yield of ^{99m}Tc varies from generator to generator and usually ranges from 80% to 90% of the theoretical value. The concentration of ^{99m}Tc activity in the eluate initially increases, then reaches a maximum, and finally decreases with increasing volume of the eluate (Fig. 5.4).

It is important to note that in a Moly generator, $(A_{Tc})_0$ is zero at the time of loading ^{99}Mo on the generator column. Afterward, if it is eluted only once daily, the amount of $(A_{Tc})_0$ ($\sim$5–15%) would have decayed to less than 1% in 24 hr and would not be significant enough to be considered in the calculation of the theoretical yield of ^{99m}Tc the next day. However, if the

FIGURE 5.4. Elution profile of the ^{99m}Tc activity expressed as concentration of radioactivity versus eluate volume. The profile may be broader or narrower depending on the type of generator. For generators using fission-produced ^{99}Mo, the eluate volume is about 2 to 3 ml due to the smaller alumina column.

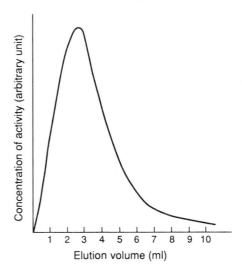

time difference between the two successive elutions is only several hours, the contribution of $(A_{Tc})_0$ could be appreciable and must be taken into account. If $(A_{Tc})_0$ is neglected in the daily elution of a generator, then the maximum activity of ^{99m}Tc is achieved in about four half-lives (i.e., in approximately 24 hr). Thereafter, the transient equilibrium between ^{99}Mo and ^{99m}Tc will be reached and Eq. (5.3) becomes

$$A_{Tc} = 0.957 \, (A_{Mo})_t \tag{5.4}$$

where

$$(A_{Mo})_t = (A_{Mo})_0 e^{-0.0105t} \tag{5.5}$$

It should be pointed out that ^{99m}Tc decays by 140-keV γ transition (90%) and via internal conversion (10%). Therefore, one has to multiply the above A_{Tc} values by 0.90 in order to estimate the number of photons available for imaging.

Usually the amount of ^{99}Mo along with the date and time of calibration is recorded on the generator by the commercial supplier. Different suppliers use different days of the week for calibration. As required by the Food and Drug Administration (FDA), ^{99}Mo radioactivity is calibrated as of the day of shipping and must be so stated on the label posted on the generator. The amount of calibrated ^{99}Mo activity in a given generator can vary from 0.22 to 3 Ci (8.1–111 GBq) depending on the manufacturer. In a 3-Ci (111-GBq) Mallinckrodt generator calibrated for Friday 8:00 P.M. (shipping day), the ^{99}Mo activity reduces to 600 mCi (22.2 GBq) at 8:00 A.M. the following Friday. One manufacturer uses 8.3 to 16.6 Ci (307–614 GBq) ^{99}Mo in generators. These generators are used by large institutions in lieu of two to three 2–3-Ci (74–111 GBq) generators. An institution or a commercial nuclear pharmacy purchases a given size Moly generator depending on its need so that enough ^{99m}Tc activity is available on the last day of the work-week.

Problem 5.1

A 2.6-Ci (96.2-GBq) Moly generator calibrated for Wednesday noon was received on Tuesday before. What would be the total ^{99m}Tc activity eluted at 8:00 A.M. on Friday?

Answer

It is assumed that by the time the generator is received, the equilibrium between ^{99}Mo and ^{99m}Tc has been reached and still exists at 8:00 A.M. on Friday. The time from Wednesday noon to Friday 8:00 A.M. is 44 hr.

$$^{99}\text{Mo activity on Wednesday noon} = 2.6\,\text{Ci}\,(96.2\,\text{GBq})$$

$$^{99}\text{Mo activity at 8:00 A.M. on Friday} = 2.6 \times \exp(-0.0105 \times 44)$$

$$= 1.64\,\text{Ci}\,(61\,\text{GBq})$$

Assuming complete elution, according to Eq. (5.4), ^{99m}Tc activity at 8:00 A.M. on Friday will be

$$^{99m}\text{Tc activity} = 0.957 \times 1.64\,\text{Ci} = 1.57\,\text{Ci}(58.1\,\text{GBq})$$

Problem 5.2

A 3000-mCi (111-GBq) Moly generator calibrated for Friday 8:00 P.M. was eluted at 8:00 A.M. the following Wednesday. Assuming that 80% of ^{99m}Tc activity was eluted, what would be the theoretical activity of ^{99m}Tc on the column at 1:00 P.M. on the same day (Wednesday)?

Answer

The time from Friday 8:00 P.M. to Wednesday 8:00 A.M. is 108 hours. Therefore, ^{99}Mo activity at 8:00 A.M. on Wednesday

$$= 3000 \times \exp(-0.0105 \times 108) = 965\,\text{mCi}\,(35.7\,\text{GBq})$$

Assuming transient equilibrium, according to Eq. (5.4),

$$^{99m}\text{Tc activity} = 0.957 \times 965 = 923\,\text{mCi}\,(34.2\,\text{GBq})$$

With 80% elution, 20% remained in the generator; i.e., $0.2 \times 923 = 184.6$ mCi (6.83 GBq) ^{99m}Tc remained on the column. This is $(A_{Tc})_0$ in Eq. (5.3.).

The time from 8:00 A.M. to 1:00 P.M. on Wednesday is 5 hr. From Eq. (5.3),

$$A_{Tc} = 0.957 \times 965[\exp(-0.0105 \times 5) - \exp(-0.1155 \times 5)]$$

$$+ 184.6 \times \exp(-0.1155 \times 5)$$

$$= 923 \times (0.9489 - 0.5613) + 103.6$$

$$= 461.4\,\text{mCi}(17.1\,\text{GBq})$$

^{99m}Tc Content in ^{99m}Tc-Eluate

Both ^{99}Mo (13%) and ^{99m}Tc decay to ^{99}Tc and, therefore, both ^{99}Tc and ^{99m}Tc are present in the Tc-eluate from the Moly generator. Because of the rapid decay of ^{99m}Tc, the fraction of ^{99m}Tc in the generator eluate decreases and that of ^{99}Tc increases over time after elution and as the time between generator elutions increases. Since ^{99}Tc competes with ^{99m}Tc in chemical binding, it can reduce the labeling efficiency in radiopharmaceutical kits containing small amounts of stannous ion. This situation becomes critical when the generators are left without elution over the weekend and then first eluted on Monday or Tuesday. In some rediopharmaceutical preparations, limits on the content of ^{99}Tc in the Tc-eluate are implicitly specified in that only the ^{99m}Tc eluted at specific times can be used. For example, in ^{99m}Tc-HMPAO preparation for brain imaging, the ^{99m}Tc eluate must not be more than 2 hr old and also must be obtained from a generator that was eluted at least once in the past 24 hr.

The ^{99m}Tc content in the Tc-eluate is given by the mole fraction (F) of ^{99m}Tc expressed as follows:

$$F = \frac{N_A}{N_A + N_B} \tag{5.6}$$

where N_A and N_B are the number of atoms of ^{99m}Tc and ^{99}Tc, respectively. The F at any time t can be calculated from the following expression (Lamson et al. 1975):

$$F = \frac{0.87\, \lambda_1 (\exp(-\lambda_1 t) - \exp(-\lambda_2 t))}{(\lambda_2 - \lambda_1)(1 - \exp(-\lambda_1 t))} \tag{5.7}$$

where λ_1 and λ_2 are decay constants of ^{99}Mo and ^{99m}Tc, respectively, and the factor 0.87 indicates that 87% of ^{99}Mo decays to ^{99m}Tc. Using $\lambda_1 = 0.0105$ hr^{-1} and $\lambda_2 = 0.1155$ hr^{-1}, the values of F at various times are calculated, and tabulated in Table 5.2. It can be seen that, for example, at 24 hr aftr elution, only 27.9% of ^{99m}Tc atoms are present in the ^{99m}Tc eluate.

Since the total number (N) of Tc atoms affects the labeling yield of ^{99m}Tc

TABLE 5.2. Mole fractions of ^{99m}Tc in Tc-eluate at different times after elution.

Days after elution	Hours after elution							
	0	3	6	9	12	15	18	21
0		0.7346	0.6254	0.5366	0.4641	0.4044	0.3550	0.3138
1	0.2791	0.2498	0.2249	0.2035	0.1851	0.1691	0.1551	0.1428
2	0.1319	0.1222	0.1136	0.1059	0.0990	0.0927	0.0869	0.0817
3	0.0770	0.0726	0.0686	0.0649	0.0614	0.0583	0.0553	0.0526
4	0.0500	0.0476	0.0454	0.0432	0.0413	0.0394	0.0377	0.0360

radiopharmaceuticals, its prior knowledge is important in many preparations. It can be calculated by the following formula using F from Table 5.2.

$$N_{(Total)} = \frac{{}^{99m}\text{Tc Activity}}{0.1155 \times F} \tag{5.8}$$

Quality Control of ^{99m}Tc-Eluate

Since ^{99m}Tc activity is used for humans, several quality control tests of the ^{99m}Tc-eluate are mandatory. These tests are discussed below in some detail.

^{99}Mo Breakthrough

This is ^{99}Mo contamination in the ^{99m}Tc-eluate and originates from the small quantity of ^{99}Mo that may be eluted with ^{99m}Tc. The *US Pharmacopeia* (*USP* 26) limit [also the Nuclear Regulatory Commission (NRC) limit] is 0.15 μCi ^{99}Mo/mCi (0.15 kBq/MBq) ^{99m}Tc per administered dosage at the time of administration. The ^{99}Mo contamination is measured by detecting 740-keV and 780-keV photons of ^{99}Mo in a dose calibrator or a NaI (Tl) detector coupled to a pulse height analyzer. The eluate vial is shielded in a lead pot (about 6 mm thick) to stop all 140-keV photons from ^{99m}Tc and to count only 740-keV and 780-keV photons from ^{99}Mo. The shielded vial is then assayed in the dose calibrator using the ^{99}Mo setting. Molybdenum-99 along with ^{98}Mo (from the molybdenum target) can also be detected by adding phenylhydrazine to the eluate and observing the color change due to the Mo-phenylhydrazine complex by the use of a colorimeter.

The A_{Mo}/A_{Tc} ratio increases with time because ^{99}Mo ($t_{1/2} = 66$ hr) decays more slowly than ^{99m}Tc ($t_{1/2} = 6$ hr). The time at which the A_{Mo}/A_{Tc} ratio will exceed 0.15 can be calculated by

$$0.15 = \frac{(A_{Mo})_o e^{-0.0105t}}{(A_{Tc})_o e^{-0.1155t}}$$

where $(A_{Mo})_o$ is the activity of ^{99}Mo in microcurie, $(A_{Tc})_o$ is the activity of ^{99m}Tc in millicurie at the time of elution, and t is the time after initial elution. Rearranging the equation, t in hours can be calculated as

$$t = \frac{-\ln[(A_{Mo})_o/(A_{Tc})_o]}{0.105} - 18.07 \tag{5.9}$$

^{99m}TcO$_4{}^-$ obtained from the Moly generator has an expiration period of 12 hr for clinical use. For valid use of ^{99m}TcO$_4{}^-$ for 12 hr, the $(A_{Mo})_o/(A_{Tc})_o$ ratio at the initial elution can be calculated by Eq. (5.9) to be 0.043 μCi of ^{99}Mo/mCi of ^{99m}Tc or 0.043 kBq of ^{99}Mo/MBq of ^{99m}Tc.

Other Radionuclide Contamination

In generators using fission-produced molybdenum, a number of extraneous activities such as those of ^{103}Ru, ^{132}Te, ^{131}I, ^{99}Zr, ^{124}Sb, ^{134}Cs, ^{89}Sr, ^{90}Sr, and ^{86}Rb may remain in the eluate as contaminants. The *USP* 26 limits of these radionuclides in ^{99m}Tc eluate are ^{131}I:0.05 μCi/mCi (0.05 Bq/kBq) ^{99m}Tc; ^{103}Ru : 0.05 μCi/mCi (0.05 Bq/kBq) ^{99m}Tc; ^{89}Sr:0.0006 μCi/mCi (0.0006 Bq/kBq) ^{99m}Tc; ^{90}Sr:0.00006 μCi/mCi (0.00006 Bq/kBq) ^{99m}Tc; other β- and γ-emitting radionuclides: not more than 0.01% of all activity at the time of administration; gross α-particle impurity: not more than 0.001 nCi/mCi (0.001 Bq/MBq)^{99m}Tc. These contaminants can be checked by a multichannel pulse height analyzer after allowing ^{99m}Tc, ^{99}Mo, and other relatively short-lived radionuclides to decay completely. Usually these tests are performed by the manufacturer.

Aluminum Breakthrough

The aluminum contamination originates from the alumina bed of the generator. The presence of aluminum in the ^{99m}Tc-eluate interferes with the preparation of ^{99m}Tc-sulfur colloid; particularly phosphate buffer in colloid preparations tends to precipitate with excessive aluminum. It also inteferes with the labeling of red blood cells with ^{99m}Tc, causing their agglutination. The *USP* 26 limit is 10 μg Al/ml ^{99m}Tc for fission-produced ^{99}Mo.

The presence of aluminum can be detected by the colorimetric method using aurin tricarboxylic acid or methyl orange, and can be quantitated by comparison with a standard solution of aluminum. Test kits are commercially available for the determination of aluminum. In these kits, strips containing a color complexing agent are provided along with a standard solution of aluminum ($\sim$10 μg/ml). In a routine test, one drop each of the ^{99m}Tc-eluate and the standard aluminum solution are spotted on a test strip and the intensities of the colors of the two spots are visually compared. If the ^{99m}Tc-eluate spot is denser than the standard aluminum spot, then the amount of aluminum is considered excessive and the ^{99m}Tc-eluate should be discarded. Excessive amounts of aluminum in the eluate indicate lack of stability of the column.

pH

The pH of the eluate should be between 4.5 and 7.5; this can be checked quantitatively with a pH meter or qualitatively with pH paper. The actual pH of the ^{99m}Tc-eluate from the generator is about 5.5. The pH of the ^{99m}Tc solution obtained by methyl ethyl ketone extraction is slightly higher ($\sim$6–7).

Radiochemical Purity

The radiochemical impurities of the ^{99m}Tc eluate are different chemical forms of radioactivity other than ^{99m}TcO$_4^-$. These impurities should be checked by suitable analytical methods. These methods are described in Chapter 8.

$^{113}Sn{-}^{113m}In$ Generator

In the ^{113}Sn–^{113m}In generator system, the ^{113}Sn has a half-life of 117 days and decays by electron capture, and the daughter ^{113m}In decays by 393-keV isomeric transition with a half-life of 100 min. The generator has a long shelf life due to the long half-life of ^{113}Sn.

The generator is made up of hydrous zirconium oxide contained in a plastic or glass column. Tin-113 in the stannic form is adsorbed on the column, and the daughter ^{113m}In is eluted with 0.05N HCl. The common contaminants are ^{113}Sn, ^{117m}Sn, and ^{125}Sb, and the eluate should be checked for these contaminants. The nonradioactive zirconium atoms could be present in the eluate and must be checked for by analytical methods.

$^{68}Ge{-}^{68}Ga$ Generator

Germanium-68 decays by electron capture with a half-life of 271 days, and ^{68}Ga, with a half-life of 68 min, decays by positron emission and hence 511-keV annihilation radiations. This generator is made up of alumina loaded in a plastic or glass column. Carrier-free ^{68}Ge in concentrated HCl is neutralized in EDTA solution and adsorbed on the column. Then ^{68}Ga is eluted from the column with 0.005M EDTA solution. Alternatively, ^{68}Ge is adsorbed on a stannous dioxide column and ^{68}Ga is eluted with 1N HCl. This generator can be eluted quite frequently because the maximum yield is obtained in a few hours. Because of the equilibrium between ^{68}Ge and ^{68}Ga, ^{68}Ge is routinely used as standard sealed sources for calibration of PET cameras. However, its clinical use is very limited.

$^{82}Sr{-}^{82}Rb$ Generator (Cardiogen-82)

Strontium-82 has a half-life of 25 days and decays to ^{82}Rb by electron capture. Rubidium-82 decays by β^+ emission (95%) with a half-life of 75 s. The ^{82}Sr is loaded on a SnO$_2$ column and ^{82}Rb is eluted with 0.9% NaCl solution. Because of its short half-life, ^{82}Rb can be eluted repeatedly every 10 to 15 min with maximum yield. Because of its short half-life, ^{82}Rb is administered to the patient using an infusion system for myocardial perfusion imaging by the PET technique. Bracco Diagnostics supplies this generator under the brand name Cardiogen-82 to the customers on a monthly basis. Normally 100 to 110 mCi (3.7 to 41.1 GBq) ^{82}Sr is supplied in each generator. However, the fivefold (about 500 mCi or 18.5 GBq) amount of ^{85}Sr ($t_{1/2} = 65$ days) is also present, which is produced during the cyclotron production of ^{82}Sr. ^{85}Sr emits 510 keV photons.

Questions

1. Describe the principles of a radionuclide generator.
2. List the ideal characteristics of a radionuclide generator.

3. Describe in detail the construction of a Moly generator. What are the common radionuclide contaminants in this generator?

4. A 1700-mCi (62.9-GBq) Moly generator calibrated for Friday noon was eluted at 9:00 A.M. on the following Tuesday. (a) Calculate the activity of ^{99m}Tc assuming 90% yield. (b) Calculate the activity of ^{99}Mo at 1:00 P.M. on the following Wednesday.

5. A 10-mCi (370-MBq) sample of the ^{99m}Tc-eluate is found to contain 20 μCi (0.74 MBq) ^{99}Mo. Can this preparation be used for injection into humans?

6. A 100-mCi (3.7-GBq) sample of ^{99m}Tc-DTPA contains 60 μCi (2.22 MBq) ^{99}Mo. If a brain scan requires 10 mCi (370 MBq) ^{99m}Tc-DTPA, can you use this for the patient?

7. Suppose an institution regularly purchases a 2200-mCi (81.4-GBq) Moly generator calibrated for Friday noon and the elution volume of the eluent as provided by the supplier is 5 ml. On the following Wednesday morning at 8:00 A.M, what volumes of activity would you draw from the ^{99m}Tc eluate in order to prepare (a) 50 mCi (1.85 GBq) ^{99m}Tc-methylene diphosphonate, (b) 30 mCi (1.11 GBq) ^{99m}Tc-sulfur colloid, and (c) 20 mCi (740 MBq) ^{99m}Tc-labeled macroaggregated albumin (assume 80% elution)?

8. Why is aluminum undesirable in the ^{99m}Tc eluate? What is the permissible limit of aluminum concentration in the ^{99m}Tc eluate?

9. A 50 mCi (1.85 GBq) ^{99m}Tc-DISIDA sample contains 5 μCi (0.185 MBq) ^{99}Mo. If a patient is to be injected with 5 mCi (185 MBq) ^{99m}Tc-DISIDA for hepatobiliary studies 6 hr later, can you administer this radiopharmaceutical to the patient?

10. A 1350-mCi (50-GBq) ^{99}Mo–^{99m}Tc generator calibrated for Wednesday 8:00 A.M. was eluted daily at 7:00 A.M. for 3 days starting from the calibration day. What would be the ^{99m}Tc activity in the generator at 12:00 noon on the fifth day after calibration?

References and Suggested Reading

Baker RJ. A system for routine production of concentrated technetium-99m by solvent extraction of molybdenum. *Int J Appl Radiat Isot.* 1971; 22:483.

Colombetti LG. Radionuclide generators. In: Rayudu GVS, ed. *Radiotracers for Medical Applications.* Boca Raton, Fla: CRC Press; 1983:133.

Eckelman WC, Coursey BM, eds. Technetium-99m: generators, chemistry and preparation of radiopharmaceuticals. *Int J Appl Radiat Isot.* 1982; 33:793.

Guillaume M, Brihaye C. Generators for short-lived gamma and positron emitting radionuclides: Current status and prospects. *Nucl Med Biol.* 1986; 13:89.

Holland ME, Deutsch E, Heineman HR. Studies on commercially available ^{99}Mo/^{99m}Tc radionuclide generators: I. Comparison of five analytical procedures for determination of total technetium in generator eluants. *Appl Radiat Isot.* 1986; 37:165.

Holland ME, Deutsch E, Heineman HR. Studies on commercially available ^{99}Mo/^{99m}Tc radionuclide generators: II. Operating characteristics and behavior of ^{99}Mo/^{99m}Tc generators. *Appl Radiat Isot*. 1986; 37:173.

Knapp FF, Jr, Butler TA, eds. *Radionuclide Generators: New Systems for Nuclear Medicine Applications*. American Chemical Society. Advances in chemistry series, No. 241. Washington, DC: Am Chem Soc, 1984.

Lambrecht RM, Sajjad M. Accelerator-derived radionuclide generators. *Radiochim Acta*. 1988; 43:171.

Lamson ML III, Kirschner AS, Hotte CE, et al. Generator-produced ^{99m}TcO$_4^-$: carrier free? *J Nucl Med*. 1975; 16:639.

Noronha OPD, Sewatkar AB, Ganatra RD, et al. Fission-produced ^{99}Mo–^{99m}Tc generator system for medical use. *J Nucl Biol Med*. 1976; 20:32.

Richards P, O'Brien MJ. Rapid determination of ^{99}Mo in separated ^{99m}Tc. *J Nucl Med*. 1964; 10:871.

Saha GB, Go RT, MacIntyre WJ, et al. Use of the ^{82}Sr/^{82}Rb generator in clinical PET studies. *Nucl Med Biol*. 1990; 17:763.

U.S. Pharmacopeia 26 & National Formulary 21. Rockville, MD: United States Pharmacopeial Convention; 2003.

Yano Y, Anger HO. A gallium-68 positron cow for medical use. *J Nucl Med*. 1964; 5:485.

6
Radiopharmaceuticals and Methods of Radiolabeling

Definition of a Radiopharmaceutical

A radiopharmaceutical is a radioactive compound used for the diagnosis and therapeutic treatment of human diseases. In nuclear medicine nearly 95% of the radiopharmaceuticals are used for diagnostic purposes, while the rest are used for therapeutic treatment. Radiopharmaceuticals usually have minimal pharmacologic effect, because in most cases they are used in tracer quantities. Therapeutic radiopharmaceuticals can cause tissue damage by radiation. Because they are administered to humans, they should be sterile and pyrogen free, and should undergo all quality control measures required of a conventional drug. A radiopharmaceutical may be a radioactive element such as ^{133}Xe, or a labeled compound such as ^{131}I-iodinated proteins and ^{99m}Tc-labeled compounds.

Although the term *radiopharmaceutical* is most commonly used, other terms such as *radiotracer, radiodiagnostic agent*, and *tracer* have been used by various groups. We shall use the term *radiopharmaceutical* throughout, although the term *tracer* will be used occasionally.

Another point of interest is the difference between radiochemicals and radiopharmaceuticals. The former are not usable for administration to humans due to the possible lack of sterility and nonpyrogenicity. On the other hand, radiopharmaceuticals are sterile and nonpyrogenic and can be administered safely to humans.

A radiopharmaceutical has two components: a radionuclide and a pharmaceutical. The usefulness of a radiopharmaceutical is dictated by the characteristics of these two components. In designing a radiopharmaceutical, a pharmaceutical is first chosen on the basis of its preferential localization in a given organ or its participation in the physiologic function of the organ. Then a suitable radionuclide is tagged onto the chosen pharmaceutical such that after administration of the radiopharmaceutical, radiations emitted from it are detected by a radiation detector. Thus, the morphologic structure or the physiologic function of the organ can be assessed. The pharmaceutical of choice should be safe and nontoxic for human administration. Radiations from the radionuclide of choice should be easily detected by nuclear instruments, and the radiation dose to the patient should be minimal.

Ideal Radiopharmaceutical

Since radiopharmaceuticals are administered to humans, and because there are several limitations on the detection of radiations by currently available instruments, radiopharmaceuticals should possess some important characteristics. The ideal characteristics for radiopharmaceuticals are elaborated below.

Easy Availability

The radiopharmaceutical should be easily produced, inexpensive, and readily available in any nuclear medicine facility. Complicated methods of production of radionuclides or labeled compounds increase the cost of the radiopharmaceutical. The geographic distance between the user and the supplier also limits the availability of short-lived radiopharmaceuticals.

Short Effective Half-Life

A radionuclide decays with a definite half-life, which is called the physical half-life, denoted T_p (or $t_{1/2}$). The physical half-life is independent of any physicochemical condition and is characteristic for a given radionuclide. It has been discussed in detail in Chapter 2.

Radiopharmaceuticals administered to humans disappear from the biological system through fecal or urinary excretion, perspiration, or other mechanisms. This biologic disappearance of a radiopharmaceutical follows an exponential law similar to that of radionuclide decay. Thus, every radiopharmaceutical has a biologic half-life (T_b). It is the time needed for half of the radiopharmaceutical to disappear from the biologic system and therefore is related to a decay constant, $\lambda_b = 0.693/T_b$.

Obviously, in any biologic system, the loss of a radiopharmaceutical is due to both the physical decay of the radionuclide and the biologic elimination of the radiopharmaceutical. The net or effective rate (λ_e) of the loss of radioactivity is then related to the physical decay constant λ_p and the biologic decay constant λ_b. Mathematically, this is expressed as

$$\lambda_e = \lambda_p + \lambda_b \tag{6.1}$$

Since $\lambda = 0.693/t_{1/2}$, it follows that

$$\frac{1}{T_e} = \frac{1}{T_p} + \frac{1}{T_b} \tag{6.2}$$

or

$$T_e = \frac{T_p \times T_b}{T_p + T_b} \qquad (6.3)$$

The effective half-life T_e is always less than the shorter of T_p or T_b. For a very long T_p and a short T_b, T_e is almost equal to T_b. Similarly, for a very long T_b and a short T_p, T_e is almost equal to T_p.

Problem 6.1
The physical half-life of ^{111}In is 67 hr and the biologic half-life of ^{111}In-DTPA used for measurement of the glomerular filtration rate is 1.5 hr. What is the effective half-life of ^{111}In-DTPA?

Answer
Using Eq. (6.3),

$$T_e = \frac{1.5 \times 67}{67 + 1.5} = \frac{100.5}{68.5} = 1.47 \text{ hr}$$

Radiopharmaceuticals should have a relatively short effective half-life, which should not be longer than the time necessary to complete the study in question. The time to start the imaging of the tracer varies with different studies depending on the in vivo pharmacokinetics of the tracer. The faster the accumulation of the tracer, the sooner imaging should start. However, the duration of imaging depends primarily on the amount of activity administered, the fraction thereof accumulated in the target organ, and the window setting of the gamma camera.

Particle Emission

Radionuclides decaying by α- or β-particle emission should not be used as the label in diagnostic radiopharmaceuticals. These particles cause more radiation damage to the tissue than do γ rays. Although γ-ray emission is preferable, many β-emitting radionuclides, such as ^{131}I-iodinated compounds, are often used for clinical studies. However, α emitters should never be used for in vivo diagnostic studies because they give a high radiation dose to the patient. But α and β emitters are useful for therapy, because of the effective radiation damage to abnormal cells.

Decay by Electron Capture or Isomeric Transition

Because radionuclides emitting particles are less desirable, the diagnostic radionuclides used should decay by electron capture or isomeric transition without any internal conversion. Whatever the mode of decay, for diagnostic studies the radionuclide must emit a γ radiation with an energy preferably between 30 and 300 keV. Below 30 keV, γ rays are absorbed by tissue

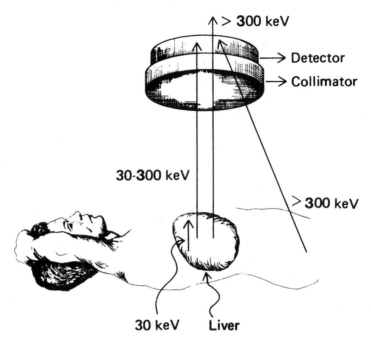

FIGURE 6.1. Photon interaction in the NaI(T1) detector using collimators. A 30-keV photon is absorbed by the tissue. A > 300-keV photon may penetrate through the collimator septa and strike the detector, or may escape the detector without any interaction. Photons of 30 to 300 keV may escape the organ of the body, pass through the collimator holes, and interact with the detector.

and are not detected by the NaI(Tl) detector. Above 300 keV, effective collimation of γ rays cannot be achieved with commonly available collimators. However, recently manufacturers have made collimators for 511-keV photons, which have been used for planar or SPECT imaging using ^{18}F-FDG. The phenomenon of collimation with 30- to 300-keV photons is illustrated in Fig. 6.1. γ-Rays should be monochromatic and have an energy of approximately 150 keV, which is most suitable for present-day collimators. Moreover, the photon abundance should be high so that imaging time can be minimized due to the high photon flux.

High Target-to-Nontarget Activity Ratio

For any diagnostic study, it is desirable that the radiopharmaceutical be localized preferentially in the organ under study since the activity from nontarget areas can obscure the structural details of the picture of the target organ. Therefore, the target-to-nontarget activity ratio should be large.

An ideal radiopharmaceutical should have all the above characteristics to provide maximum efficacy in the diagnosis of diseases and a minimum radiation dose to the patient. However, it is difficult for a given radio-pharmaceutical to meet all these criteria and the one of choice is the best of many compromises.

Design of New Radiopharmaceuticals

General Considerations

Many radiopharmaceuticals are used for various nuclear medicine tests. Some of them meet most of the requirements for the intended test and therefore need no replacement. For example, ^{99m}Tc–methylene diphosphonate (MDP) is an excellent bone imaging agent and the nuclear medicine community is fairly satisfied with this agent such that no further research and development is being pursued for replacing ^{99m}Tc-MDP with a new radiopharmaceutical. However, there are a number of other radiopharmaceuticals that offer only minimal diagnostic value in nuclear medicine tests and thus need replacement. Continual effort is being made to improve or replace such radiopharmaceuticals.

Upon scrutiny, it is noted that the commonly used radiopharmaceuticals involve one or more of the following mechanisms of localization in a given organ:

1. Passive diffusion: ^{99m}Tc-DTPA in brain imaging, ^{99m}Tc-DTPA aerosol and ^{133}Xe in ventilation imaging, ^{111}In-DTPA in cisternography.
2. Ion exchange: uptake of ^{99m}Tc-phosphonate complexes in bone.
3. Capillary blockage: ^{99m}Tc-macroaggregated albumin (MAA) particles trapped in the lung capillaries.
4. Phagocytosis: removal of ^{99m}Tc-sulfur colloid particles by the reticuloendothelial cells in the liver, spleen, and bone marrow.
5. Active transport: ^{131}I uptake in the thyroid, ^{201}Tl uptake in the myocardium.
6. Cell sequestration: sequestration of heat-damaged ^{99m}Tc-labeled red blood cells by the spleen.
7. Metabolism: ^{18}F-FDG uptake in myocardial and brain tissues.
8. Receptor binding: ^{11}C-dopamine binding to the dopamine receptors in the brain.
9. Compartmental localization: ^{99m}Tc-labeled red blood cells used in the gated blood pool study.
10. Antigen-antibody complex formation: ^{131}I-, ^{111}In-, and ^{99m}Tc-labeled antibody to localize tumors.
11. Chemotaxis: ^{111}In-labeled leukocytes to localize infections.

Based on these criteria, it is conceivable to design a radiopharmaceutical to evaluate the function and/or structure of an organ of interest. Once a radiopharmaceutical is conceptually designed, a definite protocol should be developed based on the physicochemical properties of the basic ingredients to prepare the radiopharmaceutical. The method of preparation should be simple, easy, and reproducible, and should not alter the desired property of the labeled compound. Optimum conditions of temperature, pH, ionic strength, and molar ratios should be established and maintained for maximum efficacy of the radiopharmaceutical.

Once a radiopharmaceutical is developed and successfully formulated, its clinical efficacy must be evaluated by testing it first in animals and then in humans. For use in humans, one has to have a Notice of Claimed Investigational Exemption for a New Drug (IND) from the U.S. Food and Drug Administration (FDA), which regulates the human trials of drugs very strictly. If there is any severe adverse effect in humans due to the administration of a radiopharmaceutical, then the radiopharmaceutical is discarded.

Factors Influencing the Design of New Radiopharmaceuticals

The following factors need to be considered before, during, and after the preparation of a new radiopharmaceutical.

Compatibility

When a labeled compound is to be prepared, the first criterion to consider is whether the label can be incorporated into the molecule to be labeled. This may be assessed from a knowledge of the chemical properties of the two partners. For example, ^{111}In ion can form coordinate covalent bonds, and DTPA is a chelating agent containing nitrogen and oxygen atoms with lone pairs of electrons that can be donated to form coordinated covalent bonds. Therefore, when ^{111}In ion and DTPA are mixed under appropriate physicochemical conditions, ^{111}In-DTPA is formed and remains stable for a long time. If, however, ^{111}In ion is added to benzene or similar compounds, it would not label them. Iodine primarily binds to the tyrosyl group of the protein. Mercury radionuclides bind to the sulfhydryl group of the protein. These examples illustrate the point that only specific radionuclides label certain compounds, depending on their chemical behavior.

Stoichiometry

In preparing a new radiopharmaceutical, one needs to know the amount of each component to be added. This is particularly important in tracer level chemistry and in ^{99m}Tc chemistry. The concentration of ^{99m}Tc in the ^{99m}Tc-eluate is approximately $10^{-9}\,M$. Although for reduction of this trace amount of ^{99m}Tc only an equivalent amount of Sn^{2+} is needed, 1000 to 1 million times more of the latter is added to the preparation in order to ensure complete reduction. Similarly, enough chelating agent, such as DTPA or MDP, is also added to use all the reduced ^{99m}Tc. The stoichiometric ratio of different components can be obtained by setting up the appropriate equations for the chemical reactions. An unduly high or low concentration of any one component may sometimes affect the integrity of the preparation.

Charge of the Molecule

The charge on a radiopharmaceutical determines its solubility in various solvents. The greater the charge, the higher the solubility in aqueous solution. Nonpolar molecules tend to be more soluble in organic solvents and lipids.

Size of the Molecule

The molecular size of a radiopharmaceutical is an important determinant in its absorption in the biologic system. Larger molecules (mol. wt. $> \sim 60,000$) are not filtered by the glomeruli in the kidney. This information should give some clue as to the range of molecular weights of the desired radiopharmaceutical that should be chosen for a given study.

Protein Binding

Almost all drugs, radioactive or not, bind to plasma proteins to variable degrees. The primary candidate for this type of binding is albumin, although many compounds specifically bind to globulin and other proteins as well. Indium, gallium, and many metallic ions bind firmly to transferrin in plasma. Protein binding is greatly influenced by a number of factors, such as the charge on the radiopharmaceutical molecule, the pH, the nature of protein, and the concentration of anions in plasma. At a lower pH, plasma proteins become more positively charged, and therefore anionic drugs bind firmly to them. The nature of a protein, particularly its content of hydroxyl, carboxyl, and amino groups and their configuration in the protein structure, determines the extent and strength of its binding to the radiopharmaceutical. Metal chelates can exchange the metal ions with proteins because of the stronger affinity of the metal for the protein. Such a process is called "transchelation" and leads to in vivo breakdown of the complex. For example, ^{111}In-chelates exchange ^{111}In with transferrin to form ^{111}In-transferrin.

Protein binding affects the tissue distribution and plasma clearance of a radiopharmaceutical and its uptake by the organ of interest. Therefore, one should determine the extent of protein binding of any new radiopharmaceutical before its clinical use. This can be accomplished by precipitating the proteins with trichloroacetic acid from the plasma after administration of the radiopharmaceutical and then measuring the activity in the precipitate.

Solubility

For injection, the radiopharmaceutical should be in aqueous solution at a pH compatible with blood pH (7.4). The ionic strength and osmolality of the agent should also be appropriate for blood.

In many cases, lipid solubility of a radiopharmaceutical is a determining factor in its localization in an organ; the cell membrane is primarily composed of phospholipids, and unless the radioparmaceutical is lipid soluble, it will hardly diffuse through the cell membrane. The higher the lipid solubility of a radiopharmaceutical, the greater the diffusion through the cell membrane and hence the greater its localization in the organ. Protein binding reduces the lipid solubility of a radiopharmaceutical. Ionized drugs are less lipid soluble, whereas nonpolar drugs are highly soluble in lipids and hence easily diffuse through cell membranes. The radiopharmaceutical ^{111}In-oxine is highly soluble in lipid and is therefore used specifically for labeling leukocytes and platelets. Obviously, lipid solubility and protein binding of a drug play a key role in its in vivo distribution and localization.

Stability

The stability of a labeled compound is one of the major concerns in labeling chemistry. It must be stable both in vitro and in vivo. In vivo breakdown of a radiopharmaceutical results in undesirable biodistribution of radioactivity. For example, dehalogenation of radioiodinated compounds gives free radioiodide, which raises the background activity in the clinical study. Temperature, pH, and light affect the stability of many compounds and the optimal range of these physicochemical conditions must be established for the preparation and storage of labeled compounds.

Biodistribution

The study of the biodistribution of a radiopharmaceutical is essential in establishing its efficacy and usefulness. This includes tissue distribution, plasma clearance, urinary excretion, and fecal excretion after administration of the radiopharmaceutical.

In tissue distribution studies, the radiopharmaceutical is injected into animals such as mice, rats, and rabbits. The animals are then sacrificed at different time intervals, and different organs are removed. The activities in these organs are measured and compared. The tissue distribution data will tell how good the radiopharmaceutical is for imaging the organ of interest. At times, human biodistribution data are obtained by gamma camera imaging.

The rate of localization of a radiopharmaceutical in an organ is related to its rate of plasma clearance after administration. The plasma clearance half-time of a radiopharmaceutical is defined by the time required to reduce its initial plasma activity to one half. It can be measured by collecting serial samples of blood at different time intervals after injection and measuring the plasma activity. From a plot of activity versus time, one can determine the half-time for plasma clearance of the tracer.

Urinary and fecal excretions of a radiopharmaceutical are important in its clinical evaluation. The faster the urinary or fecal excretion, the less the radiation dose. These values can be determined by collecting the urine or feces at definite time intervals after injection and measuring the activity in the samples.

Toxic effects of radiopharmaceuticals must also be evaluated. These effects include damage to the tissues, physiologic dysfunction of organs, and even the death of the animal. These considerations are discussed in Chapter 8.

Methods of Radiolabeling

The use of compounds labeled with radionuclides has grown considerably in medical, biochemical, and other related fields. In the medical field, compounds labeled with β^--emitting radionuclides are mainly restricted to in vitro experiments and therapeutic treatment, whereas those labeled with γ-emitting radionuclides have much wider applications. The latter are particularly useful for in vivo imaging of different organs.

In a radiolabeled compound, atoms or groups of atoms of a molecule are substituted by similar or different radioactive atoms or groups of atoms. In any labeling process, a variety of physicochemical conditions can be employed to achieve a specific kind of labeling. There are essentially six major methods employed in the preparation of labeled compounds for clinical use (Table 6.1). These methods and various factors affecting the labeled compounds are discussed below.

TABLE 6.1. General methods of radiolabeling.

Isotope exchange	^{125}I-labeled T3 and T4
	^{14}C-, ^{35}S- and ^{3}H-labeled compounds
Introduction of a foreign label	All ^{99m}Tc-radiopharmaceuticals
	^{125}I-labeled proteins
	^{125}I-labeled hormones
	^{111}In-labeled cells
	^{18}F-fluorodeoxyglucose
Labeling with bifunctional chelating agent	^{111}In-DTPA-albumin
	^{99m}Tc-DTPA-antibody
Biosynthesis	^{75}Se-selenomethionine
	^{57}Co-cyanocobalamin
	^{14}C-labeled compounds
Recoil labeling	^{3}H-labeled compounds
	Iodinated compounds
Excitation labeling	^{123}I-labeled compounds (from ^{123}Xe decay)
	^{77}Br-labeled compounds (from ^{77}Kr decay)

Isotope Exchange Reactions

In isotope exchange reactions, one or more atoms in a molecule are replaced by isotopes of the same element having different mass numbers. Since the radiolabeled and parent molecules are identical except for the isotope effect, they are expected to have the same biologic and chemical properties.

Examples are ^{125}I-triiodothyronine (T3), ^{125}I-thyroxine (T4), and ^{14}C-, ^{35}S-, and ^{3}H-labeled compounds. These labeling reactions are reversible and are useful for labeling iodine-containing material with iodine radioisotopes and for labeling many compounds with tritium.

Introduction of a Foreign Label

In this type of labeling, a radionuclide is incorporated into a molecule that has a known biologic role, primarily by the formation of covalent or co-ordinate covalent bonds. The tagging radionuclide is foreign to the molecule and does not label it by the exchange of one of its isotopes. Some examples are ^{99m}Tc-labeled albumin, ^{99m}Tc-DTPA, ^{51}Cr-labeled red blood cells, and many iodinated proteins and enzymes. In several instances, the in vivo stability of the material is uncertain and one should be cautious about any alteration in the chemical and biologic properties of the labeled compound.

In many compounds of this category, the chemical bond is formed by chelation, that is, more than one atom donates a pair of electrons to the foreign acceptor atom, which is usually a transition metal. Most of the ^{99m}Tc-labeled compounds used in nuclear medicine are formed by chelation. For example, ^{99m}Tc binds to DTPA, gluceptate, and other ligands by chelation.

Labeling with Bifunctional Chelating Agents

In this approach, a bifunctional chelating agent is conjugated to a macro-molecule (e.g., protein, antibody) on one side and to a metal ion (e.g., Tc) by chelation on the other side. Examples of bifunctional chelating agents are DTPA, metallothionein, diamide dimercaptide (N_2S_2), hydrazinonico-tinamide (HYNIC) and dithiosemicarbazone.

There are two methods—the preformed ^{99m}Tc chelate method and the indirect chelator-antibody method. In the preformed ^{99m}Tc chelate method, ^{99m}Tc chelates are initially preformed using chelating agents such as dia-midodithiol, cyclam, and so on, which are then used to label macro-molecules by forming bonds between the chelating agent and the protein. In contrast, in the indirect method, the bifunctional chelating agent is initially conjugated with a macromolecule, which is then allowed to react with a metal ion to form a metal-chelate-macromolecule complex. Various anti-bodies are labeled by the latter method. Because of the presence of the che-lating agent, the biological properties of the labeled protein may be altered and must be assessed before clinical use. Although the prelabeled chelator approach provides a purer metal-chelate complex with a more definite structural information, the method involves several steps and the labeling yield often is not optimal, thus favoring the chelator-antibody approach.

Biosynthesis

In biosynthesis, a living organism is grown in a culture medium containing the radioactive tracer, the tracer is incorporated into metabolites produced by the metabolic processes of the organism, and the metabolites are then chemically separated. For example, vitamin B_{12} is labeled with ^{60}Co or ^{57}Co by adding the tracer to a culture medium in which the organism *Streptomyces griseus* is grown. Other examples of biosynthesis include ^{14}C-labeled carbohydrates, proteins, and fats.

Recoil Labeling

Recoil labeling is of limited interest because it is not used on a large scale for labeling. In a nuclear reaction, when particles are emitted from a nucleus, recoil atoms or ions are produced that can form a bond with other molecules present in the target material. The high energy of the recoil atoms results in poor yield and hence a low specific activity of the labeled product. Several tritiated compounds can be prepared in the reactor by the ^{6}Li$(n, \alpha)^3$H reaction. The compound to be labeled is mixed with a lithium salt and irradiated in the reactor. Tritium produced in the above reaction labels the compound, primarily by the isotope exchange mechanism, and then the labeled compound is separated.

Excitation Labeling

Excitation labeling entails the utilization of radioactive and highly reactive daughter ions produced in a nuclear decay process. During β decay or electron capture, energetic charged ions are produced that are capable of labeling various compounds of interest. Krypton-77 decays to ^{77}Br and, if the compound to be labeled is exposed to ^{77}Kr, then energetic ^{77}Br ions label the compound to form the brominated compound. Similarly, various proteins have been iodinated with ^{123}I by exposing them to ^{123}Xe, which decays to ^{123}I. The yield is considerably low with this method.

Important Factors in Labeling

The majority of radiopharmaceuticals used in clinical practice are relatively easy to prepare in ionic, colloidal, macroaggregated, or chelated forms, and many can be made using commercially available kits. Several factors that influence the integrity of labeled compounds should be kept in mind. These factors are described briefly below.

Efficiency of the Labeling Process

A high labeling yield is always desirable, although it may not be attainable in many cases. However, a lower yield is sometimes acceptable if the product is pure and not damaged by the labeling method, the expense involved is minimal, and no better method of labeling is available.

Chemical Stability of the Product

Stability is related to the type of bond between the radionuclide and the compound. Compounds with covalent bonds are relatively stable under various physicochemical conditions. The stability constant of the labeled product should be large for greater stability.

Denaturation or Alteration

The structure and/or the biologic properties of a labeled compound can be altered by various physicochemical conditions during a labeling procedure. For example, proteins are denatured by heating, at pH below 2 and above 10, and by excessive iodination, and red blood cells are denatured by heating.

Isotope Effect

The isotope effect results in different physical (and perhaps biologic) properties due to differences in isotope weights. For example, in tritiated compounds, H atoms are replaced by ^3H atoms and the difference in mass numbers of ^3H and H may alter the property of the labeled compounds. It has been found that the physiologic behavior of tritiated water is different from that of normal water in the body. The isotope effect is not as serious when the isotopes are heavier.

Carrier-Free or No-Carrier-Added (NCA) State

Radiopharmaceuticals tend to be adsorbed on the inner walls of the containers if they are in a carrier-free or NCA state. Techniques have to be developed in which the labeling yield is not affected by the low concentration of the tracer in a carrier-free or NCA state.

Storage Conditions

Many labeled compounds are susceptible to decomposition at higher temperatures. Proteins and labeled dyes are degraded by heat and therefore should be stored at proper temperatures; for example, albumin should be stored under refrigeration. Light may also break down some labeled compounds and these should be stored in the dark. The loss of carrier-free tracers by adsorption on the walls of the container can be prevented by the use of silicon-coated vials.

Specific Activity

Specific activity is defined as the activity per gram of the labeled material and has been discussed in Chapter 4. In many instances, high specific activity is required in the applications of radiolabeled compounds and appropriate methods should be devised to this end. In others, high specific activity can cause more radiolysis (see below) in the labeled compound and should be avoided.

Radiolysis

Many labeled compounds are decomposed by radiations emitted by the radionuclides present in them. This kind of decomposition is called radiolysis. The higher the specific activity, the greater the effect of radiolysis. When the chemical bond breaks down by radiations from its own molecule, the process is termed "autoradiolysis." Radiations may also decompose the solvent, producing free radicals that can break down the chemical bond of the labeled compounds; this process is indirect radiolysis. For example, radiations from a labeled molecule can decompose water to produce hydrogen peroxide or perhydroxyl free radical, which oxidizes another labeled molecule. To help prevent indirect radiolysis, the pH of the solvent should be neutral because more reactions of this nature can occur at alkaline or acidic pH.

The longer the half-life of the radionuclide, the more extensive is the radiolysis, and the more energetic the radiations, the greater is the radiolysis. In essence, radiolysis introduces a number of radiochemical impurities in the sample of labeled material and one should be cautious about these unwanted products. These factors set the guidelines for the expiration date of a radiopharmaceutical.

Purification and Analysis

Radionuclide impurities are radioactive contaminants arising from the method of production of radionuclides. Fission is likely to produce more impurities than nuclear reactions in a cyclotron or reactor because fission of the heavy nuclei produces many product nuclides. Target impurities also add to the radionuclidic contaminants. The removal of radioactive contaminants can be accomplished by various chemical separation methods, usually at the radionuclide production stage.

Radiochemical and chemical impurities arise from incomplete labeling of compounds and can be estimated by various analytical methods such as solvent extraction, ion exchange, paper, gel, or thin-layer chromatography, and electrophoresis. Often these impurities arise after labeling from natural degradation as well as from radiolysis. This subject is discussed in detail in Chapter 8.

Shelf Life

A labeled compound has a shelf life during which it can be used safely for its intended purpose. The loss of efficacy of a labeled compound over a period of time may result from radiolysis and depends on the physical half-life of the radionuclide, the solvent, any additive, the labeled molecule, the nature of emitted radiations, and the nature of the chemical bond between the radionuclide and the molecule. Usually a period of three physical half-lives or a maximum of 6 months is suggested as the limit for the shelf life of a labeled compound. The shelf-life of ^{99m}Tc-labeled compounds varies between 0.5 and 18 hr, the most common value being 6 hr.

Specific Methods of Labeling

In nuclear medicine, the two most frequently used radionuclides are ^{99m}Tc and ^{131}I. The ^{99m}Tc-labeled compounds constitute more than 80% of all radiopharmaceuticals used in nuclear medicine, whereas ^{123}I- and ^{131}I-labeled compounds and other nuclides account for the rest. The principles of iodination and ^{99m}Tc-labeling are discussed below.

Radioiodination

Iodination is used extensively for labeling the compounds of medical and biological interest. Iodine is a metallic element belonging to the halogen group VIIA. Its atomic number is 53 and its only stable isotope is ^{127}I. A number of iodine radioisotopes are commonly used for radioiodination, and those of clinical importance are presented in Table 4.1. Of all iodine isotopes, ^{123}I is most suitable for in vivo diagnostic procedures because it has a convenient half-life (13.2 hr) and photon energy (159 keV), and gives a low radiation dose to the patient. It is a cyclotron-produced isotope and therefore is expensive. The isotope ^{125}I is commonly used for producing radiolabeled antigens and other compounds for in vitro procedures and has the advantage of a long half-life (60 days). However, its low-energy (27- to 35-keV) photons make it unsuitable for in vivo imaging. The isotope ^{131}I has an 8-day half-life and 364-keV photons and is used for thyroid uptake and scan. However, its β^- emission gives a larger radiation dose to the patient than ^{123}I, and it is exclusively used for thyroid treatment.

In ^{123}I preparations, ^{124}I is an undesirable radionuclidic impurity that is produced by the α-particle bombardment of Te targets, because of its long half-life (4.2 days) and its annihilation and other high-energy radiations [511 keV (46%), 603 keV (61%), 723 keV (10%), and 1.69 MeV (10.4%)]. These high-energy photons degrade resolution of scintigraphic images because of their septal penetration of the collimator and also spillover of the scattered radiations in the 159-keV window of ^{123}I. Therefore, high-purity ^{123}I needs to be produced via appropriate nuclear reactions; the latter have been discussed in Chapter 4.

Principles of Iodination

Iodination of a molecule is governed primarily by the oxidation state of iodine. In the oxidized form, iodine binds strongly to various molecules, whereas in the reduced form, it does not. Commonly available iodide is oxidized to I^+ by various oxidizing agents. The free molecular iodine has the structure of $I^+–I^-$ in aqueous solution. In either case the electrophilic species I^+ does not exist as a free species, but forms complexes with nucleophilic entities such as water or pyridine.

$$I_2 + H_2O \rightleftharpoons H_2OI^+ + I^- \tag{6.4}$$

$$I_2 + OH^- \rightleftharpoons HOI + I^- \tag{6.5}$$

The hydrated iodonium ion, H_2OI^+ and hypoiodous acid, HOI, are believed to be the iodinating species in the iodination process. Iodination occurs by electrophilic substitution of a hydrogen ion by an iodonium ion in the molecule of interest, or by nucleophilic substitution (isotope exchange) where a radioactive iodine atom is exchanged with a stable iodine atom that is already present in the molecule. These reactions are represented as follows:

Nucleophilic substitution:

$$R-I + Na^{131}I \rightleftharpoons R-^{131}I + NaI + H_2O \tag{6.6}$$

Electrophilic substitution:

$$R-H + H_2O^{131}I^+ \rightleftharpoons R-^{131}I + HI + H_2O \tag{6.7}$$

In protein iodination, the phenolic ring of tyrosine is the primary site of iodination and the next important site is the imidazole ring of histidine. The pH plays an important role in protein iodination. The optimum pH is 7 to 9. Temperature and duration of iodination depend on the type of molecule to be iodinated and the method of iodination used. The degree of iodination affects the integrity of a protein molecule and generally depends on the type of protein and the iodination method. Normally, one atom of iodine per protein molecule is desirable.

Methods of Iodination

There are several methods of iodination, and principles of only the important ones are described below.

Triiodide Method

The triiodide method essentially consists of adding radioiodine to the compound to be labeled in the presence of a mixture of iodine and potassium iodide:

$$I_2 + KI + {}^{131}I_2 + 2RH \rightarrow R^{131}I + K^{131}I + RI + 2HI \qquad (6.8)$$

where RH is an organic compound being labeled. In the case of protein labeling by this method, minimum denaturation of proteins occurs, but the yield is low, usually about 10% to 30%. Because cold iodine is present, the specific activity of the labeled product is considerably diminished.

Iodine Monochloride Method

In the iodine monochloride (ICl) method, radioiodine is first equilibrated with stable ^{127}I in iodine monochloride in dilute HCl, and then the mixture is added directly to the compound of interest for labeling at a specific pH and temperature. Yields of 50% to 80% can be achieved by this process. However, cold iodine of ICl can be introduced in the molecule, which lowers the specific activity of the labeled compound, and the yield becomes unpredictable, depending on the amount of ICl added.

Chloramine-T Method

Chloramine-T is a sodium salt of N-monochloro-p-toluenesulfonamide and is a mild oxidizing agent. In this method of iodination, first the compound for labeling and then chloramine-T are added to a solution of ^{131}I-sodium iodide. Chloramine-T oxidizes iodide to a reactive iodine species, which then labels the compound. Since cold iodine need not be introduced, high specific activity compounds can be obtained by this method and the labeling efficiency can be very high ($\sim 90\%$). However, chloramine-T is a highly reactive substance and can cause denaturation of proteins. Sometimes milder oxidants such as sodium nitrite and sodium hypochlorite can be used in lieu of chloramine-T. This method is used in iodination of various compounds.

Electrolytic Mehod

Many proteins can be radioiodinated by the electrolytic method, which consists of the electrolysis of a mixture of radioiodide and the material to be labeled. In the electrolytic cell, the anode and cathode compartments are separated by a dialyzing bag that contains the cathode immersed in saline, whereas the anode compartment contains the electrolytic mixture. Electrolysis releases reactive iodine, which labels the compound. Slow and steady liberation of iodine causes uniform iodination of the compound, and in the absence of any carrier iodine, a labeling yield of almost 80% can be achieved.

Enzymatic Method

In enzymatic iodination, enzymes, such as lactoperoxidase and chloroperoxidase, and nanomolar quantities of H_2O_2 are added to the iodination mixture containing radioiodine and the compound to be labeled. The hydrogen peroxide oxidizes iodide to form reactive iodine, which in turn iodinates the compound. Denaturation of proteins or alteration in organic molecules is minimal because only a low concentration of hydrogen peroxide is added. Yields of 60% to 85% and high specific activity can be obtained by this method. This method is very mild and useful in the iodination of many proteins and hormones.

Conjugation Method

In the conjugation method, initially *N*-succinimidyl-3(4-hydroxyphenyl)-propionate (*N*-SHPP) is radioiodinated by the chloramine-T method and separated from the reaction mixture. The radioiodinated *N*-SHPP in dry benzene is available commercially. Proteins are labeled by this agent by allowing it to react with the protein molecule, resulting in an amide bond with lysine groups of the protein. The labeling yield is not very high, but the method allows iodination without alteration of protein molecules whose tyrosine moieties are susceptible to alteration, although in vivo dehalogenation is encountered in some instances.

Demetallation Method

To improve the in vivo stability of iodinated proteins, various organometallic intermediates such as organothallium, organomercury, organosilane, organoborane, and organostannane have been used to iodinate the aromatic ring of the precursor. The carbon-metal bond is cleaved by radioiodination in the presence of oxidizing agents such as chloramine-T and iodogen. Of all these, organostannane [succinimidyl para-tri-n-butylstannyl benzoate (SBSB)] is most attractive because of the ease of preparation, stability, and easy exchange reaction with radioiodine. SBSB is first radioiodinated by a suitable method whereby tributyl stannyl group is substituted by radioiodine. Protein is then coupled to SBSB by mixing the two at alkaline pH. Tamoxifen, vinyl estradiol, and phenyl fatty acids are iodinated by this technique.

Iodogen Method

Proteins and cell membranes can be radioiodinated by the iodogen method. Iodogen or chloramide (1, 3, 4, 6-tetrachloro-3α, 6α-diphenylglycoluril) dissolved in methylene chloride is evaporated in tubes in order to obtain a uniform film coating inside the tube. The radioidide and protein are mixed together in the tube for 10 to 15 min, and the mixture is removed by decantation. Iodogen oxidizes iodide, and iodine then labels the protein. The unreacted iodide is separated by column chromatography of the mixture using Sephadex gel or DEAE ion exchange material. The denaturation of protein is minimal, because the reaction occurs on a solid phase and iodogen is poorly soluble in water. The labeling yield is of the order of 70% to 80%.

Iodo-bead Method

In the iodo-bead method, iodo-beads are used to iodinate various peptides and proteins containing a tyrosine moiety. Iodo-beads consist of the oxidant N-chlorobenzenesulfonamide immobilized on 2.8-mm diameter nonporous polystyrene spheres. These spheres are stable for at least 6 months if stored in an amber bottle at 4 °C. Radioiodination is carried out by simply adding five to six iodo-beads to a mixture of protein ($\sim 100\ \mu g$) and ^{131}I-sodium iodide in 0.5 ml of phosphate buffer solution contained in a capped polystyrene tube. The reaction is allowed to proceed for 15 min at room temperature. The iodination mixture can be removed by pipetting and iodinated protein is then separated by conventional techniques. This method has been claimed to be very successful with little denaturation of the protein. The labeling yield is almost 99%.

Radioiodinated Compounds

After radioiodination the residual free iodide is removed by precipitation, anion exchange, gel filtration, or dialysis; the particular method of choice depends on the iodinated compound. Many iodinated compounds can be sterilized by autoclaving, but sterilization of labeled proteins must be carried out by membrane filtration because autoclaving denatures proteins.

In general, iodine binds firmly and irreversibly to aromatic compounds, but its binding to aliphatic compounds is rather reversible. Iodine binds with amino and sulfhydryl groups, but these reactions are reversible. Partially unsaturated aliphatic fatty acids and neutral fats (e.g., oleic acid and triolein) can be labeled with radioiodine. However, iodination saturates the double bond in these molecules and thus alters their chemical and perhaps biological properties.

Various examples of radioiodinated compounds are ^{125}I-, or ^{131}I-labeled human serum albumin, fibrinogen, insulin, globulin, and many hormones, antibodies and enzymes. The major drawback of ^{131}I-labeled compounds is the high radiation dose to the patient and high-energy photons (364 keV). The radiation characteristics of ^{123}I are suitable for use in vivo, and with their increasing availability many ^{123}I-radiopharmaceuticals are prepared for clinical use in nuclear medicine. In many institutions, ^{123}I-sodium iodide is used routinely for thyroid studies.

Labeling with ^{99m}Tc

General Properties of Technetium-99m

As previously mentioned, more than 80% of radiopharmaceuticals used in nuclear medicine are ^{99m}Tc-labeled compounds. The reason for such a pre-eminent position of ^{99m}Tc in clinical use is its favorable physical and radiation characteristics. The 6-hr physical half-life and the little amount of electron emission permit the administration of millicurie amounts of ^{99m}Tc radioactivity without significant radiation dose to the patient. In addition, the monochromatic 140-keV photons are readily collimated to give images of superior spatial resolution. Furthermore, ^{99m}Tc is readily available in a sterile, pyrogen-free, and carrier-free state from ^{99}Mo–^{99m}Tc generators.

Chemistry of Technetium

Technetium is a transition metal of silvery gray color belonging to group VIIB (Mn, Tc, and Re) and has the atomic number 43. No stable isotope of technetium exists in nature. The ground state ^{99}Tc has a half-life of 2.1×10^5 years. The electronic structure of the neurtal technetium atom is $1s^2 2s^2 2p^6 3s^2 3p^6 3d^{10} 4s^2 4p^6 4d^6 5s^1$. Technetium can exist in eight oxidation states, namely, $1-$ to $7+$, which result from the loss of a given number of electrons from the 4d and 5s orbitals or gain of an electron to the 4d orbital. The stability of these oxidation states depends on the type of ligands and chemical environment. The $7+$ and $4+$ states are most stable and exist in oxides, sulfides, halides, and pertechnetates. The lower oxidation states, $1-$, $1+$, $2+$, and $3+$, are normally stabilized by complexation with ligands, for example, Tc^{1+} complexed with six isonitrile groups in ^{99m}Tc-sestamibi (see Chapter 7). Otherwise, they are oxidized to the $4+$ state and finally to the $7+$ state. The Tc^{5+} and Tc^{6+} species frequently disproportionate into Tc^{4+} and Tc^{7+} states:

$$3Tc^{5+} \longrightarrow 2Tc^{4+} + Tc^{7+} \tag{6.9}$$

$$3Tc^{6+} \longrightarrow Tc^{4+} + 2Tc^{7+} \tag{6.10}$$

The coordination number of ^{99m}Tc-complexes can vary between 4 and 9.

The low concentration of carrier-free ^{99m}Tc($\sim 10^{-9} M$) in many ^{99m}Tc-labeled compounds presents a difficult problem in determining its chemistry. Most of the information regarding the chemistry of technetium has been obtained from that of ^{99}Tc, which is available in concentrations of 10^{-4} to 10^{-5} M, by applying various analytic techniques such as polarography, mass spectrometry, x-ray crystallography, chromatography, and so on.

The principles of dilute solutions play an important role in the chemistry of ^{99m}Tc, because the concentration of ^{99m}Tc in ^{99m}Tc-radiopharmaceuticals is very low. For example, a 3-Ci (111-GBq) sample of the ^{99m}Tc eluate from the Moly generator would have a ^{99m}Tc concentration of about $2.8 \times$

10^{-7} M. Because ^{99}Tc competes with ^{99m}Tc in all chemical reactions, the chemistry of ^{99m}Tc radiopharmaceuticals is further complicated by the presence of ^{99}Tc, which arises from the 13% direct decay of ^{99}Mo and the decay of ^{99m}Tc over time. In preparations containing only a limited amount of Sn^{2+}, the total amount of both ^{99m}Tc and ^{99}Tc may be too high to undergo complete reduction by Sn^{2+}, thus lowering the labeling yield. For example, the tin content in HMPAO kits is limited, and therefore freshly eluted ^{99m}Tc is required for maximum labeling yield. Thus it is essential to have knowledge of the relative proportions of ^{99m}Tc and ^{99}Tc in the Tc-eluate to estimate the labeling yield of a ^{99m}Tc-radiopharmaceutical.

It has been found that the amount of Sn^{2+} available for ^{99m}Tc labeling in typical lyophilized kits is much lower than expected from the original amount added to the formulation. This has been attributed to the likely formation of colloidal tin oxide during the later phase of lyophilization. At present, there is no method to prevent this loss of Sn^{2+}.

Reduction of ^{99m}TcO$_4^-$

The chemical form of ^{99m}Tc available from the Moly generator is sodium pertechnetate (^{99m}Tc-NaTcO$_4$). The pertechnetate ion, ^{99m}TcO$_4^-$, having the oxidation state 7+ for ^{99m}Tc, resembles the permanganate ion, MnO_4^-, and the perrhenate ion, ReO_4^-. It has a configuration of a pyramidal tetrahedron with Tc^{7+} located at the center and four oxygen atoms at the apex and corners of the pyramid. Chemically, ^{99m}TcO$_4^-$ is a rather nonreactive species and does not label any compound by direct addition. In ^{99m}Tc-labeling of many compounds, prior reduction of ^{99m}Tc from the 7+ state to a lower oxidation state is required. Various reducing agents that have been used are stannous chloride ($SnCl_2 \cdot 2H_2O$), stannous citrate, stannous tartrate, concentrated HCl, sodium borohydride ($NaBH_4$), dithionite, and ferrous sulfate. Among these, stannous chloride is the most commonly used reducing agent in most preparations of ^{99m}Tc-labeled compounds. Another method of reduction of ^{99m}Tc^{7+} involves the electrolysis of a mixture of sodium pertechnetate and the compound to be labeled using an anode of zirconium.

The chemical reactions that occur in the reduction of technetium by stannous chloride in acidic medium can be stated as follows:

$$3Sn^{2+} \rightleftharpoons 3Sn^{4+} + 6e^- \tag{6.11}$$

$$2\,^{99m}TcO_4^- + 16H^+ + 6e^- \rightleftharpoons 2\,^{99m}Tc^{4+} + 8H_2O \tag{6.12}$$

Adding the two equations, one has

$$2\,^{99m}TcO_4^- + 16H^+ + 3Sn^{2+} \rightleftharpoons 2\,^{99m}Tc^{4+} + 3Sn^{4+} + 8H_2O \tag{6.13}$$

Equation (6.12) indicates that ^{99m}Tc^{7+} has been reduced to ^{99m}Tc^{4+}. Other reduced states such as ^{99m}Tc^{3+} and ^{99m}Tc^{5+} may be formed under different physicochemical conditions. It may also be possible for a mixture of these species to be present in a given preparation. Experiments with millimolar quantities of ^{99}Tc have shown that Sn^{2+} reduces ^{99}Tc to the 5+ state and then slowly to the 4+ state in citrate buffer at pH 7. Technetium-99 is reduced to the 4+ state by Sn^{2+} in concentrated HCl.

The amount of ^{99m}Tc atoms in the ^{99m}Tc-eluate is very small ($\sim 10^{-9}\ M$), and therefore only a minimal amount of Sn^{2+} is required for reduction of such a small quantity of ^{99m}Tc; however, enough Sn^{2+} is added to ensure complete reduction. The ratio of Sn^{2+} ions to ^{99m}Tc atoms may be as large as 10^6.

Labeling with Reduced Technetium

The reduced ^{99m}Tc species are chemically reactive and combine with a wide variety of chelating agents. A schematic reaction would be

$$\text{Reduced } ^{99m}\text{Tc} + \text{chelating agent} \rightleftharpoons {}^{99m}\text{Tc-chelate} \qquad (6.14)$$

The chelating agent usually donates lone pairs of electrons to form coordinate covalent bonds with reduced ^{99m}Tc. Chemical groups such as—COO^-,—OH^-,—NH_2, and—SH are the electron donors in compounds such as DTPA, gluceptate, and various proteins. Several investigators proposed that tin is incorporated into the ^{99m}Tc-chelate, for example, ^{99m}Tc-Sn-dimethylglyoxime. However, it has been shown by experiments that ^{99m}Tc-labeled DTPA, $N[N'$-(2,6-dimethylphenyl)carbamoylmethyl] imminodiacetic acid (HIDA), methylene diphosphonate (MDP), pyrophosphate (PYP), hydroxyethylidene diphosphonate (HEDP), and gluconate do not contain any tin in the structure of the complex.

Free Pertechnetate in ^{99m}Tc-Radiopharmaceuticals

In a typical preparation of ^{99m}Tc-radiopharmaceutical in the kit vial, the quantity of free pertechnetate usually remains within the acceptable limit. However, the presence of oxygen in the vial, particularly before the addition of ^{99m}Tc, can cause oxidation of the stannous ion to stannic ion whereby the amount of stannous ion available for reduction of Tc^{7+} decreases. This results in an increase in free $^{99m}TcO_4^-$ in ^{99m}Tc-radiopharmaceuticals. Further, the high activity of ^{99m}Tc in the presence of oxygen can cause radiolysis of water or other products in the sample producing hydroxy($OH\cdot$), alkoxy($RO\cdot$), and peroxy($RO_2\cdot$) free radicals. These species interact with ^{99m}Tc-chelates producing free $^{99m}TcO_4^-$ in the sample. However, limits of ^{99m}Tc activity suggested for adding to the commercial kits are sufficiently low such that the radiolytic effects are normally negligible.

The above effects can be mitigated by using sufficient quantity of stannous ion and by avoiding oxygen, air, or any oxidizing agent in the vial throughout its shelf life. It is a common practice to flush the kit vials with N_2 gas to maintain inert gas atmosphere in them. In some kits such as MDP and HDP kits, antioxidants (e.g., ascorbic acid and gentisic acid) are added to prevent oxidation.

Hydrolysis of Reduced Technetium and Tin

There is a possibility that reduced ^{99m}Tc may undergo hydrolysis in aqueous solution. In this case, reduced ^{99m}Tc reacts with water to form various hydrolyzed species depending on the pH, duration of hydrolysis, and presence of other agents. An analysis of chemical reactions shows that hydrolyzed technetium is a compound of ^{99m}TcO$_2$ complexed with other ingredients (e.g., SnO, MoO$_3$ or Al). This hydrolysis competes with the chelation process of the desired compound and thus reduces the yield of the ^{99m}Tc-chelate. The hydrolyzed species can also interfere with the diagnostic test in question if they are present in large quantities in the radiopharmaceutical.

The use of stannous chloride has a disadvantage in that the Sn^{2+} ion also readily undergoes hydrolysis in aqueous solution at pH 6 to 7 and forms insoluble colloids. These colloids bind to reduced ^{99m}Tc and thus compromise the labeling yield. For this reason, an acid is added to prevent the hydrolysis of Sn^{2+} before the reduction of technetium if the preparation is made using basic ingredients rather than a kit.

These two disadvantages, namely, the hydrolysis of reduced ^{99m}Tc and Sn^{2+}, can be circumvented by adding enough chelating agents. The latter will bind to reduced ^{99m}Tc and Sn^{2+}, and thus prevent their hydrolysis. The ratio of the chelating agent to Sn^{2+} should be large enough to ensure complete binding. Binding between the chelating agent and reduced ^{99m}Tc or Sn^{2+} is highly dependent on the affinity constant of the chelating agent. If it is a weak chelating agent (e.g., phosphate compounds), then hydrolyzed species in the ^{99m}Tc-labeled preparation tend to be relatively high. However, if the chelating agent has a high-affinity constant (e.g., DTPA), then the amount of hydrolyzed species will be minimal.

At any rate, in a preparation of a ^{99m}Tc-labeled compound, three ^{99m}Tc species may be present:

1. "Free" ^{99m}Tc as ^{99m}TcO$_4^-$ that has not been reduced by Sn^{2+}.
2. "Hydrolyzed" ^{99m}Tc, such as ^{99m}TcO$_2$ that did not react with the chelating agent; this includes reduced ^{99m}Tc bound to hydrolyzed Sn^{2+} (Sn(OH)$_2$).
3. "Bound" ^{99m}Tc-chelate, which is the desired compound formed by binding of reduced ^{99m}Tc to the chelating agent.

In most routine preparations, the major fraction of radioactivity is in the bound form. The free and hydrolyzed fractions are undesirable and must be removed or reduced to a minimum level so that they do not interfere significantly with the diagnostic text in question. Analysis of ^{99m}Tc- and ^{99}Tc-HEDP samples by high-performance liquid chromatography has revealed that there are at least seven Tc-containing species of unknown oxidation states. The distribution of different components in these mixtures depends on reaction time and the presence of molecular oxygen.

Formation of ^{99m}Tc-Complexes by Ligand Exchange

The ligand exchange method, also termed the *transchelation*, involves first forming a ^{99m}Tc-complex with a weak ligand in aqueous media and then allowing the complex to react with a second ligand that is relatively more stable. Because of the difference in stability of the two ligands, a ligand exchange occurs, forming a more stable ^{99m}Tc-complex with the second ligand. For example, in the preparation of ^{99m}Tc-labeled mercaptoacetyl-glycylglycylglycine (MAG3), ^{99m}Tc-tartrate or ^{99m}Tc-gluconate is first formed by reduction of ^{99m}TcO$_4^-$ with stannous ion in the presence of sodium tartrate or gluconate. Subsequent heating with MAG3 results in ^{99m}Tc-MAG3. The following are the sequences of reactions for ^{99m}Tc-MAG3:

$$^{99m}\text{TcO}_4^- + \text{Sn}^{2+} \rightleftharpoons \text{Reduced } ^{99m}\text{Tc} + \text{Sn}^{4+} \qquad (6.15)$$

$$\text{Reduced } ^{99m}\text{Tc} + \text{tartrate} \rightleftharpoons \,^{99m}\text{Tc-tartrate} \qquad (6.16)$$

$$^{99m}\text{Tc-tartrate} + \text{MAG3} \longrightarrow \,^{99m}\text{Tc-MAG3} + \text{tartrate} \qquad (6.17)$$

Stronger ligands such as MAG3, isonitrile, and ECD are less soluble in aqueous solution and require heating or a long time to dissolve. In contrast, weaker ligands such as tartrate, citrate, and EDTA are highly soluble in aqueous solution. In kits containing both weak and strong ligands, stannous ions primarily remain bound to weaker ligands rather than stronger ligands because of the ready solubility of the former. After the addition of ^{99m}TcO$_4^-$, Tc^{7+} is reduced by Sn^{2+} ions and the reduced Tc readily forms ^{99m}Tc-chelate with the weaker ligands. Upon heating or with a long reaction time, stronger ligands readily dissolve and ligand exchange occurs between the stronger ligand and ^{99m}Tc-chelate.

The addition of a weaker chelating agent is necessary to stabilize the reduced Tc, particularly in the lower oxidation states. Because the reaction between the stronger ligand and the reduced Tc is slow due to poor solubility of the ligand, the stronger ligand alone, in the absence of a weaker ligand, would tend to precipitate most of the reduced Tc as colloid.

Based on these principles, several kits for ^{99m}Tc-labeling have been formulated containing both weak and stronger ligands along with stannous ions. Examples are tartrate and MAG3 for renal imaging, EDTA and ethyl cysteine dimer(ECD) for brain imaging, and hexakis-methoxyisobutyl isonitrile and sodium citrate for myocardial imaging.

Structure of ^{99m}Tc-Complexes

The oxidation state of technetium in many ^{99m}Tc-complexes are not known with certainty. Polarographic measurements and iodometric titrations have been employed to determine the oxidation state of technetium in these compounds. In ^{99m}Tc-DTPA, the oxidation state of technetium has been reported to be ^{99m}Tc^{4+}, whereas in ^{99m}Tc-labeled albumin it has been suggested to be ^{99m}Tc^{5+}. Various physicochemical factors influence the reduction of ^{99m}Tc^{7+} and thus the oxidation state of technetium in a ^{99m}Tc-complex.

Various methods such as electronic and vibrational spectroscopy, x-ray crystallography, solvent extraction, electrophoresis, and mass spectrometry are currently employed in the separation and characterization of ^{99m}Tc-complexes. It has been shown that many ^{99m}Tc-complexes studied thus far have technetium in the 5+ oxidation state. It has also been found that most of these compounds are stabilized by oxo groups and contain oxotechnetium (^{99m}Tc $= O$) cores such as ^{99m}TcO^{3+}, $trans$-^{99m}TcO$_2^+$, and ^{99m}Tc$_2$O$_3^{4+}$ (Jones and Davison, 1982). The structures of ^{99m}TcO^{3+} and $trans$-^{99m}TcO$_2^+$ are illustrated in Figure 6.2. In the figure, "L" represents ligands in the cis position that form coordinate covalent bonds with technetium of the ^{99m}Tc $= O$ core. In Figure 6.2b, there is an oxygen atom in the $trans$ position to the ^{99m}Tc $= O$ core. Figure 6.2a is an illustration of a five-coordinate complex and Figure 6.2b represents a six-coordinate complex. The oxygen in the $trans$ position may become labile by the influence of the electronic structure of the cis ligands and can easily undergo solvolysis in alcohols and water.

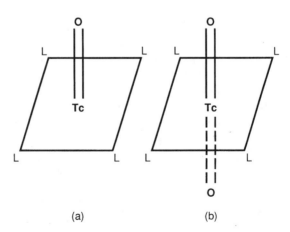

FIGURE 6.2. Structures of oxotechnetium cores: (a) TcO^{3+} and (b) TcO$_2^+$ in ^{99m}Tc-labeled complexes.

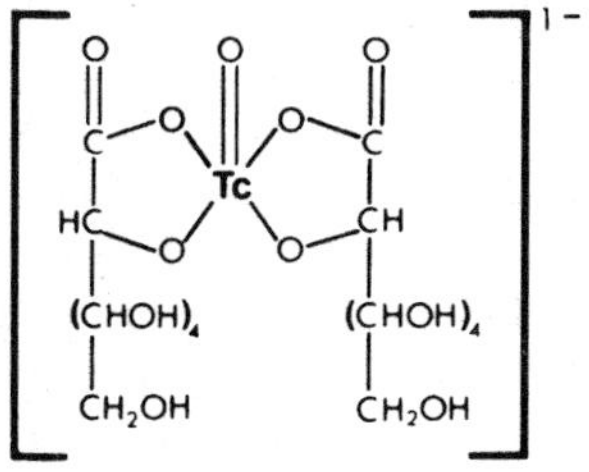

FIGURE 6.3. Proposed structure of ^{99m}Tc-gluceptate.

The charge of a ^{99m}Tc-complex is determined by adding the charges of the ligands to that of the ^{99m}Tc = O core. The coordination number of ^{99m}Tc-complexes can vary from four to nine depending on the nature of the ligands. The structure of ^{99m}Tc-gluceptate with an ionic charge of 1– and coordination number 5 is shown in Figure 6.3.

The biodistribution and in vivo kinetics of ^{99m}Tc-radiopharmaceuticals are influenced by their stereochemical structures. The latter depend on the ligand stereochemistry, the number, type and arrangement of donor atoms, chelate ring size and conformation, the coordination geometry of the metal, and the number of possible ways a ligand can arrange around the metal. The majority of stereochemical studies on ^{99m}Tc radiopharmaceuticals have been made with six-coordinate octahedral complexes containing two or more bidentate ligands and five-coordinate square pyramidal Tc = O complexes. For example, ^{99m}Tc-hexamethylpropyleneamine oxime (HMPAO) is an octahedral complex having the d, l stereoisomer as well as the meso-isomer, and ^{99m}Tc-ECD has the five-coordinate square pyramidal structure giving rise to l,l, d,d, and mesoisomers. However, d,l HMPAO and l,l ECD isomers only are used for clinical purposes, because of their preferential localization in the brain.

Oxidation States of ^{99m}Tc in ^{99m}Tc-Radiopharmaceuticals

As already mentioned, technetium can exist in various oxidation states from 1– to 7+. The Tc^{5+} oxidation state is most common in ^{99m}Tc-complexes, although compounds containing ^{99m}Tc in other oxidation states exist and are being developed in increasing numbers. Various ^{99m}Tc-complexes in different oxidation states are discussed below. No useful Tc^{6+}, Tc^{2+}, and Tc^{0} complexes have been developed for clinical use and, therefore, these complexes have been omitted.

Tc^{7+}

This state is most stable and is found in pertechnetate (^{99m}TcO$_4^-$) and technetium heptasulfide (^{99m}Tc$_2$S$_7$).

Tc^{5+}

This oxidation state exists in ^{99m}Tc-citrate, ^{99m}Tc-gluconate, and ^{99m}Tc-gluceptate prepared by the $SnCl_2$ reduction of pertechnetate in aqueous solution. Tc^{5+} forms complexes with various dithiols (containing sulfur) in which the coordination number of the complex is 5 in the solid state. The four sulfur atoms occupy the four corners of the square base plane and an oxygen atom at the apex of the square pyramid. In solution, six-coordinate compounds are formed, in which case the octahedral structure renders the molecule more labile. One example of this type is diaminodithiol (DADT) compounds. The oxidation state of ^{99m}Tc in these complexes is 5+ and the complexes are neutral, stable, and lipophilic. Other Tc^{5+} complexes include EDTA, pyridine, and imidazole ligands containing nitrogen bases. X-ray crystallography of the ^{99m}Tc-HMPAO complex shows Tc^{5+} to have five-coordinate groups with an oxo group at the apex and four nitrogen atoms at the corners of the square base of a pyramid. Loss of a hydrogen atom from two amine groups and an oxime group in the ligand results in a neutral complex.

Tc^{4+}

The common examples of the Tc^{4+} oxidation state are found in TcO_2 and hexahalo complexes. $^{99m}TcO_2 \cdot xH_2O$ is produced by reduction of pertechnetate with zinc in HCl. But in this process, 20% of the technetium is reduced to metal. Hydrolysis of hexaiodo complex results in a pure $TcO_2 \cdot xH_2O$ product. Hexahalo complexes are stable only in a nonaqueous solution, whereas they undergo hydrolysis in aqueous solution.

The oxidation state of ^{99m}Tc in ^{99m}Tc-hydroxyethylidene diphosphonate (HEDP) has been reported to be variable, depending on the pH of the preparation. The Tc^{3+} state exists at acidic pH, the Tc^{5+} in alkaline solution, and the Tc^{4+} at neutral pH. Since a slight variation of pH can cause a change in the oxidation state, ^{99m}Tc may exist in a mixture of 3+, 4+, and 5+ states in ^{99m}Tc-HEDP.

Tc^{3+}

^{99m}Tc complexes of DTPA, EDTA, dimercaptosuccinic acid (DMSA), and HIDA all are found to have the Tc^{3+} state when prepared in acid solutions. However, the Tc^{4+} state is found in both alkaline and neutral solutions of DTPA and EDTA.

Various arsine and phosphine complexes of Tc^{3+} have been prepared mostly for myocardial imaging. These complexes are of the type $[TcD_2X_2]^+$ where D stands for a chelating diphosphine ligand and X represents a halogen. The organic ligands include [1, 2 bis-diphenylphosphino] ethane (DPPE), [bis (1,2-dimethylphosphino) ethane] (DMPE), and [o-phenylene bis (dimethylarsine)], whereas the halogen and halogen-like ligands are Cl, Br, and SCN. The structure of DPPE is found to be octahedral, in which the centrally located Tc is coordinated with four equatorial phosphorus atoms and two transaxial halogen atoms. The electrochemistry of these compounds shows that complexes with Cl^- and Br^- are highly stable.

The Tc^{3+} state exists in ^{99m}Tc-labeled oxime complex and the most common example of this type is ^{99m}Tc-labeled dimethylglyoxime, which is prepared by Sn^{2+} reduction of $^{99m}TcO_4^-$ in the presence of dimethylglyoxime. In this compound, Sn^{2+} is found to be incorporated in the structure of the complex.

Another class of compounds, called BATOs (boronic acid adducts of technetium dioxime complexes), is found to contain the Tc^{3+} state in the structure, when complexed with ^{99m}Tc. ^{99m}Tc-teboroxime (Cardiotec; Bracco, Princeton, NJ) belongs to this group and was once used for myocardial imaging. In the structure of ^{99m}Tc-teboroxime, technetium is coordinated to three N-bonded dioxime molecules and one Cl atom in an axial position. However, its very rapid washout from the myocardium made it impossible to collect meaningful data using the SPECT technique.

Tc^{1+}

This oxidation state is primarily stabilized in aqueous medium by coordination bonds with various ligands. For example, Tc^{1+} in ^{99m}Tc-sestamibi is stabilized by the isonitrile groups. Other isonitrile complexes such as tert-butyl, methyl, cyclohexile, and phenyl isocyanide groups form stable compounds with ^{99m}Tc in the 1+ oxidation state. These compounds are stable in air and water.

Oxidation States in ^{99m}Tc-Labeled Proteins

The oxidation state of technetium in ^{99m}Tc-labeled protein depends on the reducing agents used in the preparation. For example, when concentrated HCl is used as the reducing agent, Tc^{4+} is the likely oxidation state in ^{99m}Tc-albumin. However, when ascorbic acid is added to the system, Tc^{5+} is the probable oxidation state. This is true in the case of direct labeling method (described later). In the case of indirect labeling in which a bifunctional chelating agent is added as a spacer between the Tc and the protein (antibody), Tc exists primarily in the Tc^{4+} state, which binds to one end of the chelator, while the other end is bound to the protein.

Kits for ^{99m}Tc-Labeling

The introduction of kits for the formulation of many ^{99m}Tc-radiopharmaceuticals has facilitated the practice of nuclear pharmacy to a considerable extent. The kits have a long shelf life and can be purchased and stored well ahead of daily preparation; ^{99m}Tc-labeling can be accomplished simply by adding ^{99m}TcO$_4^-$ to most kits.

Kits for most ^{99m}Tc-radiopharmaceuticals are prepared from a "master" solution consisting of the compound to be labeled mixed with an acidic solution of a stannous compound in appropriate proportions. The pH of the solution is adjusted to 5 to 7 with dilute NaOH, purged with nitrogen, and aliquots of the solution are dispensed into individual kit vials. The solution is then lyophilized (freeze-dried) and the vial flushed and filled with sterile nitrogen. Lyophilization renders the dried material in the vial readily soluble in aqueous solution and thus aids in labeling by chelation. The preparation is carried out using sterile materials and under strict aseptic conditions in a laminar flow hood filled with nitrogen under positive pressure.

Various stannous compounds, such as stannous chloride, stannous fluoride, stannous citrate, stannous tartrate, stannous pyrophosphate, and so on, have been used by different commercial manufacturers, although stannous chloride is most commonly used. In the kit preparation, when the acidic solution of Sn^{2+} is added, a complex is formed between Sn^{2+} and the chelating agent:

$$Sn^{2+} + \text{chelating agent} \rightleftharpoons \text{Sn-chelate} \qquad (6.18)$$

When the pH of the solution is raised, hydrolysis of Sn^{2+} does not occur because Sn^{2+} is already chelated in the presence of a large amount of the chelating agent.

The chemistry of tin as described earlier prevails when the ^{99m}TcO$_4^-$ solution is added to the lyophilized chelating agent in the kit vial. ^{99m}Tc^{7+} is reduced by Sn^{2+} in the Sn-chelate or by the free Sn^{2+} at equilibrium in Eq. (6.18). The amount of Sn^{2+} in the latter situation should be more than sufficient to reduce the nanomolar quantity of ^{99m}Tc^{7+} added to the kit.

In each kit, the initial amounts of Sn^{2+} and chelating agent are very important. If too much tin is used, the possibility of hydrolysis of tin increases, in which case hydrolyzed tin may coprecipitate some of the reduced ^{99m}Tc to form ^{99m}Tc-Sn-colloid and other Sn-complexes, thus diminishing the yield of the labeled chelate. Too little tin may lead to incomplete reduction of ^{99m}Tc to the desired oxidation state and hence an unreliable yield of the ^{99m}Tc-complex along with unreacted ^{99m}TcO$_4^-$. A large excess of the chelating agent should be used to keep the tin complexed. This prevents the hydrolysis of tin and technetium at pH 6 to 7 after the addition of ^{99m}TcO$_4^-$ to the kit, and thus results in an improved yield of ^{99m}Tc-complex. For a weak chelating agent, the ratio of chelating agent to tin should be even higher. However, the optimum value of this ratio must be established for each kit by trial and error.

Colloids and Labeled Particles

In true solutions, such as those of sucrose, sodium chloride, and so on, the particles of a solute dissolved in the solvent are believed to be of molecular size. The particle size is less than 1 nanometer ($1 \text{ nm} = 10^{-9}$ meter) and the particles are not visible under the microscope. On the other hand, a suspension or emulsion contains particles large enough to be visible to the naked eye or at least under the light microscope. These particles are greater than 1 micrometer ($1 \text{ } \mu\text{m} = 10^{-6} \text{ meter} = 10^{-4} \text{ cm}$). Colloidal particles fall between the two extremes of true solutions and suspensions. The size of colloidal particles ranges between 10 nm and 1 μm, and they are usually electrically charged. The surface charge of the particles (immobile) is balanced by an equal and opposite charge of the mobile layer of the solvent. The potential developed between the two layers is called the ζ-potential. Addition of electrolytes (salts, acids, or bases) to a colloid breaks down this potential and eventually causes aggregation or flocculation of colloids.

Stabilizing agents such as gelatin, polyvinylpyrrolidone, or carboxymethylcellulose are added to many colloidal preparations to prevent aggregation. The stability and characteristics of a colloid depend on many factors such as size, primary charge, ζ-potential, valence of the ions, surface tension, viscosity, and polarity of the dispersion medium. Colloidal particles are not visible under the light microscope but can be detected under the ultramicroscope or electron microscope. Colloids are sometimes referred to as "microaggregates," although many investigators define the latter as having a size range of 0.5 to 5 μm. An example of a colloid used in nuclear medicine is ^{99m}Tc-sulfur colloid. These particles are removed by reticuloendothelial cells and therefore can be used for imaging the liver, spleen, and bone marrow. Colloids of smaller sizes, such as ^{99m}Tc-antimony sulfide colloid, have been used for lymphoscintigraphy.

Larger particles, or macroaggregates as they are often called, are larger than 5 μm and can be seen under the light microscope. The size of these particles can be measured using a hemocytometer under a light microscope. Examples of larger particles are ^{99m}Tc-MAA particles, which range in size between 15 and 100 μm. These particles are trapped in the capillary bed of the lungs and are used widely for imaging the lungs.

Additives and Preservatives

Additives, or preservatives as they are sometimes called, are added to many radiopharmaceuticals or labeled compounds to preserve their integrity and efficacy. As previously mentioned, labeled compounds are prone to degradation by radiolysis and there is a possibility of bacterial growth in many radiopharmaceuticals. In many cases additives prevent these complications. A preservative can function as a stabilizer, an antioxidant, or a bactericidal agent, and some additives can perform all these functions simultaneously. Additives must not react with any ingredient of the radiopharmaceutical preparation.

Stabilizers are added to maintain the integrity of a radiopharmaceutical or a labeled compound in its original state. They are very important in radiopharmaceutical preparations, particularly if the preparations are to be preserved for a long time. Ascorbic acid, gentisic acid, citrates, and acetates are all stabilizers for many ^{99m}Tc-labeled preparations. Gelatin is a widely used stabilizer for colloidal preparations, but its property as a growth medium tends to encourage bacterial growth. For this reason, proper sterilization and aseptic handling of preparations containing gelatin are essential.

Bactericidal agents are used to prevent bacterial growth in a solution. Benzyl alcohol in a concentration of 0.9% is widely used for this purpose. Such a low concentration of this compound is used because it has a vasodilating effect. Benzyl alcohol also reduces radiolysis in the radiopharmaceutical preparation. Sometimes ethanol (2.0%) is used as a bactericidal agent. These agents are not usually added to ^{99m}Tc-radiopharmaceuticals.

The pH of a radiopharmaceutical is very important for its stability and biological properties; maintenance of the proper pH of the solution is achieved by adding acid, alkali, or suitable buffers such as Tris buffer or phosphate buffers to the radiopharmaceutical preparation.

The loss of radioiodine due to oxidation of iodide in an iodide solution is often prevented by the addition of a reducing agent such as sodium thiosulfate, sodium sulfite, or ascorbic acid, or by maintaining an alkaline pH.

Questions

1. Discuss various factors that should be considered in the labeling procedure.
2. (a) What is the oxidation state of ^{131}I required for iodination? (b) What is the optimum pH for protein labeling? (c) What is the binding site in iodination of protein? (d) What is believed to be the iodinating species? (e) What are the two types of iodination reactions?
3. Describe various methods of iodination and their merits and disadvantages.
4. What is the most common reducing agent used in ^{99m}Tc-labeling?
5. In ^{99m}Tc-labeling, it is often desirable that the chelating agent be added in excess. Explain.
6. What are the three species of ^{99m}Tc present in a ^{99m}Tc-MDP prepara-

tion? Explain how the hydrolyzed ^{99m}Tc originates in the sample. Can you suggest a method to prevent this?
7. Oxygen or oxidizing agents should not be present in ^{99m}Tc-preparations. Why?
8. Write the general chemical equations for ^{99m}Tc-labeling of a chelating agent. Describe the preparation of kits for ^{99m}Tc-labeled compounds.
9. State the oxidation states of ^{99m}Tc in the following compounds: (a) ^{99m}Tc-DTPA, (b) ^{99m}Tc-labeled albumin, and (c) ^{99m}Tc-HIDA.
10. What are colloids? What are they used for? Name the common additive used in ^{99m}Tc-sulfur colloid.
11. Discuss the importance of the oxotechnetium core in the structure of ^{99m}Tc-complexes.

Suggested Reading

Billinghurst MW, Rempel S, Westendorf BA. Radiation decomposition of technetium-99m radiopharmaceuticals. *J Nucl Med.* 1979; 20:138.

Clark MJ, Podbielski L. Medical diagnostic imaging with complexes of Tc-99m. *Coord Chem Rev.* 1987; 78:253.

Deutsch E, Nicolini M, Wagner HN, Jr eds. *Technetium in Chemistry and Nuclear Medicine.* Verona: Cortina International; 1983.

Dewanjee MK. The chemistry of ^{99m}Tc-labeled radiopharmaceuticals. *Semin Nucl Med.* 1990; 20:5.

Dewanjee MK. *Radioiodination: Theory, Practice and Biomedical Application.* Boston: Kluwer Academic; 1992

Eckelman WC, Steigman J, Paik CH. Radiopharmaceutical chemistry. In: Harpert J, Eckelman WC, Neumann RD, eds. *Nuclear Medicine: Diagnosis and Therapy.* New York: Thieme Medical; 1996:213.

Jones AG, Davison A. The relevance of basic technetium chemistry to nuclear medicine. *J Nucl Med.* 1982; 23:1041.

Kotegov KV, Pavlov ON, Shvedov VP. Technetium. In: *Advances in Inorganic Chemistry and Radiochemistry.* New York: Academic Press; 1968:2.

Lathrop KA, Harper PV, Rich BH, et al. Rapid incorporation of short-lived cyclotron produced radionuclides into radiopharmaceuticals. In *Radiopharmaceuticals and Labeled Compounds.* Vienna: IAEA; 1973: 471.

Nicolini M, Bandoli G, Mazzi U, eds. *Technetium in Chemistry and Nuclear Medicine.* Verona: Cortina International; 1986.

Richards P, Steigman J. Chemistry of technetium as applied to radiopharmaceuticals. In: Subramanian G, Rhodes BA, Cooper JF, Sodd VJ, eds. *Radiopharmaceuticals.* New York: Society of Nuclear Medicine; 1975:23.

Srivastava SC, Meinken G, Smith TD, Richards P. Problems associated with stannous ^{99m}Tc-radiopharmaceutical. In: Welch MJ, ed. *Radiopharmaceuticals and Other Compounds Labelled with Short-Lived Radionuclides.* New York: Pergamon Press; 1977:83.

Steigman J, Eckelman WC. *The Chemistry of Technetium in Medicine*. Nuclear Medicine Series. NAS-NS-3204. Washington: National Head Press; 1992.

Wilbur DS, Hadley SW, Hylarides MD, et al. Development of a stable radio-
iodinating reagent to label monoclonal antibodies for radiotherapy of cancer. *J
Nucl Med*. 1989; 30:216.

Yalow RS, Berson SA. Labeling of proteins—Problems and practices. *NY Acad Sci*.
1966; 28:1033.

7
Characteristics of Specific Radiopharmaceuticals

In Chapter 6 the general principles of labeling methods, particularly iodination and ^{99m}Tc-labeling, have been discussed, and kit preparation for formulation of ^{99m}Tc-radiopharmaceuticals has been described. In this chapter the practical aspects of preparation, labeling yield, stability, storage conditions, and other characteristics of radiopharmaceuticals most commonly used in nuclear medicine will be discussed.

^{99m}Tc-Labeled Radiopharmaceuticals

The basic principle of ^{99m}Tc-labeling involves reduction of ^{99m}Tc^{7+} to an oxidation state that binds to a chelating molecule of interest. In most cases, kits for ^{99m}Tc-radiopharmaceuticals are commercially available for routine clinical use. These kits contain the chelating agent of interest and the reducing agent in appropriate quantities. In some kits, suitable stabilizers are added. Limits of volume and activity of ^{99m}Tc that can be added to specific kit vials and expiration time are given in the package inserts provided by the manufacturer. For most ^{99m}Tc-radiopharmaceuticals, the expiration time is 6 hr, equal to the physical half-life of ^{99m}Tc ($t_{1/2} = 6$ hr). Also included in the package inserts are storage temperatures for the kits before and after the formulation with ^{99m}Tc. The following is a description of the characteristics of the routinely used ^{99m}Tc-radiopharmaceuticals.

^{99m}Tc-Sodium Pertechnetate

^{99m}Tc-NaTcO$_4$ ($t_{1/2} = 6$ hr) is eluted from the ^{99}Mo-^{99m}Tc generator in saline solution. These generators are supplied by Mallinckrodt Medical Inc., Bristol-Myers Squibb, Amersham Health, and others. The ^{99m}TcO$_4^-$ solution obtained from the generator is tested for ^{99}Mo and Al breakthrough, and aliquots are used to prepare different kits, as described below. The self-life of ^{99m}TcO$_4^-$ is 12 hr after elution and can be stored at room temperature. The oxidation state of technetium in ^{99m}TcO$_4^-$ is 7+.

^{99m}TcO$_4^-$ is primarily used for preparation of ^{99m}Tc-labeled radio-pharmaceuticals, but is used as such for thyroid imaging and Meckel's diverticulum detection.

^{99m}Tc-Labeled Human Serum Albumin

Human serum albumin (HSA) kits containing HSA and Sn^{2+} are available commercially in multidosage vials supplied by Amersham Health. The kits should be stored at 2° to 8°C, and before labeling with ^{99m}TcO$_4^-$, the vial should be warmed up to the room temperature. Labeling is carried out by adding ^{99m}TcO$_4^-$ to the kit vial and the labeling efficiency is greater than 90%. The pH of ^{99m}Tc-HSA so obtained is 2.5 to 3.3. ^{99m}Tc-HSA should be stored at 2° to 8°C.

^{99m}Tc-HSA is good for 6 hr after formulation. Preservative-free saline should be used for diluting ^{99m}TcO$_4^-$ or ^{99m}Tc-HSA. The contents of the vial should be thoroughly mixed before drawing the patient dosage.

The oxidation state of technetium in ^{99m}Tc-HSA is not known with certainty, but has been postulated to be 5+.

^{99m}Tc-HSA is used for blood pool imaging by the first pass or gated technique.

^{99m}Tc-Macroaggregated Albumin

The macroaggregated albumin (MAA) is prepared by heating a mixture of human serum albumin (HSA) and stannous chloride or tartrate in acetate buffer (pH 5; isoelectric point of albumin) at 80° to 90°C for about 30 min. The particles are then washed with saline to remove any free stannous ion and resuspended in saline. The suspension is then aliquoted into vials for later use as kits.

Commercial kits are available in lyophilized form and usually contain MAA particles, stannous chloride dihydrate or tartrate and HCl or NaOH added for pH adjustment. In addition, different manufacturers add other inactive ingradients such as sodium acetate, HSA, succinic acid, and lactose to facilitate particle dispersion during reconstitution with pertechnetate. The number of particles varies from 1 to 12 million particles per milligram of aggregated albumin. The shape of the particles is irregular and the size ranges between 10 and 90 μm, with no particles larger than 150 μm. The kits should be stored at 2° to 8°C before labeling with ^{99m}Tc. Some kits can be stored at 20° to 25°C.

The preparation of ^{99m}Tc-MAA using a commercial kit involves initial warming up of the vial to the room temperature followed by the addition of ^{99m}TcO$_4^-$. Some kits require that the vials stand for 2 to 15 min for maximum tagging. The labeling efficiency is greater than 90%. The preparations are good for 6 to 8 hr and must be stored at 2° to 8°C after formulation.

The ^{99m}Tc-MAA preparations must be checked for particle size with a hemocytometer (grid size $= 50\,\mu$m) under a light microscope and suspensions containing particles larger than 150 μm should be discarded. Before drawing a dosage for a patient, the contents of the vial should be agitated gently to make a homogeneous suspension. Similarly, the contents of the syringe also should be thoroughly mixed before administration.

^{99m}Tc-MAA is the agent of choice for lung perfusion imaging. It is also used in venography for detecting deep vein thrombi in lower extremities.

^{99m}Tc-Phosphonate and Phosphate Radiopharmaceuticals

Phosphonate and phosphate compounds localize avidly in bone and, therefore, are suitable for bone imaging. However, phosphonate compounds are more stable in vivo than phosphate compounds because the P-O-P bond in phosphate is easily broken down by phosphatase enzyme, whereas the P-C-P bond in diphosphonate is not. For this reason, diphosphonate complexes labeled with ^{99m}Tc are commonly used for bone imaging, although ^{99m}Tc-pyrophosphate is used for myocardial infarct imaging. The three extensively studied diphosphonates are 1-hydroxyethylidene diphosphonate (HEDP), methylene diphosphonate (MDP), and hydroxymethylene diphosphonate (HMDP or HDP), of which MDP and HDP are most commonly used in nuclear medicine. The molecular structures of pyrophosphate (PYP), HEDP, MDP and HDP are shown in Figure 7.1.

Commercial kits for PYP, MDP, and HDP are available from different manufacturers. The composition of each kit varies from vendor to vendor in quantities of the chelating agent and the stannous ions. All ^{99m}Tc-diphosphonate agents are weak chelates and tend to degrade with time, producing ^{99m}TcO$_4^-$ impurity in the presence of oxygen and free radicals produced by radiations, as discussed in Chapter 6. These oxidative reactions can be prevented by increasing the amount of tin, purging the kits with nitrogen, and/or adding antioxidants. It should be noted that a suitable tin-

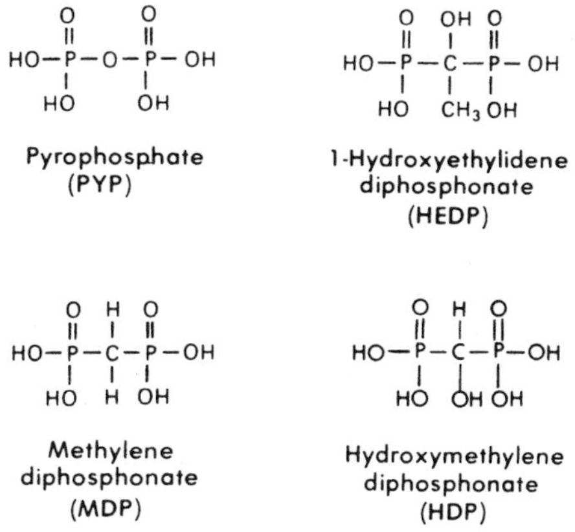

FIGURE 7.1. Molecular structures of different phosphate and phosphonate compounds used in bone imaging.

to-chelating agent ratio must be maintained for optimal bone imaging without undesirable ^{99m}Tc-Sn-colloid formation.

When bone kits containing large amounts of Sn^{2+} were used for bone imaging, subsequent brain scanning with ^{99m}TcO$_4^-$ indicated ^{99m}Tc-labeling of red blood cells for up to 2 weeks after administration of ^{99m}Tc-PYP. This mimics the situation encountered in in vivo labeling of red blood cells by first administering stannous pyrophosphate followed by pertechnetate administration. The excess Sn^{2+} ions left after the reduction of ^{99m}TcO$_4^-$ in diphosphonate kits are available in the plasma for further radiolabeling of the red blood cells. For this reason, the tin content was lowered in subsequent bone kits, which were further stabilized with nitrogen purging and using antioxidants such as gentisic acid.

The storage temperature for most kits is 15° to 30°C both before and after labeling. Labeling is carried out by simply adding ^{99m}TcO$_4^-$ to the vial and mixing. The labeling yield is greater than 95%. The ^{99m}Tc-MDP preparation is good for 6 hr after labeling, except for HDP kits for which an expiration time of 8 hr has been indicated. The oxidation state of Tc in bone kits has been reported to be 3+.

^{99m}Tc-MDP and ^{99m}Tc-HDP are used for bone imaging, whereas ^{99m}Tc-PYP is used for myocardial infarct imaging. The latter is also used in red blood cell labeling for use in gated blood pool and gastrointestinal blood loss studies.

^{99m}Tc-Sulfur Colloid

The basic principle of ^{99m}Tc-sulfur colloid (SC) preparation is to add an acid to a mixture of ^{99m}TcO$_4^-$ and sodium thiosulfate and then heat it at 95° to 100°C in a water bath for 5 to 10 min. The pH of the mixture is adjusted to 6 to 7 with a suitable buffer. The labeling yield is greater than 99%. Kits of ^{99m}Tc-SC are available from commercial manufacturers. To these kits, in addition to the basic ingredients of thiosulfate and an acid, the manufacturers add gelatin as a protective colloid and EDTA to remove by chelation any aluminum ion present in the ^{99m}Tc-eluate.

The shelf life of the kits is usually 1 year from the time of manufacture. ^{99m}Tc-SC can be stored at room temperature and dispensed within 6 to 12 hr after labeling. The particle size ranges from 0.1 to 1 μm, with a mean size of 0.3 μm, and the size distribution can vary from preparation to preparation and also from kit to kit. The presence of Al^{3+} or any other polyvalent ions interferes with colloid formation by flocculation, particularly in the presence of phosphate buffer, and the problem is remedied by the addition of EDTA to the kit. EDTA forms a complex with Al^{3+} and thus prevents flocculation of ^{99m}Tc-SC. The ^{99m}Tc-eluate containing more than 10 μg aluminum/ml should not be used. If there is aggregation, larger particles will be trapped in the pulmonary capillaries, and therefore, the preparation should be discarded.

There are two steps in the labeling process of ^{99m}Tc-SC. In the first step, the acid reacts with sodium thiosulfate in the presence of ^{99m}TcO$_4^-$ and forms colloidal ^{99m}Tc$_2$S$_7$ as given in Eq. (7.1).

$$2\,Na\,^{99m}TcO_4 + 7\,Na_2S_2O_3 + 2\,HCl \rightarrow\,^{99m}Tc_2S_7 + 7\,Na_2SO_4 + H_2O + 2\,NaCl$$

$$(7.1)$$

In the second step, colloidal sulfur is precipitated as shown in Eq. (7.2).

$$Na_2S_2O_3 + 2\,HCl \rightarrow H_2SO_3 + S + 2\,NaCl \qquad (7.2)$$

The ^{99m}Tc-SC formation is faster than the colloidal sulfur formation. It has been shown that colloidal sulfur forms at least in part on ^{99m}Tc-SC which serves as its nucleus (Eckelman et al., 1996). At the same time, colloidal sulfur can also form independently. Smaller particles generally contain relatively small quantities of colloidal sulfur but a significant amount of ^{99m}Tc-SC and conversely, larger particles contain more colloidal sulfur than ^{99m}Tc-SC. Thus, if more Tc (^{99}Tc plus ^{99m}Tc) atoms are added, as in the pertechnetate obtained from a generator that has not been previously eluted for a long period, small size particles increase in number due to an increase in the number of both ^{99}Tc- and ^{99m}Tc-SC particles and less amount of colloidal sulfur. The colloidal sulfur on the Tc-SC particles can be dissolved by heating in mild alkaline solution giving rise to smaller particles. It should be noted that the oxidation state of ^{99m}Tc in ^{99m}Tc$_2$S$_7$ is 7+, and therefore no reduction of Tc^{7+} occurs.

^{99m}Tc-sulfur colloid is most useful in liver and spleen imaging and at times in imaging bone marrow. It is also used for gastrointestinal blood loss studies and for making ^{99m}Tc-labeled egg sandwich for gastric emptying studies.

Filtered ^{99m}Tc-Sulfur Colloid

Lymphoscintigraphy is successfully performed by using smaller size ($<1\ \mu$m) ^{99m}Tc-SC. These particles are obtained by filtering the ^{99m}Tc-SC (prepared as above) through a 0.2 or 0.1 μm membrane filter. In the case of high concentration of activity, the sample is diluted to the desired concentration and then filtered. The concentration of particles in these preparations is reduced.

^{99m}Tc-Albumin Colloid (Nanocolloid)

An albumin colloid kit under the brand name of Nanocoll is supplied by the Solco Company in Europe. This kit contains the HSA colloid (also called the nanocolloid) and stannous dihydrate, and is characterized by very small size particles (almost 95% of the particles are less than 0.08 μm in size with a mean size of 0.03 μm). Labeling is carried out by adding ^{99m}TcO$_4^-$ to the kit vial and incubating the mixture for 5 to 10 min at room temperature. The labeling yield of ^{99m}Tc-nanocolloid is quantitative. Because of the smaller size of the particles, more nanocolloid localizes in the bone marrow ($\sim 15\%$) relative to ^{99m}Tc-SC (2–5%). The kit is stored at 2° to 8°C before reconstitution and at room temperature after reconstitution. ^{99m}Tc-nanocolloid is useful for 6 hr after formulation.

^{99m}Tc-nanocolloid is useful for bone marrow imaging, inflammation scintigraphy and lymphoscintigraphy.

^{99m}Tc-Pentetate (DTPA)

The commercial DTPA kits are usually made up of pentasodium or calcium trisodium salt of DTPA containing an appropriate amount of stannous chloride dihydrate in lyophilized form under nitrogen atmosphere. Labeling is performed by adding oxidant-free ^{99m}TcO$_4^-$ to the kit vial and mixing. The labeling yield is greater than 95%. ^{99m}Tc-DTPA has a shelf life of 6 hr after reconstitution. The recommended storage temperature for the kit is 15° to 30°C before and after labeling.

Using ^{99}Tc in millimolar quantities, it has been shown that in ^{99}Tc-DTPA prepared by stannous ion reduction, the oxidation state of technetium is 4+. It is not known, however, if these data can be extrapolated to the tracer level of ^{99m}Tc in ^{99m}Tc-DTPA.

The primary use of ^{99m}Tc-DTPA is for renal flow study, glomerular filtration rate (GFR) measurement, and aerosol preparation in lung ventilation studies. It is also used in stress and rest radionuclide ventriculography. For GFR measurement, ^{99m}Tc-DTPA should be used within 1 hr of preparation, because the breakdown of ^{99m}Tc-DTPA may raise the blood background and thus give an erroneous GFR. It has also been used for the study of cerebral shunt patency and cerebrospinal fluid leaks. For such use, however, ^{99m}Tc-DTPA must be tested specifically for pyrogens after reconstitution, because the cerebrospinal system is very sensitive to pyrogens.

^{99m}Tc-Labeled Red Blood Cells

The basic principle of labeling of red blood cells (RBCs) with ^{99m}Tc involves mixing RBCs with Sn^{2+} ions followed by the addition of ^{99m}TcO$_4^-$. The Sn^{2+} ion enters into the red blood cell and subsequently ^{99m}TcO$_4^-$ ion diffuses into it, whereupon Sn^{2+} reduces Tc^{7+} to a lower oxidation state, nearly 80% of which then binds to the beta chain of the globin part of hemoglobin and 20% to heme. Although various chelates of Sn^{2+} have been proposed, stannous citrate, stannous gluceptate, and stannous pyrophosphate are almost exclusively used for ^{99m}Tc labeling of RBCs. Direct addition of RBCs to a mixture of ^{99m}TcO$_4^-$ and Sn^{2+} does not cause labeling of RBCs.

There are three methods currently employed in the labeling of RBCs with ^{99m}Tc: the in vitro method, the in vivo method, and the modified in vivo method. Each method has its own merits and disadvantages and they are described below.

In Vitro Method

In the in vitro method, blood is drawn from the subject and RBCs are separated by centrifugation and washing. The packed cells are incubated with appropriate amount of Sn^{2+} (usually stannous citrate) and washed to remove excess tin. The "tinned" RBCs are then incubated with an appropriate amount of $^{99m}TcO_4^-$ to yield ^{99m}Tc-RBCs. The labeling efficiency is higher than 97%.

The commercially available kit suppiled by Mallinckrodt Medical consists of a lyophilized mixture of stannous citrate along with acid citrate dextrose (ACD). One ml of heparinized blood is incubated initially for 5 min in the kit and then a sodium hypochlorite solution is added, followed by ACD solution. Hypochlorite oxidizes excess Sn^{2+} to Sn^{4+} and citrate removes plasma-bound tin as Sn-citrate complex. ^{99m}Tc-RBCs are obtained by adding $^{99m}TcO_4^-$ and incubating for 15 min. The labeling efficiency is better than 97%. This kit is marketed under the trade name of Ultratag RBC.

The in vitro method is useful in the gastrointestinal blood loss study, hemangioma study, gated blood pool study, and also for imaging the spleen. In the latter case, the cells are denatured by heating the labeled cells at 50°C for about 20 min and then injected into patients.

In Vivo Method

In the in vivo method, the Sn-PYP kit is reconstituted with isotonic saline, and a sufficient volume of the solution to give 10 to 20 μg/kg Sn^{2+} ion is injected intravenously into the patient. After 20 to 30 min waiting, 20 to 30 mCi (0.74–1.11 GBq) $^{99m}TcO_4^-$ is injected, which tags the RBCs immediately. The tagging efficiency is somewhat lower (80–90%), partly due to extravascular distribution such as thyroid trapping, gastric secretion, and renal excretion. Certain drugs such as heparin, dextran, doxorubicin, penicillin, hydralazine, and iodinated contrast contrast media often inhibit Sn^{2+} transport through the RBC membrane and diminish ^{99m}Tc-labeling of RBCs. In these subjects, in vitro labeling methods should be employed.

This method is commonly used in the gated blood pool study. It has the added advantage of injecting $^{99m}TcO_4^-$ in a small volume as a bolus to perform the first pass radionuclide ventriculography followed by gated blood pool study (discussed in Chapter 13).

Modified In Vivo Method

The modified in vivo method is a modification of the above in vivo method (Callahan et al., 1982). A butterfly infusion set containing heparinized saline (10 units/ml of blood) is secured into the vein of the patient, while the open end is connected to a three-way stopcock. One port of the stopcock is connected to a syringe containing 20 to 30 mCi (740–1111 MBq) $^{99m}TcO_4^-$ and the other to a syringe containing heparinized saline. Residual heparin in the infusion line acts as anticoagulant. Twenty min after injection of Sn-PYP, 3 ml of blood is drawn into the ^{99m}Tc syringe and incubated for 10 min with gentle shaking. The labeled cells are then injected back into the patient followed by flushing with saline. This method gives better labeling yield (>95%) and is useful in gastrointestinal blood loss studies and gated blood pool studies.

^{99m}Tc-Iminodiacetic Acid Derivatives

The first iminodiacetic acid (IDA) derivative employed in nuclear medicine was 2,6-dimethylphenylcarbamoylmethyl iminodiacetic acid, or HIDA (its generic name is lidofenin). HIDA is synthesized by refluxing a mixture of equal molar quantities of ω-chloro-2,6-dimethylacetanilide and disodium iminodiacetate in ethanol: water (3:1) solvent (Loberg et al., 1976). Since the first use of HIDA for hepatobiliary imaging, several N-substituted iminodiacetic acid derivatives have been prepared, among which 2,6-diethyl (DIDA or etilfenin), paraisopropyl (PIPIDA or iprofenin), parabutyl (BIDA or butilfenin), diisopropyl (DISIDA or disofenin), and bromo-trimethyl (mebrofenin) analogs have undergone considerable clinical and experimental research. The chemical structures of some derivatives and a ^{99m}Tc-IDA complex are illustrated in Figure 7.2.

Kits for DISIDA (Hepatolite; CIS-US, Inc.) and mebrofenin (Choletec, Bracco Diagnostics) are commercially available and usually contain the IDA derivative and stannous chloride or fluoride dihydrate as the reducing agent. Labeling is accomplished by adding ^{99m}TcO$_4^-$ to the kit and mixing well. The labeling yield is greater than 95%. The shelf life for ^{99m}Tc-DISIDA is given to be 6 hr after reconstitution, whereas ^{99m}Tc-mebrofenin has a shelf life of 18 hr after preparation. The storage temperature for DISIDA and mebrofenin is recommended to be 15° to 30°C both before and after labeling.

The ^{99m}Tc-labeled IDA derivatives are commonly used as hepatobiliary agents to evaluate hepatic function, biliary duct patency, and mainly in cholescintigraphy. Of all IDA complexes, DISIDA and mebrofenin are claimed to be the hepatobiliary agents of choice.

^{99m}Tc-Hexamethylpropylene Amine Oxime (Ceretec)

Hexamethylpropylene amine oxime (HMPAO) is a lipophilic substance that forms a neutral complex with ^{99m}Tc after reduction with Sn^{2+} ion. The USAN (United States Adopted Names) uses the term *exametazime* for this substance. HMPAO exists in two stereoisomers: d,l-HMPAO and meso-HMPAO. The cerebral uptake of the former isomer is much higher than that of the latter, and so the d,l form must be separated from the meso form by repeated crystallization before complexation with ^{99m}TcO$_4^-$.

Commercial kits are available from Amersham Health under the brand

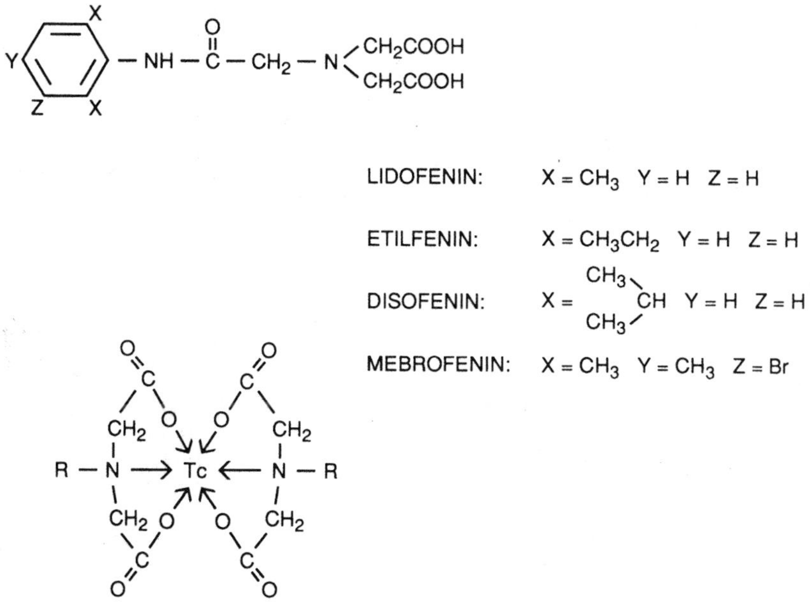

LIDOFENIN: $X = CH_3$ $Y = H$ $Z = H$

ETILFENIN: $X = CH_3CH_2$ $Y = H$ $Z = H$

DISOFENIN: $X = \underset{CH_3}{\overset{CH_3}{\diagdown}} CH$ $Y = H$ $Z = H$

MEBROFENIN: $X = CH_3$ $Y = CH_3$ $Z = Br$

FIGURE 7.2. Molecular structures of different IDA derivatives and their ^{99m}Tc-complexes.

name of Ceretec. The kit is made up of a lyophilized mixture of exametazime (pure d,l-HMPAO) and stannous chloride. Addition of ^{99m}TcO$_4^-$ to the kit vial gives greater than 80% labeling yield of ^{99m}Tc-HMPAO. There are conditions on the quality of ^{99m}TcO$_4^-$ to be used. ^{99m}TcO$_4^-$ must not be older than 2 hr after elution from the generator and must be eluted from a generator that has been eluted in the past 24 hr.

The primary ^{99m}Tc-HMPAO complex that is formed after the addition of ^{99m}TcO$_4^-$ to the kit is lipophilic and crosses the blood–brain barrier. However, it breaks down with time to a secondary complex that is less lipophilic and shows little brain uptake. As a result, ^{99m}Tc-HMPAO must be used within 30 min after preparation. Also, a strict quality control measure using thin layer chromatography must be performed to ascertain the labeling efficiency (>80%).

The instability of ^{99m}Tc-HMPAO has been attributed to three factors: (1) high pH (9 to 9.8) after reconstitution, (2) the presence of radiolytic intermediates such as hydroxy free radicals, and (3) excess stannous ions. To offset these factors, a phosphate buffer and methylene blue have been included separately in the new version of Ceretec kits. These agents are added after the normal preparation of ^{99m}Tc-HMPAO. Phosphate buffer lowers the pH around 6 at which the decomposition of ^{99m}Tc-HMPAO is minimal. Methylene blue acts as a scavenger of free radicals and oxidizes excess stannous ions. Even though decomposition still occurs to some extent

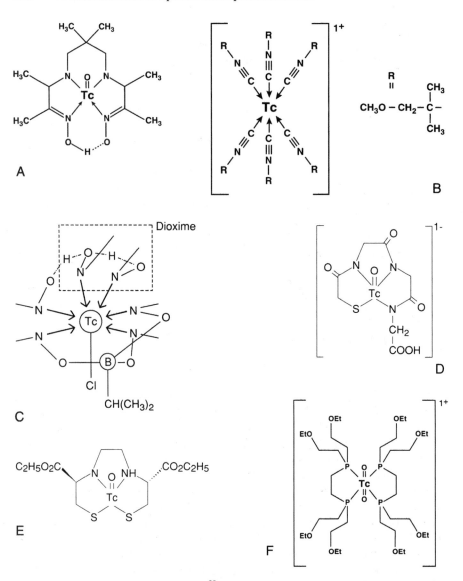

FIGURE 7.3. Molecular structures of ^{99m}Tc-labeled complexes. **A:** Tc-HMPAO. **B:** Tc-sestamibi. **C:** Tc-teboroxime. **D:** Tc-MAG3. **E:** Tc-ECD. **F:** Tc-tetrofosmin.

at pH 6 in the presence of a phosphate buffer, the combination of both phosphate buffer and methylene blue together reduces the decomposition significantly. The shelf life of these new kits is 4 hr after reconstitution.

The molecular structure of ^{99m}Tc-HMPAO is shown in Figure 7.3. X-ray crystallography of the complex shows Tc^{5+} to have five coordinate groups with an oxo group at the apex and four nitrogen atoms at the corners of the base of a square pyramid (Troutner et al., 1984). Loss of hydrogen atoms from two amine groups and one oxime group in the ligand results in a neutral complex.

The primary use of ^{99m}Tc-HMPAO is in brain perfusion imaging. Since it is lipophilic, it is used for labeling of leukocytes, substituting for ^{111}In-oxine. However, phosphate buffer and methylene blue are excluded from the formulation of ^{99m}Tc-HMPAO, when used for leukocyte labeling.

^{99m}Tc-Sestamibi (Cardiolite; Miraluma)

^{99m}Tc-sestamibi is a lipophilic cationic complex used as a substitute for ^{201}Tl for myocardial perfusion imaging and is supplied by Bristol-Myers Squibb under the brand name of Cardiolite for myocardial imaging and of Miraluma for breast tumor imaging. Sestamibi is methoxyisobutylisonitrile (MIBI) with an isonitrile group that forms a complex with ^{99m}Tc after reduction with stannous ions. Initially ^{99m}Tc-citrate is formed, which then undergoes ligand exchange with sestamibi to form ^{99m}Tc-sestamibi.

Sestamibi is supplied in a kit containing a lyophilized mixture of the chelating agent in the form of a copper (I) salt of tetrakis(2-MIBI)tetrafluoroborate, stannous chloride, sodium citrate, mannitol, and l-cysteine hydrochloride monohydrate. Labeling is carried out by adding a sufficient amount of ^{99m}TcO$_4^-$ to the kit vial and heating the mixture in a boiling water bath for 10 min. The pH of the reconstituted product is 5.5. The labeling efficiency is greater than 90%. The kit is stored at 15° to 30°C before and after reconstitution. ^{99m}Tc-sestamibi is good for 6 hr after formulation.

^{99m}Tc-sestamibi has the structure shown in Figure 7.3 and has a net charge of 1+. It has a coordination number of 6 with six isonitrile ligand groups (Abrams et al., 1983).

^{99m}Tc-sestamibi is used primarily for detection of myocardial perfusion abnormalities in patients, particularly for detection of myocardial ischemia and infarcts. It is also useful for the assessment of myocardial function using the first pass radionuclidic ventriculographic technique. ^{99m}Tc-sestamibi is also used for the detection of breast tumors (miraluma) and hyperparathyroidism.

^{99m}Tc-Teboroxime (Cardiotec)

^{99m}Tc-teboroxime is a boronic acid adduct of technetium dioxime (BATO) complex supplied by Bracco Diagnostics, under the brand name of Cardiotec. The kit vial contains a lipophilic mixture of cyclohexanedione dioxime, methyl boronic acid, stannous chloride, citric acid, pentetic acid, cyclodextrin, and sodium chloride. ^{99m}Tc-teboroxime is produced by template synthesis by adding ^{99m}TcO$_4^-$ to the vial and heating it at 100°C in a water bath for 15 min. The pH of the ^{99m}Tc-teboroxime preparation is about 3.7. The labeling yield should be greater than 90%. The kit should be stored at 15° to 30°C before and after reconstitution. The kit is good for 6 hr after preparation.

[99mTc]-teboroxime is a neutral lipophilic technetium-containing complex. It is a hepta coordinate complex in which the technetium is bound to six nitrogen atoms of the three vicinal dioximes and an axial chloride ligand (Nunn, 1990). The oximes are capped at one end through the oxygens by a tetrahedrally coordinated boron atom and at the other end by the three oxygens held together by a two-proton bridge. In [99mTc]-teboroxime, the oxime is cyclohexanedione dioxime and the fourth coordinate site of the boron is occupied by a methyl group. The molecular structure of [99mTc]-teboroxime is shown in Figure 7.3.

[99mTc]-teboroxime is a myocardial perfusion agent used for distinguishing between normal and abnormal myocardium in patients with suspected coronary diseases. Because of its rapid washout from the myocardium, it is not used routinely.

[99mTc]-Tetrofosmin (Myoview)

Tetrofosmin [6,9-bis(2-ethoxyethyl)-3,12-dioxa-6,9-diphospha-tetradecane] is supplied by Amersham Health in a kit form under the brand name of Myoview and is used for myocardial imaging. The kit contains tetrofosmin, stannous chloride dihydrate, disodium sulfosalicylate, sodium D-gluconate, and sodium hydrogen carbonate.

Labeling is carried out by adding [99mTc]TcO_4^- to the kit vial and incubating the mixture for 15 min at room temperature. [99mTc]-gluconate is initially formed with reduced Tc which is obtained by stannous ion reduction, and then ligand exchange between [99mTc]-gluconate and the tetrofosmin group gives [99mTc]-tetrofosmin. The pH should be 8.3 to 9.1 and the labeling yield should exceed 90%. The kit is stored at room temperature before and after reconstitution and [99mTc]-tetrofosmin is good for 8 hr after formulation.

[99mTc]-tetrofosmin is a lipophilic cationic complex and has the structure shown in Fig. 7.3. The chemical formula of the [99mTc]-complex is $[^{99m}Tc(tetrofosmin)_2O_2]^+$ with a charge of 1+. The oxidation state of Tc in the complex is 5+. The structure shows a linear trans-oxo core, with the four phosphorus atoms of the two bidentate diphosphine ligands forming a planar array (Kelly et al., 1993).

[99mTc]-tetrofosmin is indicated for the detection of reversible myocardial ischemia and myocardial infarction.

[99mTc]-Mercaptoacetylglycylglycylglycine (MAG3)

The MAG3 kit supplied by Mallinckrodt Medical contains a lyophilized mixture of betiatide (N-N-N-(benzoylthio)acetylglycylglycylglycine), stannous chloride dihydrate, sodium tartrate dihydrate, and lactose monohydrate under argon atmosphere. Labeling is carried out by adding [99mTc]TcO_4^- to the kit vial followed by introduction of filtered air, and heating at 100°C in a water bath for 10 min followed by cooling for 15 min. Air is introduced to oxidize the excess Sn^{2+}. The reactions involve initial reduction of pertechnetate by Sn^{2+} followed by the formation of ^{99m}Tc-tartrate. Subsequent heating of this complex in the presence of MAG3 ligand results in the formation of ^{99m}Tc-mertiatide (disodium (N-(N-(N-(mercaptoacetyl)glycyl)-glycyl) glycyl) glycinato(2−)-N, N′, N″, S′) oxotechnetate (2−)) (^{99m}Tc-MAG3) by ligand exchange. The pH of the preparation is 5 to 6. The labeling efficiency should be greater than 90%. The kit is recommended for 6 hr of use after reconstitution. The storage temperature is 15° to 30°C both before and after labeling. MAG3 is light sensitive and therefore the kits should be protected from light until use.

The structure of ^{99m}Tc-MAG3 is shown in Figure 7.3. It has a core of Tc = ON_3S with a carboxylic group on the third nitrogen (Fritzberg et al., 1986). ^{99m}Tc has a coordination number of 5 and the complex has a negative charge of 1−.

^{99m}Tc-MAG3 is used routinely for assessment of renal function, particularly in renal transplants.

^{99m}Tc-Ethyl Cysteinate Dimer (Neurolite)

Ethyl cysteinate dimer (ECD), also known as bicisate, exists in two stereoisomers, l,l-ECD and d,d-ECD. Both l,l-ECD and d,d-ECD isomers diffuse into the brain by crossing the blood–brain barrier, but l,l-ECD only is metabolized by an enzymatic process to a polar species that is trapped in the human brain. Thus, only purified l,l-ECD is used for ^{99m}Tc-ECD formulation.

The kit for ^{99m}Tc-ECD supplied by Bristol-Myers Squibb under the brand name of Neurolite contains two vials. Vial A contains a lyophilized mixture of l,l-ECD·2HCl, stannous chloride dihydrate, sodium edetate, and mannitol under nitrogen atmosphere. Vial B contains phosphate buffer, pH 7.5, under air atmosphere. To prepare ^{99m}Tc-ECD, isotonic saline is added to dissolve the contents in vial A. Labeling is carried out by adding ^{99m}TcO$_4^-$ to vial B followed by the addition of an aliquot from vial A and allowing the mixture to incubate for 30 min at room temperature.

The reaction involves initial reduction of ^{99m}Tc^{7+} to a lower oxidation state followed by the formation of the ^{99m}Tc-EDTA complex. Subsequent incubation causes ligand exchange between ^{99m}Tc-EDTA and ECD to form ^{99m}Tc-ECD (Dewanjee, 1990). The yield is consistently greater than 90% as determined by instant thin layer chromatography. The kits should be stored at 15° to 30°C before and after labeling with ^{99m}Tc. ^{99m}Tc-ECD remains stable for 6 hr after formulation.

The molecular structure of ^{99m}Tc-l,l-ECD is shown in Figure 7.3. It has the core structure of Tc = ON_2S_2, with a coordination number of 5. It is a neutral lipophilic complex (Edwards et al., 1990).

The clinical use of ^{99m}Tc-ECD is mainly for brain perfusion imaging.

^{99m}Tc-Dimercaptosuccinic Acid (Succimer)

Dimercaptosuccinic acid (DMSA) contains about 90% meso-isomer and 10% d,l-isomer in the kit supplied by Amersham Health. Each kit vial contains DMSA and stannous chloride dihydrate in lyophilized form. Labeling is accomplished by adding an appropriate amount $^{99m}TcO_4^-$ to the kit vial and incubating the mixture for 10 min at room temperature. The labeling yield is greater than 95% and the product is good for use up to 6 hr after preparation. Due to the sensitivity to light, the kits should be stored in the dark at 15° to 30°C.

^{99m}Tc-DMSA is prepared in acidic pH and the oxidation state of Tc is 3+ in this complex. When ^{99m}Tc-DMSA is prepared in alkaline pH, the oxidation state of Tc in the complex is 5+ and the biological behavior of the complex is different from that of the Tc^{3+} complex. The pentavalent Tc is coordinated by four thiolates of two DMSA ligands and an apical oxo group, and the complex has the formula $[TcO(DMSA)_2]^{-1}$.

$^{99m}Tc^{3+}$ DMSA is used for renal cortical imaging, whereas $^{99m}Tc^{5+}$ DMSA is used for the detection of medullary thyroid cancer.

^{99m}Tc-Gluceptate

^{99m}Tc-gluceptate is supplied by Draximage Inc., Canada and contains sodium gluceptate and stannous chloride in lyophilized form under nitrogen atmosphere. Labeling occurs when $^{99m}TcO_4^-$ is added to the vial and allowed to mix for 15 min. The labeling efficiency is greater than 95%. The labeled product is good for 6 hr after formulation. The kit is recommended for storage at 2° to 30°C before formulation and at 2° to 8°C after formulation.

^{99m}Tc-gluceptate is useful for renal imaging.

^{99m}Tc-Technegas

^{99m}Tc-Technegas is a radiolabeled aerosol and is prepared by first evaporating ^{99m}Tc-eluate in 0.1 to 0.3 ml saline to dryness in a graphite crucible at 1500°C (this stage is called the "simmer" stage) followed by heating at 2500°C in an atmosphere of argon (this stage is called the "burn" stage). The entire process of production is accomplished by the use of a commercially available Technegas generator. The particle size varies from 5 to 150 nm.

One theory suggests that ^{99m}Tc-Technegas is composed of ^{99m}Tc atoms attached to C_{60} molecules. Another theory suggests that salt aerosols are initially produced by the vaporization of salt at the simmer stage. At the burn stage, some graphite vaporizes, which then condenses on the salt aerosols acting as a nucleation center.

^{99m}Tc-Technegas aerosol is used for the ventilation scintigraphy of the lungs. This product is not approved by the U.S. Food and Drug Administration (FDA), whereas it is commercially available in Europe and Australia.

^{99m}Tc-N-NOET

Bis (N-ethoxy, N-ethyl)dithiocarbamato nitrido is supplied as a kit by CIS-Biointernational, France, under the name of N-NOET. The kit contains three vials: vial 1 contains stannous chloride dihydrate, 1,2-diaminopropane-N,N,N',N'-tetraacetic acid, succnyl dihydrazide, and sodium phosphate buffer, pH 7.8; vial 2 contains N-ethoxy, N-ethyl dithiocarbamate of sodium, monohydrate, and water; and vial 3 contains dimethyl B cyclodextrin and water (Vanzetto et al., 2000).

^{99m}Tc-labeling is carried out by adding 100 to 120 mCi (3.7–4.44 GBq) $^{99m}TcO_4^-$ to vial 1. After 15 min at room temperature, 1 ml from vial 2 and 1 ml from vial 3 are added to vial 1 and the reaction is allowed for 10 min at room temperature. The final volume is adjusted to 8 ml. The radiochemical purity is about 96% $\pm$ 2%. The preparation is kept at room temperature and it is good for 6 hr.

^{99m}Tc-N-NOET is a lipophilic neutral agent and is used for detecting myocardial perfusion abnormalities in patients with coronary artery disease. It is not approved by the U.S. FDA for clinical use.

Radioiodinated Radiopharmaceuticals

^{131}I-Sodium Iodide

Iodine-131 ($t_{1/2} = 8$ days) is separated in the form of sodium iodide (NaI) from the products of uranium fission or neutron irradiation of tellurium. It is available in NCA state and, according to the *USP* 26, other chemical forms of activities should not exceed 5% of the total radioactivity. It is supplied in either a capsule or a liquid form for oral administration. Capsules are prepared by evaporating an alcoholic solution of NCA ^{131}I-sodium iodide on the inner wall of a gelatin capsule. The activity remains firmly fixed, and capsules are convenient and safe to administer in both diagnostic and therapeutic dosages. ^{131}I-NaI solutions or capsules are available from CIS-US, Mallinckrodt Medical and Bracco Diagnostics.

The ^{131}I-NaI solution is clear and colorless and is made isotonic with physiologic saline. Air and radiolytic free radicals (e.g., HO_2^-) oxidize I^- to volatile I_2, which is potentially hazardous. Air oxidation is minimized by adding sodium ascorbate or thiosulfate to the solution at alkaline pH, which is maintained between 7.5 and 9.0. Radiations (β^- rays) may cause both the solution and the glass container to darken. The shelf life of a ^{131}I-NaI preparation is 4 weeks after calibration.

This agent is used mostly for the measurement of thyroid uptake and imaging after oral administration. Whether a capsule or a solution for oral administration is used is a matter of choice by the physician, although capsules are safer from radiation safety point. Another important use of ^{131}I-NaI is in the treatment of thyroid diseases such as thyroid carcinoma and hyperthyroidism.

^{123}I-Sodium Iodide

Iodine-123 ($t_{1/2} = 13.2$ hr) is available in the form of NaI after separation from other radionuclides produced in the cyclotron. The commercial suppliers are Mallinckrodt Medical, Amersham Health, Cardinal Health, formerly Syncor, and Nordion, Canada. It is supplied in a capsule or a solution for oral administration. The pH of the solution is maintained between 7.5 and 9.0. According to the *USP* 26, other chemical forms of radioactivity should not exceed 5% of the total radioactivity.

As mentioned in Chapter 4, ^{123}I may be contaminated with ^{124}I ($t_{1/2} = 4.2$ days) and ^{125}I ($t_{1/2} = 60$ days) depending on the types of target and irradiating particles used in the cyclotron. Iodine-124 is the most likely contaminant when the enriched ^{124}Te target is bombarded with protons resulting in the ^{124}Te(p, n)^{124}I reaction. At calibration time, the total amount of radiocontaminants is less than 6% of the ^{123}I activity. A 6% ^{124}I contaminiaton at calibration time results in 18.3% contamination after 24 hr of decay. Since ^{124}I emits high-energy photons that degrade scintigraphic image resolution, the ^{123}I capsule or solution should be used soon after receipt.

Iodine-125 is the primary contaminant in ^{123}I produced by the ^{127}I(p,5n) ^{123}I reaction. At calibration, its concentration does not exceed 3% of the total activity, but increases with time. However, ^{125}I does not pose a serious problem in scintigraphic imaging because of its low-energy photons, except for a higher radiation dose to the patient. When ^{123}I is produced by using the ^{124}Xe gas target, there is no ^{124}I contamination.

^{123}I-NaI is used most commonly for the measurement of thyroid uptake and imaging, and is much better than ^{131}I-NaI because ^{123}I has a photon energy of 159 keV and a half-life of 13.2 hr, and does not emit any β radiations. The shelf life of ^{123}I-NaI capsule or solution is 30 hr after calibration.

^{125}I-Albumin

Although albumin can be labeled with any radioisotope of iodine, ^{125}I-radioiodinated serum albumin (RISA) is commonly used in clinical medicine. It is prepared by iodinating human serum albumin using the chloramine-T method at 10°C in an alkaline medium. It can also be iodinated by the iodogen method. Free iodide is removed by anion-exchange resin, and membrane filtration is employed to sterilize the product. Commercial preparations contain 0.9% benzyl alcohol as a preservative. The solution must be stored at 2° to 8°C to minimize degradation. The shelf life after calibration is 60 days for ^{125}I-RISA. For dilution of RISA, one should use sterile isotonic saline containing a small quantity of human serum albumin. The latter is added to minimize adsorption of RISA on the walls of the container. Mallinckrodt Medical supplies RISA in multidosage vials or single-dosage syringes.

^{125}I-RISA appears as a clear, colorless to slightly yellow solution. Radiation may cause both the albumin solution and the container to darken with time. According to the *USP 26*, the pH of the solution should be between 7.0 and 8.5 and other forms of activity, including iodide and iodate, should not exceed 3% of the total radioactivity.

Blood volume and cardiac output are measured with ^{125}I-RISA.

^{123}I- or ^{131}I-Sodium Orthoiodohippurate

Sodium orthoiodohippurate (Hippuran) is iodinated with ^{123}I- or ^{131}I-NaI by the isotope exchange method. Iodination is carried out by refluxing the iodination mixture at 100°C for 2 hr at pH 6. Radioiodinated orthoiodohippurate is a colorless solution supplied in multidosage vials containing 1% benzyl alcohol as a preservative; ^{131}I-Hippuran should not be used more than 4 weeks after the calibration date. Its pH is maintained between 7.0 and 8.5. According to the *USP 26*, free iodide or other forms of radioactivity should not exceed 3% of the total radioactivity. It is used for the measurement of effective renal plasma flow and renography in humans. Neither ^{123}I-Hippuran nor ^{131}I-Hippuran is commercially available after the introduction of ^{99m}Tc-MAG3.

^{131}I-6β-Iodomethyl-19-Norcholesterol

The compound 6β-iodomethyl-19-norcholesterol (NP-59) is synthesized by refluxing cholest-5-en-3β, 19-diol-19-toluene-p-sulfonate in ethanol for 4 hr. NP-59 is purified and then iodinated with ^{131}I by the isotope exchange method. It is formulated in alcohol and contains Tween 80. At 4°C, ^{131}I-NP-59 is stable for 2 weeks, and deiodination occurs at room or higher temperatures.

^{131}I-labeled NP-59 is used in adrenal gland scanning and is supplied by the University of Michigan, Ann Arbor, Michigan. For human use, one has to have a physician-sponsored IND from the U.S. FDA.

^{123}I- or ^{131}I-Metaiodobenzylguanidine (MIBG)

The compound metaiodobenzylguanidine (MIBG) is labeled with ^{123}I or ^{131}I by the isotope exchange method. A mixture of ^{131}I-NaI and MIBG is refluxed for 72 hr, cooled, and then passed through an anion exchange column to remove unreacted iodide. ^{131}I-MIBG, also known as ^{131}I-Iobenguane sulfate, is commercially available. It is manufactured by CIS-US, Inc. and distributed by Cardinal Health, formerly Syncor. Its recommended storage temperature is $-20°C$ to $-10°C$, and the expiration time is 8 days after calibration.

^{123}I-MIBG is prepared by adding ^{123}I-NaI to a solution of N-chlorosuccinimide in trichloroacetic acid followed by the addition of 3-trimethylsilylbenzylguanidine in trichloroacetic acid.

Radioiodinated MIBG primarily localizes in the medulla of the adrenal gland. Its primary use is in the detection of pheochromocytoma. ^{123}I-MIBG is used to localize the myocardial regions depleted of catecholamine stores due to infarction. ^{131}I-MIBG has also been used in the treatment of neuroblastoma.

^{125}I-Sodium Iothalamate

Sodium iothalamate (Glofil) is labeled with ^{125}I ($t_{1/2} = 60$ days) by the ion exchange method in acidic medium, and is available from Questcor, Union City, California. It is supplied in a concentration of approximately 1 mg/ml sodium iothalamate with a radioactivity concentration of 250 to 300 μCi/ml (9.25–11.1 MBq). It contains 0.9% benzyl alcohol as preservative. Its expiration period is 35 to 40 days and it is stored at $2°$ to $8°C$. It is used for the measurement of glomerular filtration rate (GFR) in humans and animals.

^{123}I-d,l-N-Isopropyl-p-Iodoamphetamine Hydrochloride (IMP)

^{123}I-IMP is prepared by the isotope exchange method by heating ^{123}I-NaI and isopropyl amphetamine at $150°C$ for 30 min, followed by extraction in ether and further purification by washing with dilute HCl. It is prepared by using high-purity ^{123}I, indicating the absence of ^{124}I. The pH of the ^{123}I-IMP solution is 4 to 6. Its expiration time is 12 hr and the storage temperature is $5°$ to $30°C$. Since ^{125}I and other radiocontaminants that increase relatively with time may be present, it is advisable to administer ^{123}I-IMP to patients as soon as practical from the time of receipt. It is not available commercially in the United States.

^{123}I-IMP is useful in the evaluation of stroke and similar neurological deficits in the brain.

Miscellaneous Radiopharmaceuticals of Clinical Interest

^{111}In-DTPA

^{111}In-DTPA is prepared by adding a dilute DTPA solution to a solution of ^{111}InCl$_3$ ($t_{1/2} = 2.8$ days) in acetate buffer, pH 5, and then heating for 15 min at $100°C$ in a boiling water bath. This product is supplied by Amersham Health. This compound is primarily used for cisternography and infrequently in liquid meal for gastric emptying studies.

^{133}Xe Gas

Xenon-133 ($t_{1/2}$ = 5.3 days) is a noble gas and is chemically inert. Xenon-133 is produced by the fission of ^{235}U in the reactor. After separation and purification, the ^{133}Xe radionuclide is supplied in gaseous form in vials with diluents such as CO_2, air, or carrier xenon gas. The storage temperature for the gas is 15° to 30°C and the shelf life of ^{133}Xe is 14 days after calibration. Caution should be exercised in handling radioxenon because of the potential radiation exposure, and preferably it should be handled in the fumehood. Nuclear medicine studies using ^{133}Xe should be performed in rooms that are at negative pressure relative to the surrounding areas. It is supplied by Bristol-Myers Squibb and Mallinckrodt Medical.

Xenon-133 is indicated primarily for ventilation studies of the lungs and also for the assessment of cerebral blood flow.

^{201}Tl-Thallous Chloride

Thallium-201 ($t_{1/2}$ = 73 hr) is produced in the cyclotron and is supplied in the form of NCA thallous chloride in isotonic saline solution at pH 4.5 to 7.0 for intravenous administration. Mallinckrodt Medical, Bristol-Myers Squibb, and Amersham Health are the primary vendors of ^{201}Tl. It contains sodium chloride for isotonicity and 0.9% benzyl alcohol as a bactericidal agent. At the time of calibration, the preparation contains no more than 1% ^{200}Tl, no more than 1% ^{202}Tl, no more than 0.25% ^{203}Pb, and no less than 98% ^{201}Tl of total activity.

The shelf life of ^{201}Tl is suggested as 5 to 6 days after calibration, depending on the manufacturer. This radionuclide should be stored at room temperature.

It is used for myocardial perfusion imaging in order to delineate between ischemic and infarcted myocardium. It is also indicated for the detection of hyperparathyroidism and brain tumors.

^{67}Ga-Citrate

The ^{67}Ga-citrate complex is formed by adding a sufficient amount of sodium citrate to a ^{67}Ga chloride ($t_{1/2}$ = 78.2 hr) solution and raising the pH to 5 to 8 with sodium hydroxide. At higher pH, gallium hydroxide and gallate form at the loss of citrate. The preparation is stabilized with 0.9% benzyl alcohol. It should be stored at room temperature and used within 7 days after calibration. It is available from Mallinckrodt Medical, Cardinal Health, formerly Syncor, and Amersham Health.

Gallium-67-citrate is used primarily for detecting malignant diseases such as Hodgkin's disease, lymphomas, and bronchogenic carcinoma. It is also used for localizing acute inflammatory diseases and infections.

^{32}P-Sodium Orthophosphate

Phosphorus-32 ($t_{1/2} = 14.3$ days) is produced by irradiating sulfur with neutrons in the reactor; it is separated by leaching from the melted sulfur with NaOH solution. It is obtained as a solution of ^{32}P-disodium phosphate suitable for oral or intravenous administration. This is a clear and colorless solution with a pH of 5 to 6. It contains a 0.9% NaCl solution for isotonicity and a sodium acetate buffer. It is supplied by Mallinckrodt Medical. The primary uses of ^{32}P include the therapeutic treatment of polycythemia vera, leukemia, and other neoplastic hematologic disorders. Sometimes it is used as a diagnostic agent for certain ocular tumors.

^{32}P-Chromic Phosphate Colloid

^{32}P-chromic phosphate colloid is supplied by Mallinckrodt Medical as a sterile, nonpyrogenic aqueous suspension in a 30% dextrose solution with 2% benzyl alcohol added as a preservative. Each milliliter of the suspension contains 1 mg sodium acetate. It is primarily used for the treatment of peritoneal or pleural effusions caused by metastatic diseases.

^{89}Sr-Strontium Chloride (Metastron)

Strontium-89 ($t_{1/2} = 50.6$ days) is a reactor-produced radionuclide and supplied in the form of ^{89}SrCl$_2$ containing 4 mCi (148 MBq) in a vial or a syringe. Its pH is 4 to 7.5. It is supplied by Amersham Health under the brand name of Metastron. The product is stored at 15° to 25°C and should be used within 28 days after calibration. Since it is a β^--particle emitter, it is contained in plastic syringes or vials.

Strontium-89 is indicated for the relief of pain in patients with skeletal metastases, which must be confirmed prior to therapy.

^{153}Sm-Ethylenediaminetetramethylene Phosphonic Acid (Quadramet)

Samarium-153 ($t_{1/2} = 1.9$ days) is produced in the reactor and is chelated to ethylenediaminetetramethylene phosphonic acid (EDTMP) to form the ^{153}Sm-EDTMP complex. It is manufactured by Cytogen Corp. and distributed by Cardinal Health, formerly Synor. Its trade name is Quadramet and its USAN name is Sm-153 Lexidronam injection. The pH of the final product is 7.0 to 8.5 and the radiochemical purity is >99%. ^{153}Sm-EDTMP is stored at room temperature and retains its stability for >7 days. Because of its beta particles, it is used for the palliation of pain from metastatic bone cancer. Also its 103 keV (28%) photons allow scintigraphic imaging of the whole body.

^{57}Co- or ^{58}Co-Cyanocobalamin

Radiolabeled cyanocobalamin, or vitamin B_{12}, is prepared by biosynthesis: the organism *Streptomyces griseus* is grown in a medium containing ^{57}Co ($t_{1/2} = 271$ days) or ^{58}Co ($t_{1/2} = 71$ days) and the labeled cobalamins are then separated. The compound is supplied in a capsule for oral administration or in a solution for intravenous injection and is available from Mallinckrodt Medical, Bracco Diagnostics, and Amersham Health. The final pH of the solution should be 4.0 to 5.0. This compound is sensitive to light, heat, and high pH, and therefore it is stored at 5°C in the dark. Its shelf life is 6 months. The absorption of vitamin B_{12} in anemic patients and in other vitamin B_{12} malabsorption syndromes are studied with labeled cyanocobalamins with and without intrinsic factor.

^{51}Cr-Labeled Red Blood Cells

To label red blood cells efficiently with ^{51}Cr ($t_{1/2} = 27.7$ days), 50 to 100 μCi (1.85–3.7 MBq) ^{51}Cr-sodium chromate is added to 20 to 30 ml of human blood containing ACD solution, and the mixture is incubated in a water bath at 37°C for 20 min with occasional shaking. It is then cooled for 10 min at room temperature and ascorbic acid is added to reduce untagged Cr^{6+} to Cr^{3+} and to stop the reaction. The reason for this is that two Cr^{6+} ions bind to the globin part of hemoglobin, whereas Cr^{3+} does not label RBCs. The cells are washed and finally suspended in saline for injection. The labeling yield is almost 80% to 90%. When ^{51}Cr-labeled RBCs are used for the measurement of red cell survival, the labeling mixture is injected without washing off Cr^{3+}. Cr^{3+} is excreted in the urine in several hours.

The ^{51}Cr-labeled RBCs are commonly used for the measurement of red cell mass and its survival. These labeled cells can also be used for imaging the spleen. In this case, the cells are denatured by heating at 50°C for 20 min, whereby they become spheroidal and nondeformable, and they are then readily sequestered by the spleen after intravenous administration.

Radiolabeled Leukocytes and Platelets

Leukocyte Separation

Leukocytes are initially separated from whole blood by sedimentation, centrifugation, and washing with isotonic saline. Heparin or ACD is added as anticoagulant. Hetastarch is added to enhance the sedimentation rate of RBCs. Leukocytes are then separated by centrifugation at 200 g, and washed with isotonic saline. Leukocytes obtained by this technique are partially contaminated with RBCs and platelets, but such a level of contamination does not compromise significantly the labeling efficiency of leukocytes. Labeling is preferred in saline solution rather than in plasma, since ^{111}In binds to transferrin in the latter more avidly than to leukocytes.

Platelet Separation

Platelets are isolated by initial separation of platelet-rich plasma (PRP) after centrifugation of whole blood at 200 g to remove RBCs and leukocytes, followed by centrifugation of the PRP at 1500 g. ACD is added at a blood-to-ACD ratio of 6:1 to keep a slightly acidic pH of 6.5 to prevent platelet aggregation. Platelet labeling is preferable in plasma (mixed with ACD) suspension, rather than in saline, to preserve the platelet function, although the labeling yield is somewhat compromised.

^{111}In-Labeling

^{111}In-Oxine

^{111}In-oxine can be prepared by mixing ^{111}InCl$_3$ in acetate buffer, pH 5.0, with 8-hydroxyquinoline (oxine) in ethanol. The ^{111}In-oxine complex is extracted into chloroform or methylene chloride, which is then evaporated to dryness. The residue of ^{111}In oxine is taken up into ethanol for use in labeling (Thakur et al., 1977).

Amersham Health supplies ^{111}In-oxine in aqueous solution at pH 6.5 to 7.5, containing polysorbate 80 as the stabilizer. The radionuclide impurity is ^{114m}In, which should not exceed more than 0.25% of the total activity at expiration time of ^{111}In. ^{111}In-oxine tends to adhere to the plastic syringe and therefore should be drawn from the vial only immediately before labeling. It is stored at 15° to 30°C.

^{111}In-Labeling of Leukocytes and Platelets

The schematic diagrams showing sequential steps in ^{111}In-labeling are shown in Figure 7.4 for leukocytes and Figure 7.5 for platelets. It should be noted that leukocytes are labeled in saline suspension, while plasma mixed with ACD is used as the medium for platelet suspension. The commercial preparation of ^{111}In-oxine in aqueous solution is preferable to ethanol solution because ethanol tends to damage the cells.

Both leukocytes and platelets may be damaged to varying degrees by the labeling technique, particularly by the carrier oxine, and thus lose proper functional activity. This may result in clumping of cells, which should be checked visually. Also separated cells are mixed cells, for example, leukocytes mixed with RBCs and platelets, and platelets mixed with RBCs and leukocytes. This leads to undesirable in vivo biodistribution of labeled cells. Chemotaxis of granulocytes deteriorates during storage and this can lead to false-negative scans. For this reason, it is recommended that labeled leukocytes should be reinjected within 5 hr after initial blood drawing or within 3 hr after labeling.

Lymphocytes are very sensitive to radiations and exhibit chromosome

LEUKOCYTE LABELING WITH IN-111 OXINE

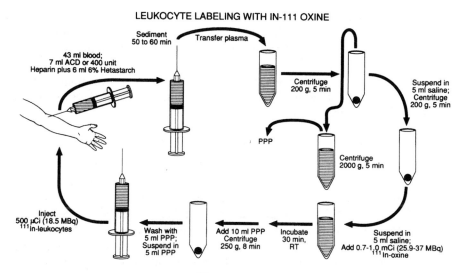

FIGURE 7.4. Method of ^{111}In-labeling of leukocytes (WBCs).

aberrations consisting of gaps and breaks induced by radiations. At 150 μCi (5.55 MBq) per 100 million lymphocytes, 93% of cells are reported to become abnormal (ten Berge et al., 1983).

The labeling yield varies with the number of leukocytes or platelets, and usually increases with the number of cells. The yield ranges between 75% and 90% for an average 100 million leukocytes, although it is somewhat lower for platelets. Metal ions such as Cu, Zn, Fe, Al, and Cd interfere with ^{111}In-labeling and should be avoided.

In vitro experiments elucidate the mechanism of ^{111}In-labeling that indium oxine is a neutral lipophilic complex that crosses the cell membrane into

PLATELET LABELING WITH IN-111 OXINE

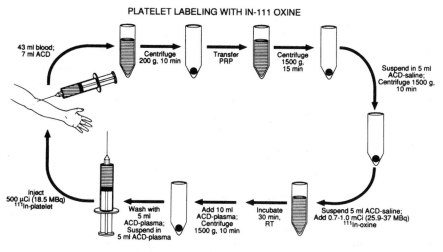

FIGURE 7.5. Method of ^{111}In-labeling of platelets.

the cell. Since indium oxine is a relatively weak chelate, ^{111}In is transchelated to macromolecular proteins in cytoplasm due to higher binding affinity and remains there for a long period of time. The released oxine diffuses out of the cell.

The primary use of ^{111}In-leukocytes is for the detection of inflammatory diseases, abscesses or other infections. ^{111}In-platelets are used for detecting actively forming deep vein thrombi.

^{99m}Tc-Labeling

As mentioned previously, ^{99m}Tc-HMPAO is a neutral lipophilic complex and thus, like ^{111}In-oxine, can serve as a labeling agent for leukocytes. Normally, separated leukocytes are suspended in plasma/ACD mixture and then ^{99m}Tc-HMPAO (freshly formulated) is added to the cell (Peters et al., 1986). The cells are incubated for 15 min at room temperature, then washed with plasma, and finally suspended in plasma for injection. The labeling yield is of the order of 50% to 60%. The cellular integrity appears to remain normal.

Several studies have shown that granulocytes can be labeled in vivo by first labeling antigranulocyte antibodies with ^{99m}Tc in vitro and then injecting the labeled antibodies into the subject. Currently, a commercial kit under the name of LeukoScan (Sulesomab) (see later) containing antigranulocyte antibody fragment is supplied by Immunomedies Inc. in Europe.

^{99m}Tc-labeling of platelets has not yet developed considerably, although some studies similar to those of leukocyte labeling have been made.

^{99m}Tc-leukocytes are used for the detection of inflammation, abscess, or other infections.

Radiolabeled Monoclonal Antibodies

Antibodies are immunoglobulins (Ig) produced in vivo in response to the administration of an antigen to animals and humans, and bind specifically to that antigen, forming an antigen–antibody complex. Antibodies are produced by the differentiation of B lymphocytes. An antigen molecule may comprise many determinants that can produce a variety of antibodies upon antigenic challenge in animals or humans. Such antibodies are called polyclonal antibodies because they are heterogeneous and nonspecific in nature.

The structural model of a typical antibody molecule is illustrated in Figure 7.6. It is a Y-shaped molecule composed of two identical heavy and two identical light polypeptide chains that are covalently linked by disulfide bonds. The light chain has one variable region (V_L) and a constant region (C_L), whereas the heavy chain has one variable region (V_H) and three constant regions (C_{H1}, C_{H2}, C_{H3}). The combined region of V_L, C_L, V_H, and C_{H1} is called the Fab portion of the molecule. The C_{H2} and C_{H3} regions are collectively called the Fc portion. The variable regions of the molecule are responsible for binding to the antigen, whereas the Fc region binds to Fc

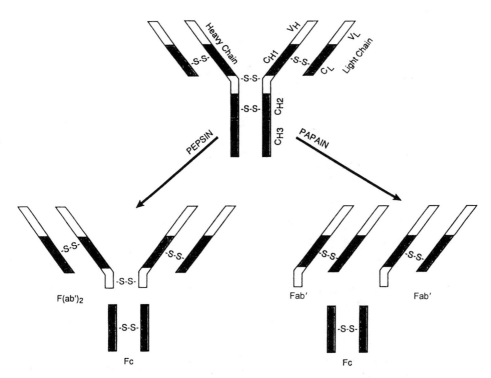

FIGURE 7.6. Molecular structure of antibody and the fragments of antibody obtained after enzymatic digestion with papain and pepsin.

receptors of phagocytic cells, activates the complement cascade, and metabolizes the Ig molecules.

By digestion of the antibody molecule with the proteolytic enzyme papain, two Fab′ fragments and one Fc fragment are obtained, whereas digestion of antibody with pepsin results in the production of one $F(ab′)_2$ fragment and one Fc fragment (Fig. 7.6).

Production of Monoclonal Antibody

The polyclonal antibodies labeled with ^{131}I and ^{125}I were used originally to detect tumors, and success was limited because of the heterogeneity and nonspecific binding of the antibodies. Köhler and Milstein (1975) introduced the hybridoma technology to produce monoclonal antibodies (Mab), which are homogeneous and highly specific for a particular antigen. A comprehensive review on monoclonal antibodies has been reported by Zuckier et al. (1990).

A schematic diagram for the production of Mabs is illustrated in Figure 7.7. The hybridoma technology involves the initial immunization of a mouse with a particular antigen. The spleen cells from the immunized mouse are then mixed with myeloma cells in the presence of polyethylene glycol (PEG) whereby some immune cells (B lymphocytes) fuse to the myeloma cells forming hybrid cells. The cell mixture is suspended in HAT (hypoxanthine–

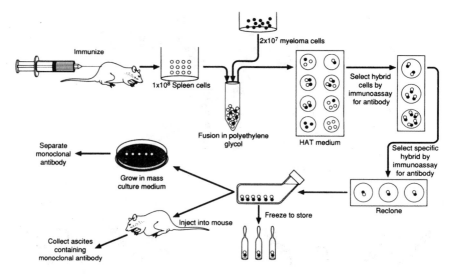

FIGURE 7.7. A basic scheme for the production of hybrid cells that are used to make monoclonal antibodies.

aminopterin–thymidine) selective media in which unfused B lymphocytes will die and unfused myeloma cells are killed. The hybrid cells are then cloned further and ultimately screened for hybrids, producing Mabs that react with the antigen used for immunizing the mouse. The hybridoma cells can be grown in tissue culture media or by administering the cells to mice intra-peritoneally and obtaining their ascites fluid. Large quantities of Mabs are produced by the hybrid cells in the culture medium, hollow fiber matrix, and ascites fluid, and are separated by chromatographic methods such as affinity chromatography or ion-exchange chromatography. An important advantage of the hybridoma technology is that the hybridoma cells can be safely stored by freezing, and the production of antibody can be renewed as needed by growing the cells in tissue culture media or injecting them into mice.

There are several problems associated with the hybridoma technology that need attention for the production of Mabs. The efficiency of fusion between the immune cell and the myeloma cell is very low, and even in suc-cessful fusions, only 1 in 20,000 fused cells is ultimately converted into a viable hybridoma to produce specific Mab. This is largely due to weak anti-gens or small quantities of antigens used in the immunization process. This problem can be overcome by selective association and fusion of cells to produce highly specific Mabs.

A major difficulty exists in making human Mabs that are desirable for parenteral administration to patients. The use of murine Mabs in humans elicits human antimurine antibody (HAMA) response depending on the administered dosages and immune status of the patient, and must be moni-tored carefully. The difficulty in making human Mabs also lies in the lack of appropriate fusion partner (myeloma cell) and in the problem of obtaining sensitized B lymphocytes. Fusion partners, called heteromyelomas, have been constructed by fusing human and mouse myeloma cells, giving only limited success in producing human hybridoma. It is generally impossible to immunize humans with an antigen of interest to produce immune B lymphocytes. However, in some instances, peripheral B lymphocytes from immunized patients have been used for generating hybridomas.

Recombinant DNA techniques have been developed in which the variable region (V) of the mouse monoclonal antibody is coupled to the constant region (C) of human monoclonal antibody, resulting in a chimeric molecule. These restructured molecules are then transfected into mouse myeloma cell lines that produce antibodies that are less immunogenic in humans than murine antibodies. This method is used particularly for antibodies to be used for treatment in high dosages and repeated administrations.

Radiolabeling of Monoclonal Antibody

Radiolabeling of Mabs can be accomplished with several radionuclides, among which ^{131}I, ^{123}I, ^{125}I, ^{111}In, and ^{99m}Tc are most commonly used in nuclear medicine. An excellent review on radiolabeling of antibodies has been reported by Hnatowich (1990). Following is a brief description of the techniques of labeling with iodine isotopes, ^{111}In and ^{99m}Tc.

Radioiodination of Antibody

Approximately 100 to 500 μg of antibody is dissolved in 50 to 100 μl phosphate buffered saline (PBS), pH 7, in a tube coated with iodogen (see Radioiodination). An appropriate amount of iodine isotope [1–5 mCi (37–185 MBq) ^{131}I-NaI] in 50 μl solution is added to the reaction tube. After 12 to 15 min of incubation at room temperature, the mixture is transferred to a separate tube. The iodinated antibody is separated from unreacted iodide by either dialysis against saline overnight at 2°C or by gel chromatography using a Sephadex G-25 gel. The yield is 60% to 80%. Other methods of iodination described previously can be adopted, although the labeling yield may vary and the protein may lose immunoreactivity.

^{111}In- or ^{90}Y-Labeling of Antibody

Mabs are labeled with ^{111}In or ^{90}Y using bifunctional chelating agents (BFC) such as DTPA, GYK-DTPA, SCN-Bz-DTPA, and DOTA. Initially, the chelating agent is conjugated to the antibody and then ^{111}In binds to the conjugated Mab via coordinate bonds with the chelating agent.

A typical ^{111}In-labeling method for Mab using DTPA anhydride as the chelator is briefly described here. The DTPA cyclic anhydride is dissolved in chloroform and the solution is evaporated in a reaction tube with N_2. Mab is then added so that the molar ratio of Mab to DTPA is 1:1. The antibody is dissolved in bicarbonate buffer, pH 8.2, in the tube. After incubation for 30 min at room temperature, the free DTPA is removed by either dialysis or gel chromatography. The resulting conjugated Mab is labeled by adding ^{111}InCl$_3$ in acetate buffer, pH 5.5, or in citrate buffer, pH 5.0, or ^{90}YCl$_3$ in appropriate buffer to the Mab solution. In many cases, incubation for 30 min at room temperature suffices for quantitative labeling, obviating the need for further purification by dialysis or gel chromatography.

Increasing the number of DTPA molecules coupled to the antibody molecule diminishes the immunoreactivity of Mab and usually not more than one chelating molecule per Mab molecule is essential for optimal labeling. DTPA is linked to the antibody via amide bonds between an amino group of the lysine residue of the antibody and one carboxylate group of DTPA. In this instance, four carboxylate groups are available for chelation with ^{111}In. However, in the case of SCN-Bz-DTPA, the chelator is linked to the antibody via a thiourea bond formed between the isothiocyanate group and an amino group of the lysine residue. This leaves all its five carboxylate groups available for chelation with ^{111}In for improved stability of the complex (Hnatowich, 1990).

Antibodies labeled with ^{111}In via the macrocyclic chelator, DOTA, have shown high stability in vivo without any transchelation to other serum proteins. But all chelating agents have shown increased liver uptake, which is the major drawback with ^{111}In-labeled Mabs.

The U.S. FDA has approved ^{111}In-capromab pendetide (Prostasint) and ^{111}In- and ^{90}Y-ibritumomab tiuxetan (Zevalin) for clinical use.

^{111}In-Capromab Pendetide (ProstaScint)

The single dosage kit, ProstaScint, supplied by Cytogen Corporation contains Mab 7E11.C5.3, a murine monoclonal antibody produced against prostate carcinoma and prostate hypertrophy. In the kit, the antibody is chelated to GYK-DTPA and lypophilized to give capromab pendetide. Labeling with ^{111}In is carried out by adding ^{111}InCl$_3$ to the vial and incubating for 30 min at room temperature. The mixture is then filtered through a 0.22 μm Millex GV filter to remove any particulate matter. The labeling yield should be more than 90%. ^{111}In-capromab pendetide should be stored at room temperature and dispensed within 8 hr of labeling.

^{111}In-capromab pendetide is used for detecting primary and metastatic prostate cancer.

^{111}In- and ^{90}Y-Ibritumomab Tiuxetan (Zevalin)

This single dosage kit is supplied by IDEC Pharmaceuticals Corp. under the brand name Zevalin. It consists of a murine monoclonal anti-CD20 antibody covalently conjugated to the metal chelator DTPA, which forms a stable complex with ^{111}In for imaging and with ^{90}Y for therapy.

The kit is supplied with four vials—a vial containing 3.2 mg of conjugated antibody in 2 ml saline, a vial containing 2 ml 50 mM sodium acetate, a vial containing phosphate buffer, and a fourth empty reaction vial. Prior to labeling, a volume of sodium acetate buffer equivalent to 1.2 times the volume of the tracer solution is transferred to the reaction vial. Then 5.5 mCi (203.5 MBq) ^{111}In or 40 mCi (1.48 GBq) ^{90}Y is added to the reaction vial and mixed thoroughly without shaking. Next 1.3 ml of conjugated antibody is added. The mixture is incubated for exactly 30 min for ^{111}In-labeling and for 5 min for ^{90}Y labeling, followed by the addition of enough phosphate buffer to make the final volume to 10 ml. The labeling yield is determined by instant thin-layer liquid chromatography using ITLC-SG strips and 0.9% NaCl solvent and should be greater than 95% for both radionuclides.

^{90}Y-ibritumomab tiuxetan is used for the treatment of relapsed or refractory low-grade, follicular or CD20 transformed non-Hodgkin's lymphoma (NHL). ^{111}In-ibritumomab tiuxetan is used as an imaging agent to predict the distribution within the body of the subsequent therapeutic dosage of ^{90}Y-ibritumomab. An earlier version of anti-CD20 antibody, rituximab, has also been approved under the brand name Rituxan for the treatment of NHL.

^{99m}Tc-Labeling of Antibody

There are three methods of ^{99m}Tc labeling of antibodies or their fragments: (1) direct method; (2) indirect method by first preparing a preformed ^{99m}Tc-chelate, which is then attached to the antibody; and (3) the indirect labeling using a bifunctional chelating (BFC) agent that is attached to the antibody on one side and ^{99m}Tc to the other (Eckelman et al., 1996).

Direct Method

In the direct method, also called the pretinning method, the antibody and a solution of stannous chloride, potassium phthalate, and sodium potassium tartrate are incubated for 21 hr at room temperature. The pretinned antibody can be stored frozen at $-20°C$ for future use. To radiolabel the antibody, ^{99m}TcO$_4^-$ is added to the pretinned kit and incubated for 1 hr at room temperature. ^{99m}Tc remains firmly bound to immunoglobulin G (IgG) as shown by high-performance liquid chromatography (HPLC) following transchelation challenge with various agents.

In the pretinning process, sulfhydryl groups are freed by the reduction of disulfide bonds of the antibody by stannous ions. Use of high concentration of stannous ions often leads to the formation of ^{99m}Tc-labeled Fab' and F(ab')$_2$ fragments due to the breakdown of the disulfide bonds in the region between C_{H1} and C_{H2} segments of the heavy chain (Hnatowich, 1990). In this method, chromatographic separation of the ^{99m}Tc-labeled antibody or fragment from free or reduced ^{99m}Tc is essential to achieve maximum purity.

To prevent the breakdown of the antibody into smaller fragments, milder agents such as 2-mercaptoethanol and dithiothreitol have been used in place of stannous ions. In these cases, postlabeling purification may be avoided if proper conditions are applied to achieve maximum labeling.

Indirect Method Using Preformed ^{99m}Tc-Chelate

In this technique, initially a ^{99m}Tc-chelate is formed using a BFC such as diamidodithio or a cyclam derivative, and then the complex is allowed to react with the antibody to obtain the ^{99m}Tc-labeled antibody. The disadvantage of this method is that it requires several steps rather than one or two simple steps, and the labeling yield is poor. For these reasons, this method is not widely favored.

Indirect Labeling using Bifunctional Chelating Agent

In this approach, a BFC is conjugated to the antibody on one side of the BFC and a radiometal ion by chelation on the other side. In practice, the antibody is first reacted with the BFC to form a BFC-antibody complex that is then separated from the reaction mixture. ^{99m}Tc-labeling is carried out by adding ^{99m}TcO$_4^-$ to the BFC-antibody complex in the presence of a reducing agent (e.g., Sn^{2+} ions), or by ligand exchange using a weak ^{99m}Tc-chelate such as ^{99m}Tc-gluceptate, ^{99m}Tc-tartrate, or ^{99m}Tc-citrate.

A number of BFCs have been utilized to label antibodies with ^{99m}Tc, and of these, cyclic anhydride of DTPA is the most common one. Other chelating agents include metallothionein, dithiosemicarbazone, and diamine dimercaptide (N$_2$S$_2$), the latter being the very popular. However, nonspecific binding with the antibody leads to the in vivo breakdown of the ^{99m}Tc complex and thus reduces the clinical utility of the ^{99m}Tc-labeled antibody.

Some newer BFCs have been introduced for use in ^{99m}Tc labeling of different antibodies, antibody fragments, peptides, and other small molecules useful for imaging. Among them, 6-hydrazinopyridine-3-carboxylic acid or hydrazinonicotinamide (HYNIC) has been very promising for this purpose. The active ester of HYNIC is used to derivatize the amino groups of lysine residues in proteins or peptides. Incubation of these conjugates with simple Tc^{5+} oxo core such as in ^{99m}Tc-gluceptate(GH) yields quantitative labeling of proteins or peptides.

In this method, an excess of freshly prepared HYNIC solution (3 to 4:1 molar ratio) is added dropwise to a stirred solution of a protein or peptide in phosphate buffer at slightly alkaline pH ($\sim$pH 7.8). After continuous stirring for 5 hr in the dark at room temperature, the solution is dialyzed against citrate buffer. After dialysis, the solution is filtered to give HYNIC-conjugated protein or peptide. Approximately three HYNIC molecules are present per protein or peptide molecule.

^{99m}Tc-labeling is accomplished by adding an appropriate amount of freshly prepared ^{99m}Tc-GH that has the Tc^{5+} oxo group and incubating the mixture for 60 min at room temperature. The reaction involves ligand exchange. The labeling yield is more than 90%, as determined by ITLC-SG method using 0.1 M sodium citrate as the solvent (described in Chapter 8). The plasma incubation shows that the labeled product is stable.

Since HYNIC can occupy only two sites of the technetium coordination sphere, there may be other sites for binding additional ligands. Based on this hypothesis, investigators have used the so-called co-ligands for adding more stability to ^{99m}Tc-labeled HYNIC conjugate of protein or peptide. Many co-ligands, namely tricine, ethylenediaminediacetic acid (EDDA), tricine plus trisodium triphenylphosphinetrisulfonate (TPPTS), tricine plus nicotinic acid (NIC), and tricine plus isonicotinic acid (ISONIC), have been evaluated to enhance the labeling yield; however, tricine has been the co-ligand of choice in many cases. The addition of a co-ligand in ^{99m}Tc-labeling enhances the elimination of the labeled product from the blood and thus improves the target to nontarget activity ratio in organ imaging.

In co-ligand labeling, tricine in water is added to the HYNIC conjugate in ammonium acetate buffer at pH 5.2. ^{99m}TcO$_4^-$ solution with appropriate activity is then added to the mixture, followed by SnCl$_2$ solution in HCl. The solution is incubated for 30–60 min at room temperature, and finally the labeled product is purified by dialysis or P4 column chromatography. The yield is almost 90% with added stability of the labeled product.

Radiolabeled antibodies are used for detecting a variety of pathophysiological conditions depending on the type and characteristics of the antibody. Many antibodies have been developed against various cancer antigens and used for their detection by the radiolabeling technique. Use of radioiodinated antibodies is limited, because ^{131}I gives higher radiation dose to the patients, ^{123}I is expensive, and in vivo dehalogenation causes a high blood background. ^{111}In-labeled antibodies are useful for tumor imaging in that the half-life is reasonably long enough to localize in the tumor and the photon energy (171 keV and 245 keV) is optimally acceptable for imaging. However, the amount to be administered is restricted due to higher radiation dose to the patient. In clinical situations, the half-life of ^{99m}Tc is somewhat short to allow for sufficient localization of ^{99m}Tc-labeled antibodies in tumors. However, using higher activity, tumors have been successfully detected with ^{99m}Tc-labeled antibodies.

^{99m}Tc-Arcitumomab (CEA-Scan)

This single dosage kit, also called the CEA-Scan, contains the Fab' fragment of arcitumomab, a murine monoclonal antibody IMMU-4, and Sn^{2+} ions along with potassium sodium tartrate, sodium acetate, and other inactive ingredients in lyophilized form. This kit is manufactured by Immunomedics, Inc. and distributed by Mallinckrodt Medical. Labeling is carried out by adding ^{99m}TcO$_4^-$ to the reaction vial and incubating the mixture for 5 min at room temperature. The labeling yield should be more than 90%. ^{99m}Tc-arcitumomab should be stored at room temperature and dispensed within 4 hr after preparation. The nonradioactive kits should be stored at 2° to 8°C.

The IMMU-4 antibody is targeted against the carcinoembryonic antigens of the colorectal tumors and, therefore, ^{99m}Tc-arcitumomab is used for detecting these tumors. The fragment Fab' has the advantage of rapid plasma clearance and urinary excretion due to its small size, compared to the whole antibody.

^{99m}Tc-Sulesomab (LeukoScan)

This single-dosage kit is manufactured by Immunomedics, Inc. Morris Plains, New Jersey, under the brand name of LeukoScan. It is approved for human use in Europe and other countries, but not in the U.S. The kit vial contains the Fab′ fragment, called sulesomab, obtained from the murine monoclonal antigranulocyte antibody, IMMU-MN3, along with Sn^{2+} ions plus potassium sodium tartrate, sodium acetate, sodium chloride, glacial acetic acid, and sucrose. The contents are lyophilized under nitrogen atmosphere. Reconstitution of the kit is carried out by adding 0.5 ml of saline to dissolve the lyophilized product, followed by the addition of approximately 30 mCi (1110 MBq) ^{99m}TcO$_4^-$ in 1 ml volume. The reaction is allowed for 10 min and the labeling yield should be more than 90%. The kit should be shored at 2° to 8°C before and after reconstitution, and should be used within 4 hr of formulation.

^{99m}Tc-sulesomab targets the granulocytes, and therefore is primarily used to detect infection and inflammation. Although repeated administration of LeukoScan can cause HAMA in vivo, no case has been reported to have HAMA from a single injection.

Radiolabeled Peptides

Imaging with radiolabeled antibodies encounters the difficulty of higher background due to slow plasma clearance and tumor uptake. This problem is somewhat mitigated by the use of peptides whose molecular size is smaller than those of proteins. The plasma clearance of the peptides is much faster. They exhibit rapid target tissue uptake and rapid excretion mainly due to the degradation of the peptides by peptidases. Based on these facts, various peptides have been introduced for targeting specific tumors and actively forming thrombi. Various derivatives of native peptides have also been synthesized to improve their biological characteristics and thus to enhance their binding to biological targets.

Peptides have been labeled with both ^{111}In and ^{99m}Tc. The basic principles of labeling of peptides are identical to those of antibodies described above and, therefore, are not discussed here. High specific activity of radiolabeled peptides can be achieved, particularly with ^{99m}Tc. However, due to the small size of the peptide molecules, ^{99m}Tc-labeling is likely to alter the regions of the peptide that interact with the biological target and consequently to result in the loss of their binding affinity. Direct labeling of peptides with ^{99m}Tc using Sn^{2+} as the reducing agent may cause damage to the molecule by breaking open the disulfide bonds. So the indirect labeling method using BFCs is preferable for ^{99m}Tc-labeling of peptides.

The radiolabeled peptides that have been approved by the U.S. FDA for clinical use are briefly discussed below.

[111]In-Pentetreotide (OctreoScan)

The single dosage kit, also known as OctreoScan, is supplied by Mallinckrodt Medical. It consists of a reaction vial containing a lyophilized mixture of octreotide conjugated to DTPA (pentetreotide), gentisic acid, trisodium citrate, citric acid, and inositol. Also included in the kit is a 3 mCi (111 MBq) [111]InCl$_3$ solution. Labeling is carried out by adding [111]InCl$_3$ to the reaction vial and incubating the mixture for 30 min at room temperature. The labeling yield should be more than 90%. ^{111}In-pentetreotide should be stored at a temperature below 25°C and be dispensed within 6 hr after preparation.

Octreotide is a synthetic analog of the human hormone somatostatin, and therefore ^{111}In-pentetreotide binds to somatostatin receptors on body tissues. It is particularly useful in detecting primary and metastatic neuroendocrine tumors such as carcinoids, gastrinomas, neuroblastomas, pituitary adenomas, and medullary thyroid carcinomas.

[99m]Tc-Peptide

^{99m}Tc-MAG3 is a peptide that has been described earlier and is used for renal imaging. There are other ^{99m}Tc-labeled peptides that have been experimentally tested for detecting thrombi, different tumors, inflammations, and infections, but none has been approved for clinical use. Among them are ^{99m}Tc-labeled P280 and P748, which bind to GPllb/llla receptors in actively forming thrombi, ^{99m}Tc-labeled P587 and P829 peptides for tumor detection, and ^{99m}Tc-labeled P483H peptide for labeling white blood cells for use in the detection of infections. Labeling is carried out via ligand exchange by adding ^{99m}Tc-gluceptate to the peptide solution and incubating. The yield is of the order of 95%.

[99m]Tc-Apcitide (AcuTect)

Diatide manufactures and Amersham Health distributes this single-dosage kit of ^{99m}Tc-apcitide under the brand name of AcuTect. The kit vial contains bibapcitide, which consists of two apcitide monomers, stannous chloride and sodium glucoheptonate. The contents are lyophilized and kept under nitrogen atmosphere. Labeling is performed by adding up to 50 mCi (1.85 GBq) [99m]TcO$_4^-$ to the kit vial and heating for 15 min in a boiling water bath. Bibapcitide is split and ^{99m}Tc-apcitide is formed in the reaction vial. The labeling yield should be greater than 90% and the product should be used within 6 hr of preparation. The cold kits must be stored at 2° to 8°C, whereas the reconstituted product can be stored at 20° to 25°C.

[99m]Tc-apcitide binds to the GP IIb/IIIa receptors on activated platelets that are responsible for aggregation in forming the thrombi, and therefore is used for the detection of acute deep vein thrombosis (DVT) in lower extremities.

^{99m}Tc-Depreotide (NeoTect)

This single-dosage kit is supplied under the brand name of NeoTect by Diatide. The kit vial contains a lyophilized mixture of depreotide, sodium glucoheptonate, stannous chloride, and sodium EDTA. Labeling is carried out by adding $^{99m}TcO_4^-$ to the reaction vial and incubating the mixture for 10 minutes in a boiling water bath followed by cooling for 15 min at room temperature. The labeling yield is determined by using ITLC-SG paper and saturated sodium chloride solution and 1:1 methanol:1M ammonium acetate (MAM) solvents, and should be more than 90%. The nonradioactive kit is stored at $<10°C$, whereas the reconstituted solution is stored at room temperature and should be used within 5 hr of preparation.

Depreotide is a synthetic peptide that binds with high affinity to somatostatin receptors (SSTR) in normal as well as abnormal tissues. This agent is used to detect SSTR-bearing pulmonary masses in patients proven or suspected to have pulmonary lesions by CT and/or chest x-ray.

Other Radiopharmaceuticals of Clinical Importance

The compound ^{111}In-indium chloride is supplied as a sterile solution in HCl at pH below 2.5; acidic pH is needed because it precipitates as hydroxide at pH above 5.5. It is used for bone marrow imaging and for labeling different antibodies and peptides. The compound ^{51}Cr-sodium chromate is supplied as a sterile solution at pH 7.5 to 8.5, and is used for labeling RBCs for use in the study of red cell survival and spleen imaging. Colloidal ^{32}P-chromic phosphate suspended in saline is used for the treatment of malignant pleural and peritoneal effusion.

PET Radiopharmaceuticals

^{18}F-Sodium Fluoride

Fluorine-18 is produced by irradiation of ^{18}O-water with protons in a cyclotron and recovered as ^{18}F-sodium fluoride by passing the irradiated water target mixture through a carbonate type anion exchange resin column. The water passes through, whereas $^{18}F^-$ is retained on the column, which is removed by elution with potassium carbonate solution. Its pH should be between 4.5 to 8.0. While ^{18}F-sodium fluoride is most commonly used for the synthesis of ^{18}F-fluorodeoxyglucose, it is also used for other ^{18}F-labeled PET radiopharmaceuticals. The FDA has approved it for bone scintigraphy.

^{18}F-Fluorodeoxyglucose (FDG)

^{18}F-2-fluoro-2-deoxyglucose (2-FDG) is normally produced in places where a cyclotron is locally available. Deoxyglucose is labeled with ^{18}F ($t_{1/2} = 110$ min) by nucleophilic displacement reaction of an acetylated sugar derivative followed by hydrolysis (Hamacher et al, 1986). A solution of

1,3,4,6-tetra-*O*-acetyl-2-*O*-trifluormethane-sulfonyl-*β*-D-mannopyranose   in anhydrous acetonitrile is added to a dry residue of ^{18}F-fluoride containing aminopolyether (Kryptofix 2.2.2) and potassium carbonate. The mixture is heated under reflux for about 5 min. The solution is then passed through a C-18 Sep-Pak column to elute acetylated carbohydrates with tetrahydrofuran (THF), which is then hydrolyzed by refluxing in hydrochloric acid at 130°C for 15 min. ^{18}F-2-fluoro-2-deoxyglucose (2-FDG) is obtained by passing the hydrolysate through a C-18 Sep-Pak column. The yield can be as high as 60%, and the preparation time is approximately 50 min. ^{18}F-2-FDG is routinely synthesized in an automated synthesis box in which ^{18}F-fluoride is introduced and the sequence of reactions follows to yield ^{18}F-2-FDG. The final solution diluted with saline has a pH of 7.0. The molecular structure of ^{18}F-2-FDG is shown in Fig. 7.8.

^{18}F-2-FDG is used primarily for the study of metabolism in the brain and heart and for the detection of epilepsy and various tumors. In metabolism, ^{18}F 2-FDG is phosphorylated by hexokinase to 2-FDG-6-phosphate, which is not metabolized further. It should be noted that 3-fluorodeoxyglucose (3-FDG) is not phosphorylated and hence it is not trapped and is essentially eliminated rapidly from the cell.

^{18}F-Fluorodopa

Like ^{18}F-2-FDG, ^{18}F-fluorodopa is also produced in places where a cyclotron is available locally. There are several methods of synthesizing 6-^{18}F-fluoro-3,4-dihydroxy-phenylalanine (6-^{18}F-fluorodopa), of which the method of fluorodemetallation using electrophilic fluorinating agents is the most common. Only the l-isomer is important, because the enzymes in the conversion of dopa to dopamine, which is targeted by the radiopharmaceutical, are selective for this isomer. Initially, a suitably protected organomercury

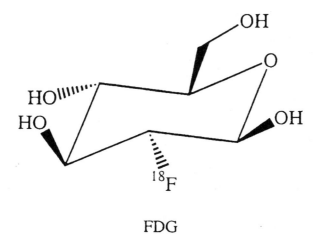

FDG

FIGURE 7.8. Molecular structure of ^{18}F-2-fluoro-2-deoxyglucose (^{18}F-FDG).

precursor of dopa is prepared. [^{18}F]-labeled acetylhypofluorite prepared in the gas phase is then allowed to react with the mercury precursor in chloroform or acetonitrile at room temperature. Acid hydrolysis with 47% HBr provides a relatively high yield (10–12%) of 1-6-^{18}F-fluorodopa (Luxen et al, 1987). Substitution at position 6 is most desirable because this does not alter the behavior of dopa, whereas substitutions at 2 and 5 do. It is supplied at pH between 4.0 and 5.0. Normally EDTA and ascorbic acid are added to the final preparation for stability. 1-6-^{18}F-fluorodopa is used for the assessment of the presynaptic dopaminergic function in the brain.

^{18}F-Fluorothymidine (FLT)

^{18}F-fluorothymidine (FLT) is prepared by nucleophilic reaction between ^{18}F-fluoride and a precursor, 2, 3′-anhydro-5′-0-benzoyl-2′-deoxythymidine, which is prepared by standard organic synthesis (Machulla et al, 2000). ^{18}F-fluoride is added to a mixture of Kryptofix 2.2.2 and potassium carbonate in acetonitrile and the mixture is dried to a residue by heating at 120°C for 5 min. The precursor in dimethyl sulfoxide (DMSO) is added to the dried residue and heated at 160°C for 10 min. Hydrolysis of the 5′-0- protecting group is performed with sodium hydroxide. ^{18}F-FLT is isolated by passing through alumina Sep-Pak and further purified by using the HPLC. The overall yield is about 45% and the radiochemical purity is more than 95%. The synthesis time is about 60 min.

Since thymidine is incorporated into DNA and provides a measure of cell proliferation, ^{18}F-FLT is commonly used for in vivo diagnosis and characterization of tumors in humans.

^{15}O-Water

^{15}O-oxygen is produced in the cyclotron by the ^{15}N (p, n) ^{15}O reaction, and the irradiated gas is transferred to a [^{15}O] water generator in which it is mixed with hydrogen and passed over a palladium/charcoal catalyst at 170°C (Meyer et al, 1986). The H$_2$^{15}O vapor is trapped in saline, which is then passed through a radiation detector for radioassay and ultimately injected into the patient in a very short time.

H$_2$^{15}O is commonly used for myocardial and cerebral perfusion studies.

n-^{15}O-Butanol

n-^{15}O-butanol is prepared by the reaction of ^{15}O-oxygen, produced by the ^{15}N(p, n) ^{15}O reaction, with tri-n-butyl borane loaded onto an alumina Sep-Pak cartridge (Kabalka et al, 1985). Carrier oxygen at a concentration of about 0.5% is added to the ^{15}N target in order to recover ^{15}O. After the reaction, n-^{15}O-butanol is eluted from the cartridge with water. It is further purified by passing through C-18 Sep-Pak and eluting with ethanol-water.

^{15}O-butanol is used for blood flow measurement in the brain and other organs. It is a better perfusion agent than ^{15}O-water because its partition coefficient is nearly 1.0 compared to 0.9 for water.

^{13}N-Ammonia

Nitrogen-13-labeled ammonia is produced by reduction of ^{13}N-labeled nitrates and nitrites that are produced by proton irradiation of water in a cyclotron. The reduction is carried out with titanium chloride in alkaline medium. ^{13}N-NH$_3$ is then distilled and finally trapped in acidic saline solution. Its pH should be between 4.5 and 7.5. The FDA has approved it for measurement of myocardial and cerebral perfusion.

^{11}C-Sodium Acetate

^{11}C-labeled acetate is produced by the reaction of the Grignard reagent, methylmagnesium bromide, with cyclotron-produced ^{11}C-carbon dioxide. After reaction, the product is hydrolyzed with water or aqueous acid, followed by further purification using solvent extraction. ^{11}C-acetate has been found to be stable at pH between 4.5 and 8.5 for up to 2 hr at room temperature. It is used for the measurement of oxygen consumption in the heart and brain.

^{11}C-Flumazenil

^{11}C-flumazenil is commonly labeled at the N-methyl position by N-methylation with ^{11}C-iodomethane, which is prepared from ^{11}C-CO$_2$, and using the freshly prepared Grignard reagent, methylmagnesium bromide. The specific activity is very important for this product and therefore is analyzed by HPLC to give an optimum value between 18.5 to 74 GBq/μmol (0.5 to 2 Ci/μmol). It remains stable for up to 3 hr at room temperature at pH 7.0.

Since it is a benzodiazepine receptor ligand, ^{11}C-flumazenil is primarily used for the neuroreceptor characterization in humans.

^{11}C-Methylspiperone (MSP)

^{11}C-labeled methylspiperone (MSP) is prepared by N-methylation of spiperone with ^{11}C-iodomethane in the presence of Grignard reagent, methylmagnesium bromide, using different solvents and bases. Since spiperones are sensitive to bases and to radiolysis at high dose, the yield of ^{11}C-MSP has been different for different investigators. Cold spiperone present in the preparation reduces its specific activity and should be controlled. Specific activity should be around 10 to 50 GBq/μmol (270 to 1350 mCi/μmol). High specific activity ^{11}C-MSP undergoes autodecomposition in saline due to radiation, and a hydroxyl radical scavenger (e.g., ethanol) is added to prevent it.

^{11}C-methylspiperone is primarily used to determine the dopamine-2 receptor density in patients with neurologic diseases.

^{11}C-L-Methionine

^{11}C-L-methionine has ^{11}C at its methyl position and has two forms: L-[1-^{11}C] methionine and L-[s-methyl-^{11}C] methionine. The former is obtained by the reaction between ^{11}C-CO_2 precursor and carbanion produced by a strong base added to the respective isonitrile, followed by hydrolysis with an acid. The latter is obtained by alkylation of the sulfide anion of L-homocysteine with ^{11}C-iodomethane. The product is purified by HPLC yielding a purity of >98%. The pH should be between 6.0 and 8.0 and it is stable for 2 hr at room temperature.

This compound is used for the detection of different types of malignancies, reflecting the amino acid utilization (transport, protein synthesis, transmethylation, etc.).

^{11}C-Raclopride

Raclopride is labeled with ^{11}C either by N-ethylation with [1-^{11}C] iodoethane or by O-methylation with [^{11}C] iodomethane, although the latter is more suitable for routine synthesis. Both ^{11}C-labeled iodoethane and iodomethane are prepared from ^{11}C-CO_2. The product is purified by HPLC giving a purity of >98%. The specific activity should be in the range of 0.5 to 2 Ci/μmol (18.5 to 74 GBq/μmol). The product at pH between 4.5 to 8.5 remains stable for more than 1 hr at room temperature.

^{11}C-raclopride is primarily used to detect various neurologic and psychiatric disorders, such as Parkinson's disease and schizophrenia.

^{82}Rb-Rubidium Chloride

^{82}Rb-rubidium chloride is available from the ^{82}Sr-^{82}Rb generator, which is manufactured and supplied monthly by Bracco Diagnostics. ^{82}Rb is eluted with saline and must be checked for ^{82}Sr and ^{85}Sr breakthrough daily before the start of its use for patient studies. Since ^{82}Rb has a short half-life of 75 s, it is administered to the patient by an infusion pump. The administered activity is the integrated activity infused at a certain flow rate for a certain period of time set by the operator, which is provided by a printer.

^{82}Rb is used for myocardial perfusion imaging to delineate ischemia from infarction.

Questions

1. What is the difference between MAA and colloid particles?
2. Twenty mCi (740 MBq) ^{99m}Tc-MAA contains 2 million MAA particles. If a patient is injected with 3 mCi (111 MBq) ^{99m}Tc-MAA for lung imaging, how many particles did he receive?
3. What are the most useful phosphonate compounds for bone imaging? Describe the general methods of ^{99m}Tc-labeling of these compounds.
4. Describe the basic principle of ^{99m}Tc-sulfur colloid preparations. Why are gelatin and EDTA added to ^{99m}Tc-sulfur colloid?
5. Name the important radiopharmaceuticals used for the study of hepatobiliary function and describe the basic methods of their preparation.
6. What are the usual expiratory periods for (a) ^{131}I-labeled compounds and (b) ^{99m}Tc-labeled compounds?

7. Describe the methods of labeling RBCs with ^{99m}Tc and ^{51}Cr. Discuss the merits and disadvantages of each method.

8. State the recommended temperatures of storage of the following compounds: (a) ^{99m}Tc-sulfur colloid, (b) ^{57}Co-cyanocobalamin, and (c) ^{131}I-NP-59.

9. Describe the methods of ^{111}In-labeling of platelets and leukocytes. What is the mechanism of labeling of platelets with ^{111}In?

10. Why is ^{111}In-indium chloride supplied at pH below 2.5?

11. Explain how the ^{99m}Tc-HMPAO kit is stabilized.

12. What is the charge of the following ^{99m}Tc-radiopharmaceuticals: (a) ^{99m}Tc-HMPAO, (b) ^{99m}Tc-MAG3, (c) ^{99m}Tc-sestamibi, (d) ^{99m}Tc-tetrofosmin?

13. What is the amount of Sn^{2+} needed for optimum labeling of RBCs by the in vivo method?

14. What are the restrictions on the quality of ^{99m}TcO$_4^-$ in the preparation of ^{99m}Tc-HMPAO?

15. Why is hetastarch added to the whole blood for leukocyte separation?

16. Describe the methods of production of monoclonal antibody and its labeling with ^{111}In and ^{99m}Tc.

17. What are the difficulties in making human monoclonal antibodies?

18. Why is SCN-Bz-DTPA better than DTPA as a bifunctional chelating agent in labeling antibodies?

19. What is the mechanism of ^{99m}Tc labeling of antibodies by the direct method?

20. Discuss the method of labeling of antibodies with HYNIC and tricine.

21. Describe the methods of preparation of ^{18}F-FDG and ^{18}F-fluorodopa.

22. What are the agents for palliation of pain due to bone metastasis and why are they used?

References and Suggested Reading

Abrams MJ, Davison A, Jones AG, et al. Synthesis and characterization of hexakis (alkylisocyanide) and hexakis (arylisocyanide complexes of Technetium (I). *Inorg Chem.* 1983; 22:2798.

Callahan RJ, Froelich JW, McKusick KA, et al. A modified method for the in vivo labeling of red blood cells with Tc-99m: concise communication. *J Nucl Med.* 1982; 23:315.

Dewanjee MK. The chemistry of ^{99m}Tc-labeled radiopharmaceuticals. *Semin Nucl Med.* 1990; 20:5.

Eckelman WC, Stiegman J, Paik CH. Radiopharmaceutical chemistry. In: Harpert J, Eckelman WC, Neumann RD, eds, *Nuclear Medicine: Diagnosis and Therapy.* New York: Thieme Medical; 1996:217.

Edwards DS, Cheeseman EH, Watson MW, et al. Synthesis and characterization of technetium and rhenium complexes of N, N'-1, 2-diethylenediylbis-L-cysteine. Neurolites and its metabolites. In: Nicolini M, Bandoli G, Mazzi U, eds. *Technetium and Rhenium in Chemistry and Nuclear Medicine.* Verona, Italy: Cortina International; 1990; 433.

Fritzberg AR, Kasina S, Eshima D, et al. Synthesis and biological evaluation of technetium-99m MAG3 as hippuran replacement. *J Nucl Med.* 1986; 27:11.

Hamacher K, Coenen HH, Stocklin G. Efficient stereospecific synthesis of NCA 2-[18F]-fluoro-2-deoxy-D-glucose using aminopolyether supported nucleophilic substitution. *J Nucl Med.* 1986; 27:235.

Hnatowich DJ. Recent developments in the radiolabeling of antibodies with iodine, indium and technetium. *Semin Nucl Med.* 1990; 20:80.

Kabalka GW, Lambrecht RM, Fowler JS, et al. Synthesis of 15O-labelled butanol via organoborane chemistry. *Appl Radiat Isot.* 1985; 36:853.

Kelly JD, Forster AM, Higley B, et al. Technetium-99m-tetrofosmin as a new radiopharmaceutical for myocardial perfusion imaging. *J Nucl Med.* 1993; 34: 222.

Köhler G, Milstein C. Continuous cultures of fused cells secreting antibody of predefined specificity. *Nature.* 1975; 256:495.

Loberg MD, Cooper M, Harvey E, et al. Development of new radiopharmaceuticals based on N-substitution of iminodiacetic acid. *J Nucl Med.* 1976; 17:633.

Luxen A, Bida GT, Phelps ME, et al. Synthesis of enantiomerically pure D and L 6-[F-18] fluorodopa and in vivo metabolites via regioselective fluorodemercuration. *J Nucl Med.* 1987; 28:624.

Machulla HJ, Blocher A, Kuntzsch M, et al. Simplified labeling approach for synthesizing 3'-dioxy-3'-[18F] fluorothymidine ([18F] FLT). *J Radioanal Nucl Chem.* 2000; 243:843.

Meyer GJ, Ostercholz A, Hundeshagen H. 15O-Water constant infusion system for clinical routine application. *J Label Comp Radiopharm.* 1986; 23:1209.

Nunn AD. Radiopharmaceutical for imaging myocardial perfusion. *Semin Nucl Med.* 1990; 20:111.

Package inserts of various kits available from commercial suppliers.

Peters AM, Danpure HJ, Osman S, et al. Clinical experience with 99mTc-hexamethyl propylene amine oxime for labeling leukocytes and imaging inflammation. *Lancet.* 1986; 2:946.

Sodd VJ, Allen DR, Hoagland DR, et al., eds. *Radiopharmaceuticals II.* New York: Society of Nuclear Medicine; 1979.

ten Berge RJM, Natarajan AT, Hardenman MR, et al. Labeling with indium-111 has detrimental effects on human lymphocytes. *J Nucl Med.* 1983; 24:615.

Thakur ML, Coleman RE, Welch MJ. Indium-111-labeled leukocytes for the localization of abscesses: preparation, analysis, tissue distribution and comparison with gallium-67 citrate in dogs. *J Lab Clin Med.* 1977; 82:217.

Troutner DR, Volkert WA, Hoffman TJ, et al. A neutral lipophilic complex of Tc-99m with a multidentate amine oxime. *Int J Appl Radiat Isot.* 1984; 35:467.

U.S. Pharmacopeia 26 & National Formulary 21. United States Pharmacopeial Convention, Rockville, MD; 2003.

Vanzelto G, Fagret D, Pasqualini R, et al. Biodistribution, dosimetry and safety of myocardial perfusion agent 99mTc-N-NOET in healthy volunteers. *J Nucl Med.* 2000; 41:141.

Welch MJ, ed. *Radiopharmaceuticals and Other compounds Labelled with Short-Lived Radionuclides.* New York: Pergamon Press; 1977.

Zuckier LS, Rodriguez LD, Scharff MD. Immunologic and pharmacologic concepts of monoclonal antibodies. *Semin Nucl Med.* 1990; 20:166.

8
Quality Control of Radiopharmaceuticals

Since radiopharmaceuticals are intended for administration to humans, it is imperative that they undergo strict quality control measures. Basically, quality control involves several specific tests and measurements that ensure the purity, potency, product identity, biologic safety, and efficacy of radiopharmaceuticals. All quality control procedures that are applied to nonradioactive pharmaceuticals are equally applicable to radiopharmaceuticals; in addition, tests for radionuclidic and radiochemical purity have to be carried out. Often these quality control tests are carried out by the manufacturers from the beginning of production all the way up to the finished product. However, the introduction of kits, the increasing use of short-lived radionuclides such as ^{99m}Tc and the on-site preparation of many radiopharmaceuticals require that most, if not all, quality control tests be performed on all in-house preparations before dispensing these products for human administration.

The quality control tests fall into two categories: physicochemical tests and biological tests. The physicochemical tests indicate the level of radionuclidic and radiochemical impurities and determine the pH, ionic strength, osmolality, and physical state of the sample, particularly if it is a colloid. The biological tests establish the sterility, apyrogenicity, and toxicity of the material. These methods are outlined in detail below.

Physicochemical Tests

Various in vitro physicochemical tests are essential for the determination of the purity and integrity of a radiopharmaceutical. Some of these tests are unique for radiopharmaceuticals because they contain radionuclides.

Physical Characteristics

The physical appearance of a radiopharmaceutical is important both on receipt and subsequently. One should be familiar with the color and state of a radiopharmaceutical. A true solution should not contain any particulate matter. Any deviation from the original color and clarity should be viewed with concern because it may reflect changes in the radiopharmaceutical that would alter its biologic behavior.

Colloidal or aggregate preparations should have a proper size range of particles for a given purpose. For example, for visualization of the reticuloendothelial system, the colloidal particle should have a mean size around 100 nm. In ^{99m}Tc-sulfur colloid preparations, the particle size (0.1 to 1 μm) may vary considerably from batch to batch. This can be checked by means of a microscope. These observations should be corroborated further by tissue distribution studies in animals, in which colloids of proper size should localize in the liver, while larger aggregated particles would deposit in the lungs.

In aggregate preparations such as ^{99m}Tc-MAA, the particle size should vary between 10 and 100 μm. The size can be checked with a hemocytometer under a light microscope. Preparations containing particles larger than 150 μm should be discarded because of the possibility of pulmonary arterial blockade by these large particles. The number of particles in a preparation is equally important and can be determined by counting the particles on a hemocytometer under a light microscope.

pH and Ionic Strength

All radiopharmaceuticals should have an appropriate hydrogen ion concentration or pH for their stability and integrity. The ideal pH of a radiopharmaceutical should be 7.4 (pH of the blood), although it can vary between 2 and 9 because of the high buffer capacity of the blood. The pH of a solution is accurately measured by a pH meter, whereas colorimetric evaluation with pH paper (litmus pper) is rather inaccurate. Any deviation from the desired pH must be treated with caution and should be remedied.

Radiopharmaceuticals must also have proper ionic strength, isotonicity, and osmolality in order to be suitable for human administration. Correct ionic strength can be achieved by adding a proper acid, alkali, or electrolyte and can be calculated from the concentrations of added electrolytes.

At this point a word of caution is in order. Since ionic strength and pH are important factors for the stability of a radiopharmaceutical, it is important to use the proper diluent, preferably the same solvent as used in the original preparation, when diluting a radiopharmaceutical.

Radionuclidic Purity

Radionuclidic purity is defined as the fraction of the total radioactivity in the form of the desired radionuclide present in a radiopharmaceutical. Impurities arise from extraneous nuclear reactions due to isotopic impurities in the target material or from fission of heavy elements in the reactor. Some examples are ^{99}Mo in ^{99m}Tc-labeled preparations (this arises due to ^{99}Mo breakthrough from the Moly generator) and many iodine isotopes in ^{131}I-labeled preparations. The undesirable radionuclides may belong to the same element as the desired radionuclide or to a different element. The presence of these extraneous radionuclides increases the undue radiation dose to the patient and may also degrade the scintigraphic images. These impurities can be removed by appropriate chemical methods, provided their chemical properties are distinctly different from those of the desired radionuclide.

Radionuclidic purity is determined by measuring the half-lives and characteristic radiations emitted by individual radionuclides. Radionuclides that emit γ rays are distinguished from one another by identification of their γ-ray energies on the spectra obtained on a NaI(Tl) detector or a lithium-drifted germanium [Ge(Li)] detector coupled to a multichannel analyzer (see Chapter 3).

Pure β emitters are not as easy to check as the γ emitters because they pose a counting problem. They may be checked for purity with a β spectrometer or a liquid scintillation counter. Since a given radiation may belong to a number of radionuclides, determination of radiation energy alone does not establish the identity of a radionuclide. Its half-life also must be established, and this can be accomplished by measuring the activity under the photopeak in question over a period of time and plotting it versus time. The time it takes for any initial radioactivity to be reduced to one half is the half-life of the radionuclide and is read from the plot.

Radionuclidic purity depends on the relative half-lives and the quantities of the desired radionuclide and other contaminants, and changes with time. The presence of small quantities of a long-lived contaminant radionuclide is difficult to detect in the presence of large quantities of a desired short-lived radionuclide. In these instances, the short-lived radionuclide is allowed to decay and then the long-lived activity is measured. Trace amounts of various radionuclidic impurities in the ^{99m}Tc-eluate from a Moly generator are usually measured by a Ge(Li) detector after allowing ^{99m}Tc to decay. The detection and determination of ^{99}Mo in the ^{99m}Tc-eluate have been described in Chapter 5.

Radiochemical Purity

The radiochemical purity of a radiopharmaceutical is the fraction of the total radioactivity in the desired chemical form in the radiopharmaceutical. Radiochemical impurities arise from decomposition due to the action of solvent, change in temperature or pH, light, presence of oxidizing or reducing agents, and radiolysis. Examples of radiochemical impurity are free ^{99m}TcO$_4^-$ and hydrolyzed ^{99m}Tc in ^{99m}Tc-labeled complexes, free ^{113}I-iodide in ^{131}I-labeled proteins, and ^{51}Cr^{3+} in a solution of ^{51}Cr-sodium chromate. The presence of radiochemical impurities in a radiopharmaceutical results in poor-quality images due to the high background from the surrounding tissues and the blood, and gives unnecessary radiation dose to the patient.

Decomposition of labeled compounds by radiolysis depends on the specific activity of the radioactive material, the type and energy of the emitted radiation, and the half-life of the radionuclide. Absorption of radiations by labeled molecules results in the formation of free radicals with unpaired electrons, which in turn leads to further decomposition of other molecules. A secondary process due to radiolysis produces H_2O_2 or HO_2 from decomposition of water (solvent), which reacts with and ultimately decomposes labeled molecules. Particles are more damaging than γ-rays due to their short range and complete local absorption in matter.

The stability of a compound is time-dependent on exposure to light, change in temperature, and radiolysis. The longer a compound is exposed to these conditions, the more it will tend to break down. For this reason, most radiopharmaceuticals are assigned an expiratory date after which they are not guaranteed for their intended use. Substances such as sodium ascorbate, ascorbic acid, and sodium sulfite are often added to maintain the stability of radiopharmaceuticals. Some radiopharmaceuticals are stored in the dark under refrigeration to lessen the degradation of the material.

A number of analytical methods are used to detect and determine the radiochemical impurities in a given radiopharmaceutical. Particularly important are precipitation, paper, thin-layer, and gel chromatography, paper and gel electrophoresis, ion exchange, solvent extraction, high performance liquid chromatography, and distillation. These methods are briefly outlined below.

Precipitation

This method involves the precipitation of one radiochemical entity from another with an appropriate chemical reagent. The precipitate is separated by centrifugation. For example, the amount of $^{51}Cr^{3+}$ present in a ^{51}Cr-sodium chromate solution may be measured by precipitating chromate as lead chromate and determining the supernatant radioactivity.

Paper and Instant Thin-Layer Chromatography

In paper and instant thin-layer chromatography, a small aliquot of the radiopharmaceutical preparation is spotted on a paper (Whatman paper strip) or an instant thin-layer chromatography (ITLC) strip [ITLC strips are made of glass fiber impregnated with silica gel (SG) or polysilicic acid (SA)] and then chromatography is carried out by dipping the spotted strip into an appropriate solvent contained in a jar or a chamber. The commonly used solvents are 85% methanol, acctone, methyl ethyl ketone(MEK), 0.9% NaCl solution, and water, the strip is dipped in such a way that the spot remains above the solvent. During the chromatographic process, different components of the sample distribute themselves between the adsorbent (paper or silica gel) and the solvent, depending on their distribution coefficients. Here the adsorbent is the stationary phase and the solvent the mobile phase. Electrostatic forces of the stationary phase tend to retard various components, while the mobile phase carries them along. This effect and varying solubilities of different components in a solvent cause the individual components to move at different speeds and to appear at different distances along the paper or ITLC strip. Polarity of the solvent also affects the chromatographic separation of different components in a sample.

Paper or ITLC chromatography can be either the ascending or descending type. In ascending chromatography, the mobile phase moves up, whereas in the descending type it moves down. Whereas some chromatography takes hours for the complete procedure, ITLC is a relatively fast method that takes only a few minutes.

In paper chromatography or ITLC, each component in a given sample is characterized by an R_f value, which is defined as the ratio of the distance traveled by the component to the distance the solvent front has advanced from the original point of application of the test material. These values are established with known components and may vary under different experimental conditions. The R_f values are used primarily for the identification of different components in a given sample.

When the solvent front moves to a desired distance, the strip is removed from the chamber, dried. and divided into several segments, usually 10, and the radioactivity of each segment is measured in an appropriate counter, particularly in a NaI(Tl) well counter. Histograms are obtained by plotting the radioactivity of each segment. Alternatively, the activity along the strip can be measured by a radiochromatographic scanner, which, with an automatic integrator device, plots the radioactivity versus the distance of the strip. Radiochemical impurity is calculated as the ratio (as a percentage) of the radioactivity of the undesirable component to the total activity applied at the origin.

As previously mentioned in Chapter 6, three ^{99m}Tc species may exist in any ^{99m}Tc-labeled preparation: free, hydrolyzed, and bound ^{99m}Tc. The ITLC method is used routinely in nuclear pharmacy to estimate the amounts of these three components and hence the labeling yield. Because the chromatographic separation depends on the type of paper and solvent, different information can be obtained with different systems. For example, in the analysis of ^{99m}Tc-pyrophosphate, the ITLC method using 85% methanol or acetone and ITLC-SG paper gives only two peaks—bound and hydrolyzed ^{99m}Tc at the origin ($R_f = 0$) and free ^{99m}Tc at the solvent front ($R_f = 1.0$), as shown in Figure 8.1. If, however, Whatman No. 1 paper and saline are used in ITLC chromatography, the three components can be separated: the bound ^{99m}Tc at the solvent front, the hydrolyzed ^{99m}Tc at the origin, and the free ^{99m}Tc at $R_f = 0.7$. It is therefore obvious that an interpretation of chromatographic results should be made with caution depending on the system used. The R_f values of different ^{99m}Tc species observed

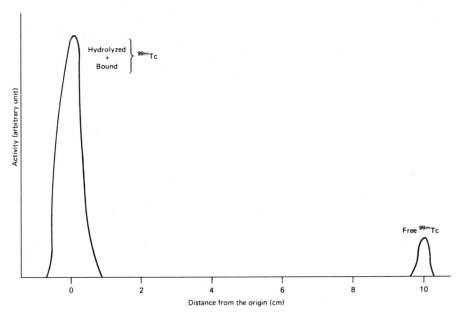

FIGURE 8.1. Typical chromatogram obtained with ITLC-SG paper and acetone, showing two peaks: one at the solvent front for free $^{99m}TcO_4^-$ and the other at the origin for both hydrolyzed and bound ^{99m}Tc-labeled compounds.

with several chromatographic systems are shown in Table 8.1. For radiopharmaceuticals other than ^{99m}Tc-labeled products, the R_f values are presented in Table 8.2.

For the sake of brevity, in nuclear medicine, 5- to 6-cm long and 1-cm wide ITLC (SG or SA) or Whatman No. 1 or 3 strips are employed for the analysis of ^{99m}Tc-labeled radiopharmaceuticals. Chromatography is usually performed with acetone or saline in a small vial fitted with a screw cap (Fig. 8.2). The total time of chromatography is only a few minutes. Afterward, the chromatogram is cut in half and the activity in each half is measured. As described in Figure 8.3, the activities of free, hydrolyzed and bound ^{99m}Tc can be determined and their percentages calculated.

For practical reasons, some ^{99m}Tc-labeled radiopharmaceuticals require only one solvent chromatography. For example, the thin-layer chromatography of ^{99m}Tc-DMSA is performed with only ITLC-SA and acetone, because DMSA does not move to the solvent front in saline. Similarly, ^{99m}Tc-SC and ^{99m}Tc-MAA require only ITLC-SG and acetone, giving free $^{99m}TcO_4^-$ and ^{99m}Tc-chelate because these radiopharmaceuticals do not dissolve in saline. ^{131}I-MIBG is checked for radiochemical purity using silica gel plated plastic and a mixture of ethylacetate and ethanol (1:1) as solvent, which gives for ^{131}I-iodide $R_f = 0.6$ and for ^{131}I-MIBG $R_f = 0.0$.

TABLE 8.1. Chromatographic data of ^{99m}Tc-labeled radiopharmaceuticals.

^{99m}Tc-labeled Radiopharmaceuticals	Stationary phase	Solvent	R_f		
			^{99m}TcO$_4^-$	^{99m}Tc-Complex	Hydrolyzed ^{99m}Tc
^{99m}Tc-PYP	ITLC-SG	Acetone	1.0	0.0	0.0
	ITLC-SG	Saline	1.0	1.0	0.0
^{99m}Tc-HDP	ITLC-SG	Acetone	1.0	0.0	0.0
	ITLC-SG	Saline	1.0	1.0	0.0
^{99m}Tc-MDP	ITLC-SG	Acetone	1.0	0.0	0.0
	ITLC-SG	Saline	1.0	1.0	0.0
^{99m}Tc-DTPA	ITLC-SG	Acetone	1.0	0.0	0.0
	ITLC-SG	Saline	1.0	1.0	0.0
^{99m}Tc-SC	ITLC-SG	Acetone	1.0	0.0	0.0
^{99m}Tc-MAA	ITLC-SG	Acetone	1.0	0.0	0.0
^{99m}Tc-Gluceptate	ITLC-SG	Acetone	1.0	0.0	0.0
	ITLC-SG	Saline	1.0	1.0	0.0
^{99m}Tc-DISIDA	ITLC-SA	20% NaCl	1.0	0.0	0.0
^{99m}Tc-Mebrofenin	ITLC-SG	Water	1.0	1.0	0.0
^{99m}Tc-DMSA	ITLC-SA	Acetone	1.0	0.0	0.0
^{99m}Tc-teboroxime	Whatman 31 ET	Saline: acetone (1:1)	1.0	1.0	0.0
	Whatman 31 ET	Saline	1.0	0.0	0.0
^{99m}Tc-sestamibi	Al$_2$O$_3$ coated plastic plate	Ethanol	0.0	1.0	0.0

TABLE 8.1, *Continued*

99mTc-labeled Radiopharmaceuticals	Stationary phase	Solvent	R_f		
			$^{99m}TcO_4^-$	^{99m}Tc-Complex	Hydrolyzed ^{99m}Tc
^{99m}Tc-HSA	ITLC-SG	Ethanol:NH$_4$OH:H$_2$O (2:1:5)	1.0	1.0	0.0
^{99m}Tc-HMPAO	Whatman 31 ET	Acetone	1.0	0.0	0.0
	ITLC-SG	Butanone (MEK)	1.0	1.0 (primary)	0.0
^{99m}Tc-tetrofosmin	ITLC-SG	Saline	1.0	0.0	0.0
	Whatman 1	50% Acetonitrile	1.0	1.0	0.0
	ITLC-SG	Acetone:dichloromethane (35:65 v/v)	1.0	0.5	0.0
^{99m}Tc-architumomab	ITLC-SG	Acetone	1.0	0.0	0.0
^{99m}Tc-MAG3	Whatman 3 MM	Acetone	1.0	0.0	0.0
	Whatman 3 MM	Water	1.0	1.0	0.0
^{99m}Tc-bicisate	Whatman 3 MM	Ethylacetate	0.0	1.0	0.0
^{99m}Tc-nanocolloid	Whatman ET-31	Saline	0.8	0.0	0.0
^{99m}Tc-apcitide	ITLC-SG	Water	0.25–1.0	0.25–1.0	0.0–0.25
		Sat'd NaCl sol	0.75–1.0	0.0–0.75	0.0–0.75
^{99m}Tc-depreotide	ITLC-SG	Sat'd NaCl solution	0.75–1.0	0.0–0.75	0.0–0.75
		1:1 Methanol:1M Ammonium acetate	0.4–1.0	0.4–1.0	0.0–0.4
^{99m}Tc-N-NOET	Whatman KCF18	Methanol: 0.5 M ammonium acetate	1.0	0.25	0.47

TABLE 8.2. Chromatographic data of radiopharmaceuticals other than ^{99m}Tc-complexes.[a]

Radiopharmaceuticals	Stationary phase	Solvent	R_f Values	
			Labeled product	Impurities
^{125}I-RISA	ITLC-SG	85% Methanol	0.0	1.0 (I^-)
^{131}I-Hippuran	ITLC-SG	$CHCl_3$: AceticAcid (9:1)	1.0	0.1 (I^-)
^{131}I-NP-59	ITLC-SG	Chloroform	1.0	0.1 (I^-)
^{131}I-MIBG	Silica gel plated plastic	Ethylacetate : Ethanol (1:1)	0.0	0.6 (I^-)
^{131}I-NaI	ITLC-SG	85% Methanol	1.0	0.2 (IO_3^-)
^{51}Cr-sodium chromate	ITLC-SG	n-butanol saturated with 1N HCl	0.9	0.2 (Cr^{3+})
^{67}Ga-citrate	ITLC-SG	$CHCl_3$: Acetic acid (9:1)	0.1	1.0
^{111}In-DTPA	ITLC-SG	10% Ammonium acetate:Methanol (1:1)	1.0	0.1 (In^{3+})
^{111}In-capromab[b] pendetide	ITLC-SG	Saline	0.0	1.0 (In^{3+})
^{18}F-FDG[b]	Silicagel	CH_3CN/H_2O (95:5)	0.37	0.0
^{90}Y-, ^{111}In-ibritumomab tiuxetan[b]	ITLC-SG	0.9% NaCl sol	0.0	1.0

[a] Data are adapted from Procedure manual—Radiochemical purity of radiopharaceuticals using Gelman Seprachrom^{TM} (ITLC^{TM}) chromatography. Gelman Science, Inc., Ann Arbor, Michigan, 1977.
[b] Data are from package insert.

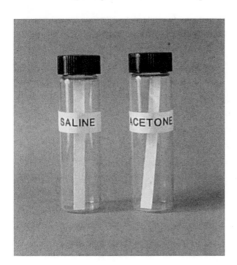

FIGURE 8.2. Chromatographic chamber type vials.

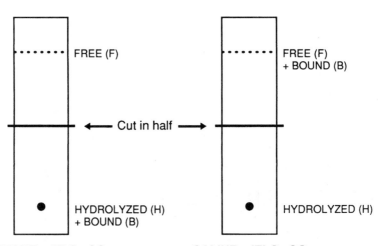

$$F\,(\%) = \frac{F \times 100}{H + B + F} \qquad\qquad H\,(\%) = \frac{H \times 100}{H + B + F}$$

$$B\,(\%) = 100 - F\,(\%) - H\,(\%)$$

FIGURE 8.3. Miniaturized ITLC system for analyzing radiochemical purity of ^{99m}Tc-labeled radiopharmaceuticals.

Some factors in thin-layer chromatography must be considered in order to avoid artifacts. The chromatographic paper should be dry. Caution should be exercised to avoid streaking of solvents along the edge of the paper strip. The sample spot should be small and long air drying should be avoided to prevent air oxidation of ^{99m}Tc-chelate.

Gel Chromatography

Gel chromatography is a very useful method for separating different components of a radiopharmaceutical preparation. In this method, a sample is spotted on the top of a column of Sephadex gel or Bio-Rad gel, soaked in an appropriate solvent, and then eluted with the same solvent. Separation of the components of a sample depends on the molecular size of the species—the larger ones are eluted faster than the smaller ones. Sequential fractions of the eluate are collected by means of an automated fraction collector and the radioactivity is measured in each fraction. The identity of different components is established by using known samples on the gel column. The radioactivity in each fraction is then plotted versus the fraction number, which gives the relative concentrations of different molecular size components in a given sample. The amount of a component is expressed as the ratio (as a percentage) of its radioactivity to the total radioactivity placed on the column.

Gel chromatography is useful in separating proteins of different molecular weights. This method is equally important in detecting impurities in ^{99m}Tc-radiopharmaceuticals. Free, bound, and unbound hydrolyzed ^{99m}Tc species can be separated and identified by this method using Sephadex gel and saline as the eluting solvent. In this case, the ^{99m}Tc-chelate is eluted first, ^{99m}TcO$_4^-$ comes through next, and the hydrolyzed ^{99m}Tc is retained by the column. In several ^{99m}Tc-labeled preparations, the chelate binds to Sephadex gel, which causes problems in the separation of the impurities. Examples are ^{99m}Tc-gluconate and ^{99m}Tc-mannitol, which are adsorbed on the Sephadex column.

Paper or Polyacrylamide Gel Electrophoresis

Paper or polyacrylamide gel electrophoresis consists of applying a radioactive sample on a paper or polyacrylamide gel soaked in a suitable buffer, and then applying an appropriate voltage across the paper or gel for a certain period of time. The components of the sample move to different positions along the paper or gel medium, depending on their charge and ionic mobility. After electrophoresis, the distribution of activity along the strip or gel column can be determined by a counter or a radiochromatographic scanner. The latter cannot be used, however, for the gel electrophoresis column because they are technically incompatible. Since protein molecules become charged in buffer solutions above or below their isoelectric pH, most proteins can be separated by this method with the use of appropriate buffers. If the amount of carrier is sufficient, color formation between the sample and a suitable reagent (e.g., ninhydrin in the case of proteins and amino acids) can be used advantageously in the development of an electrophoretogram. For example, a good separation of free iodide and radio-iodinated proteins can be achieved by electrophoresis in buffer.

Ion Exchange

Ion exchange is performed by passing a sample of a radiopharmaceutical through a column of ionic resin and eluting the column with suitable solvents. Separation of different species in a sample is effected by the exchange of ions from the solution onto the resin and their relative affinity for this exchange under certain physicochemical conditions.

Resins are polymerized, high molecular weight, insoluble electrolytes. They consist of two components: a large, heavy, polymeric ion and an oppositely charged small ion that is exchangeable with other ions in solution in contact with the resin. There are two kinds of ion-exchange resins: cation-exchange resins, which have small cations, and anion-exchange resins, which have small anions. Typical examples of cation exchange and anion exchange reactions are illustrated below:

$$\text{Cation exchange: } R - H + Na^+ \rightarrow R - Na + H^+$$

$$\text{Anion exchange: } R - OH + Cl^- \rightarrow R - Cl + OH^-$$

Cation-exchange resins contain carboxylates, silicates, and sulfonate groups. Dowex-50 is an example of this kind of resin. Anion-exchange resins include quaternary ammonium compounds, and Dowex-1 is an example of this type. Pore size and cross-linkage of the resin affect the ion-exchange separation of different components in a sample.

The ion-exchange method is useful in radiochemistry. In nuclear pharmacy, the presence of $^{99m}TcO_4^-$ in ^{99m}Tc-labeled protein can be definitely determined by this method. $^{99m}TcO_4^-$ is adsorbed on Dowex-1 resin, and ^{99m}Tc-labeled protein and hydrolyzed ^{99m}Tc come through in the eluate when the column is washed with saline. Since the hydrolyzed ^{99m}Tc activity accompanies ^{99m}Tc-labeled protein in the elution, it remains undetected by this method. Another example of an application of the ion-exchange method is the removal of unreacted iodide from an iodination mixture. Iodide is retained by the anion-exchange resin, whereas iodinated protein is eluted with the solvent.

Solvent Extraction

In solvent extraction, a solution containing one or more chemical compounds is shaken with an immiscible liquid and separation of different compounds is effected by the preferential solubility of individual compounds in one solvent or another. Thus, different solutes distribute themselves between two immiscible liquid phases. The ratio of solubilities of a component in two phases is called the distribution or partition coefficient. The efficiency of solvent extraction of a compound from one solvent into another depends primarily on this partition coefficient.

Solvent extraction of $^{99m}TcO_4^-$ with MEK from $^{99}MoO_4^{2-}$ has been a successful method of avoiding various radiocontaminants in the ^{99m}Tc-eluate. The use of the solvent extraction method is limited in nuclear pharmacy because ITLC methods are generally more convenient.

High-Performance Liquid Chromatography

High-performance liquid chromatography (HPLC) is very important in the analysis of radiopharmaceutical samples, because it provides separation of components with high resolution. The general principles of HPLC are the same as those of the regular liquid chromatography. The basic difference lies in the dimensions of the columns and the size of the packing materials through which the samples are forced by electrical pumps. High resolution, speed of separation, and high recovery of solutes are the important advantages of HPLC.

The HPLC columns are heavy-walled tubes of glass or stainless steel 2 to 5 mm in internal diameter and between 15 and 30 cm in length and are packed with appropriate packing materials. In a typical HPLC method, a sample is injected by an injection valve or by a syringe/septum arrangement and then the eluent is pumped into the column under pressure (up to 6000 psi) at a precisely controlled rate. The eluate is passed on to a sensitive detector that monitors the concentration of different solutes in the sample. The detector response (proportional to the concentration of solutes) is plotted against time after injection of the sample, which is often called the retention time.

The packing material consists of very fine microparticulates with mean diameters between 5 and 10 μm for analytical HPLC and greater than 20 μm for preparative HPLC. The sample size should be optimally small (5–250 μl) for a given size column, since larger volumes decrease the resolution of chromatographic separation. Two types of pumps are available: constant flow rate pump and constant pressure pump.

Generally, HPLC methods can be used for many types of liquid chromatography such as molecular exclusion chromatography, ion-exchange chromatography, liquid–solid adsorption chromatography, liquid–liquid partition chromatography, and liquid–solid partition chromatography, the last one being the most common. In this type of chromatography, the stationary phase is a polymer chemically bonded to the surface of silica support. This polymer layer possesses partition properties similar to those of a stationary liquid of similar composition.

The HPLC methods are of two types: normal-phase and reverse-phase. In normal-phase HPLC, the packing material is polar in nature and is prepared by reacting the—OH groups of the silica surface with various reagents to give highly stable R—Si—C, R–Si—N or R—Si—O—C bonded materials. The standard bonded phase material is the siloxane (Si—O—Si—R) packing. By varying the nature of the polar functional group on the organic side chain, different selectivity can be imparted relative to the silica packing. The commonly used solvents in normal-phase HPLC are hexane, heptane, acetone, and other hydrocarbons, often mixed with small amounts of a more polar solvent. For a given application, solvent strength is varied by changing the concentration of the more polar solvent component. Samples of moderate to strong polarity are usually well separated by normal-phase HPLC.

In reverse-phase HPLC, the stationary phase consists of fully porous, silica microparticulates chemically bonded with alkyl chains and is relatively nonpolar in nature. The octyl-(C_8) and octadecyl-(C_{18}) hydrophobic phases bonded onto silica microparticulates have been the most widely used column packing materials. The latter is commonly noted as octadecylsilane (ODS or C_{18}) packing. The common mobile phases used in reverse-phase HPLC are polar solvents such as water, to which varying concentrations of miscible organics (e.g., methanol and acetonitrile) are added. Solvent strength is usually varied by changing the composition of the solvent mixture. Nonpolar to weakly polar compounds are well separated by reverse-phase HPLC.

Of various detectors used to monitor the concentration of various solutes in the eluate, the ultraviolet (UV) monitor and the radiation detector such as NaI(Tl) detector are most common. The UV monitor measures the absorbance of light in the eluate, which is proportional to the concentration of a solute present in the eluate. The radiation detector is used for measuring the concentration of radioactive components in the eluate. In the analysis of radiopharmaceuticals, both the UV monitor and radiation detector are often used for measuring the concentration of different components in a radiopharmaceutical.

A variety of compounds such as carbohydrates, drugs, proteins, fatty acids, and so on have been separated by HPLC methods. Reverse-phase HPLC has been a strong tool in the analysis of many radiopharmaceuticals.

Distillation

Two compounds with considerably different vapor pressure can be separated by simple distillation at a specific temperature. The compound with higher vapor pressure is distilled off first, leaving the other compound in the distilling flask. For example, iodide present as a contaminant in an iodination mixture can be oxidized to iodine and separated by distillation. Noble gases (^{133}Xe, ^{81}Kr, etc.) are separated by distillation.

Chemical Purity

The chemical purity of a radiopharmaceutical is the fraction of the material in the desired chemical form, whether or not all of it is in the labeled form. Chemical impurities arise from the breakdown of the material either before or after labeling, their inadvertent addition during labeling, and their undue accompaniment in the preparation of the compound. For example, aluminum is a chemical impurity in the ^{99m}Tc-eluate. The presence of a slight amount of globulins in the preparation of albumin is indicative of impurities in the latter. However, additives, acid, alkali, and buffers are not considered impurities.

The presence of chemical impurities before radiolabeling may result in undesirable labeled molecules that may or may not interfere with the diagnostic test. Undue chemical impurities may also cause a toxic effect. Purification of radiopharmaceuticals from these impurities is often carried out by methods of chemical separation such as precipitation, solvent extraction, ion exchange, and distillation.

Radioassay

The amount of radioactivity of a radiopharmaceutical before dispensing, as well as that of each individual dosage before administration to patients, must be determined. These activity determinations are carried out by means of an isotope dose calibrator described in Chapter 3. The performance of the dose calibrator must be checked by carrying out several quality control tests.

Dose Calibrator Quality Control

According to the NRC regulations, the following quality control tests must be performed at the frequencies indicated:

1. constancy (daily)
2. accuracy (at installation, annually, and after repairs)
3. linearity (at installation, quarterly, and after repairs)
4. geometry (at installation and after repairs).

Constancy

The constancy test indicates the reproducibility of measurements by a dose calibrator, and is performed by measuring the activity of a sealed source of a long-lived radionuclide (^{226}Ra, ^{137}Cs, or ^{57}Co) on frequently used settings in the dose calibrator. A deviation of the reading by more than $\pm 10\%$ of the calculated activity may indicate the malfunction of the dose calibrator and hence repair or replacement. The constancy test must be done daily and at other times, whenever the dose calibrator is used, using at least a 10 μCi

(370 kBq) or more ^{226}Ra or a 50 μCi (1.85 MBq) or more ^{137}Cs or ^{57}Co source.

Accuracy

The accuracy of a dose calibrator is determined by measuring the activities of at least two long-lived reference sources at their respective isotope settings, and comparing the measured activity with the stated activity. The measured activity must agree with the stated activity within $\pm 10\%$. Otherwise, the dose calibrator needs repair as replacement.

The activity of the reference sources must be accurate within $\pm 5\%$ and one of them must have energy between 100 keV and 500 keV. These sources are available from the National Institute of Standards and Technology and other manufacturers whose standards are of equal accuracy. The typical reference sources are ^{57}Co, ^{133}Ba and ^{137}Cs.

Linearity

The linearity test indicates the dose calibrator's ability to measure the activity accurately over a wide range of values. Normally, dose calibrators exhibit a linear response for activities up to 200 mCi (7.4 GBq) to 2 Ci (74 GBq), depending on the chamber geometry and the electronics of the dose calibrator, and tend to underestimate at higher activities. The linearity test must be carried out over the range of activities from the higest dosage administered to the patient down to 30 μCi (1.11 MBq). Two common methods for checking the linearity of the dose calibrator are described below:

Decay Method. In this method of linearity check, a source of ^{99m}Tc is usually used, the activity of which is at least equal to the highest dosage normally administered to the patients in a given institution. The source is then assayed in the dose calibrator at 0 hr and then every 6 hr during the working hours everyday until the activity decays down to 30 μCi (1.11 MBq). The measured activities are plotted against time intervals on semilog paper and the "best fit" straight line is drawn through the data points (Fig. 8.4). The deviation of the point farthest from the line is calculated. If this deviation is more than $\pm 10\%$, the dose calibrator needs to be replaced or adjusted, or correction factors must be applied to activities when measured in nonlinear regions.

Shielding Method. This method is less time consuming and easy to perform. A commercial calibration kit used in this method contains seven concentric cylindrical tubes or "sleeves". The innermost tube is not lead-lined and therefore provides no attenuation of gamma radiations. The other six tubes are lead-lined with increasing thickness to simulate the various periods of decay. When these tubes are placed over the source of a radionuclide (normally ^{99m}Tc) in the dose calibrator, seven activity measurements

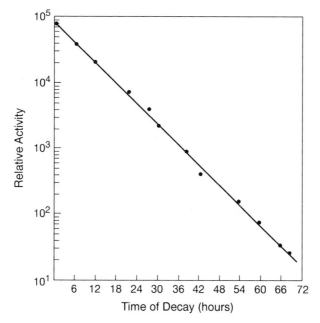

FIGURE 8.4. Plot of ^{99m}Tc activity versus time for the linearity check of the dose calibrator.

represent activities at different times. From the first time measurements, calibration factors are established for each tube by dividing the innermost tube reading by each outer tube reading. For subsequent linearity tests, identical measurements are made by the kit using a source of the same radionuclide. Each tube measurement is then corrected by the corresponding calibration factor to give identical values for all tubes. The average of these values is calculated. If each individual tube measurement falls within $\pm 10\%$ of the average value, the dose calibrator is supposed to be functioning linearly; otherwise it needs to be replaced or adjusted or to apply correction factors.

It should be pointed out that before the linearity test by the shielding method can be instituted, the dose calibrator linearity must be established first by the decay method.

Geometry

Variations in sample volumes or geometric configurations of the container can affect the accuracy of measurements in a dose calibrator because of the attenuation of radiations, particularly the weak gamma radiations such as those of ^{125}I and ^{201}Tl. Thus, the same activity in different volumes [1 mCi (37 MBq) in 1 ml or 1 mCi (37 MBq) in 30 ml], in different containers (3-cc syringe or 10-cc syringe or 10-ml vial) or in containers of different materials (glass or plastic) may give different readings in the dose calibrators. Correction factors must be established for changes in volume or container configuration while measuring the activity of the radionuclide in question and must be applied to similar measurements, if the difference exceeds $\pm 10\%$.

Measurement of Radioactivity

Radioactivity of a radiopharmaceutical is measured by placing the sample inside the dose calibrator with the appropriate isotope selector setting. The reading is displayed in appropriate units (curie or becqurel) on the dial. Corrections are applied whenever necessary.

Radioactivity can also be measured in a well-type NaI(Tl) counter. However, high-activity samples must be diluted before counting so that there is no loss of counts due to deadtime. Normally, the radioactivity should be 1 μCi (37 kBq) or less per sample. Furthermore, the well counter must be calibrated before measurement of radioactivity. Readers are referred to standard books on physics and instrumentation for details of calibration techniques.

Biological Tests

Biological tests are carried out essentially to examine the sterility, apyrogenicity, and toxicity of radiopharmaceuticals before human administration. These tests for radiopharmaceuticals are identical to those for conventional pharmaceuticals. It should be realized that it is quite possible for a particular radiopharmaceutical solution to be sterile but still be highly pyrogenic when injected into patients. While radiopharmaceuticals become asterile due to bacterial, fungal, and yeast growth, pyrogenicity arises from certain metabolic byproducts (endotoxin) of these microorganisms. The tests for sterility, pyrogenicity, and toxicity are discussed below in some detail.

Sterility

Sterility indicates the absence of any viable bacteria or microorganisms in a radiopharmaceutical preparation. As already mentioned, all preparations for human administration must be sterilized by suitable methods that depend on the nature of the product, the solvent, and various additives.

Methods of Sterilization

Autoclaving

In autoclaving, the radiopharmaceutical is sterilized by heating in steam at 121°C under a pressure of 18 pounds per square inch (psi) for 15 to 20 min. This type of terminal steam sterilization kills microorganisms present in radiopharmaceutical solutions. Autoclaving is suitable only for thermostable aqueous solutions, whereas oil-based preparations and heat-labile radiopharmaceuticals such as some ^{99m}Tc-labeled preparations and iodinated proteins cannot withstand autoclaving because the molecule is damaged by heat. Autoclaving is not suitable for short-lived radionuclides such as ^{13}N and ^{18}F because the method takes too long. Thermostable radiopharmaceuticals include ^{99m}Tc-pertechnetate, ^{111}In-DTPA, ^{67}Ga-gallium citrate, and ^{111}In-indium chloride. These compounds may also be sterilized by dry-heat sterilization and sometimes by irradiation with γ rays.

Various types of autoclaves are available commercially. For a nuclear pharmacy, autoclaving can be performed in pressure-cooker–type autoclaves equipped with a thermometer and a pressure gauge.

Membrane Filtration

Membrane filtration consists of simply filtering the radiopharmaceutical through a membrane filter that removes various organisms by a sieving mechanism. Commercially available Millipore filters are membrane filters made of cellulose esters, and are available in various pore sizes and disposable units. A typical Millipore filter is shown in Figure 8.5. The most common membrane filter size is 0.45 μm, but a smaller pore size of 0.22 μm is necessary for the sterilization of blood products and preparations suspected of contamination with smaller microorganisms.

This is the most common method of sterilization in nuclear pharmacy and is the method of choice for short-lived radionuclides and heat-labile radiopharmaceuticals. In actual practice, if the volume of the radiopharmaceutical is small, then the solution is drawn in a syringe, a membrane filter is attached to the tip of the syringe (Fig. 8.5), and the volume is discharged through the filter into an aseptic container. In the case of larger volumes of

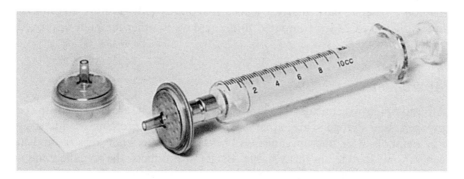

FIGURE 8.5. Millipore filter unit for sterilization of various radiopharmaceuticals. (Courtesy of Millipore Corporation, Bedford, Massachussetts.)

radiopharmaceuticals, a leak-proof cylindrical unit fitted with a membrane filter and a movable plunger is used.

Another type of filter, Nuclepore, is available and is used conveniently for the determination of particle size in colloidal preparations.

Sterility Testing

Sterility testing is performed to prove that radiopharmaceuticals are essentially free of viable microorganisms. These tests must be performed aseptically so that external bacteria are not added to the test samples during the procedure. A laminar-flow hood is preferable, and personnel performing these tests should be well trained.

According to the *USP 26*, sterility tests are performed by incubating the radiopharmaceutical sample in fluid thioglycollate medium at 30° to 35°C for 14 days. Another test uses soybean-casein digest medium for incubation at 20° to 25 °C for 14 days. The sample volume for the test should be at least as great as that for a human dosage. If bacterial growth is observed in either test, the radiopharmaceutical is considered to be asterile.

Since sterility testing frequently takes longer than the half-lives of many common short-lived radionuclides such as ^{99m}Tc, these radiopharmaceutical preparations are tested for sterility on a post hoc basis. In these cases, the product in question is released for human use provided the manufacturer has already established its sterility and apyrogenicity at the production level.

Another in vitro sterility test uses the metabolism of ^{14}C-glucose by microorganisms present in the material under test. The basic principle of the test involves the addition of the test sample to a trypticase soybroth culture medium containing ^{14}C-glucose, then incubation, and finally collection and radioassay of ^{14}CO$_2$ formed by the metabolism of microorganisms, if present, in the sample. Radioassay is done with a gas ionization chamber and both aerobic and anaerobic microorganisms can be detected by this method. Automated instruments using this principle are commercially available. This method is useful, particularly because it requires only a short amount of time, about 3 to 24 hr, compared to many days in other methods approved by the *USP*.

Apyrogenicity

All radiopharmaceuticals for human administration are required to be pyrogen free. Pyrogens are either polysaccharides or proteins produced by the metabolism of microorganisms. They are 0.05 to 1 μm in size, and in general, are soluble and heat stable. Bacterial products, the so-called endotoxins, are the prime examples of pyrogens, but various chemicals also can add pyrogens to a radiopharmaceutical solution. Following administration, pyrogens produce symptoms of fever, chills, malaise, leukopenia, pain in joints, flushing, sweating, headache, and dilation of the pupils. Pyrogenic reactions can develop in subjects within 30 min to 2 hr after administration, but usually subside in 10 to 12 hr after onset. These reactions are rarely fatal.

As already mentioned, sterility of a solution does not guarantee its apyrogenicity nor does sterilization destroy the pyrogens in a radiopharmaceutical. There is no specific method for making a sample apyrogenic. Since pyrogens arise mainly from the metabolism of bacteria, the best recourse to prevent pyrogenic contamination is to use sterile glassware, solutions, and equipment under aseptic conditions in any preparation procedure. Glassware can be made pyrogen free by hot-air sterilization at 175°C for several hours. One must use high-quality chemicals, distilled water, and glassware to avoid pyrogens. If one uses all these materials conforming to USP specifications and is absolutely meticulous in carrying out chemical manipulations, then pyrogen-free radiopharmaceuticals can be prepared without difficulty.

Pyrogenicity Testing

USP Rabbit Test

The *USP 26* bases the pyrogen test on the febrile response in rabbits within 3 hr after injection of the material. Three mature normal rabbits weighing not less than 1.5 kg are chosen for the test, and their temperatures are controlled by keeping them in an area of uniform temperature. The volume of the test sample must be an equivalent human dosage, on a weight basis, and often 3 to 10 times the human dosage by volume is used to achieve a greater safety factor. The test sample is injected into the ear vein of each of the three rabbits. The rectal temperatures of the animals are measured 1, 2, and 3 hr after injection of the test material. If the rise in temperature in individual animals is less than 0.6°C and if the sum of the temperature rises in all three animals does not exceed 1.4°C, then the test sample is considered apyrogenic. If any of the above conditions is not fulfilled, the test must be repeated with five more rabbits. If not more than three of the total eight animals show a temperature rise of 0.6°C or more individually and if the sum of the individual temperature rises does not exceed 3.7°C, the material is considered pyrogen free.

LAL Test

A more sophisticated and rapid method, called the limulus amebocyte lysate (LAL) test, is employed for the detection of endotoxin-type pyrogens. This method uses the lysate of amebocytes from the blood of the horseshoe crab, *Limulus polyphemus*. The principle of the test is based on the formation of an opaque gel by pyrogens upon incubating the sample with the LAL at 37°C. An assay mixture usually consists of 0.1 ml LAL and a test sample at pH 6 to 8. The reaction takes place within 15 to 60 min after mixing and depends on the concentration of pyrogens. The formation of a gel indicates the presence of pyrogens. The thicker the gel, the greater the concentration of pyrogens in the sample. This LAL test is officially termed as the bacterial endotoxin test (BET) in the *USP 26*.

The LAL is commercially available in lyophilized form in a kit. It should be stored at 5°C. In the kit, in addition to LAL, *Escherichia coli* endotoxin and pure water are supplied as the standards that are used to check the sensitivity of the test. The sensitivity of the test is given in endotoxin units (EU). The LAL test is conducted on unknown samples as well as on *E. coli* endotoxin and water samples. Usually 0.1 ml of the sample and LAL are incubated at 37°C for 60 min. If the *E. coli* endotoxin sample shows gel formation (positive control) and the water sample shows no gel formation (negative control), then unknown samples are considered positive or negative depending on whether they form gel or not.

The U.S. FDA has approved the LAL test for endotoxin-type pyrogens. However, two requirements must be met for acceptance of the test as official. First, a concentration limit (EU/ml or EU/mg) and a maximum dosage (ml/kg or mg/kg) to be administered to humans must be assigned to each parenteral drug including radiopharmaceuticals. For drugs without such concentration limits, manufacturers must establish the limit using proper LAL tests before FDA approval. For all radiopharmaceuticals, the endotoxin concentration limit is 175/V USP EU per ml of injection per kg, where V is the maximum recommended total dosage in ml at the expiration date or time. Second, the LAL test must be validated against an FDA-approved reference standard of endotoxin. For validation, an inhibition and enhancement test must be included in the procedure to ascertain the effect of ingredients in the sample on the LAL procedure. The maximum permissible dosage for parenteral administration (except intrathecal) is 5.0 EU/kg, whereas it is 0.2 EU/kg for intrathecal administration.

Alcoholic solvents cause precipitation of the lysate and therefore must be avoided. Several proteins at high concentrations tend to produce gel even without endotoxin and should be diluted to appropriate concentrations before the test. Calcium ions are essential for gel formation in the LAL test. When metal chelates such as chelates of ^{99m}Tc and ^{111}In are tested for pyrogens, the free chelating agents may remove by complexation calcium ions from the test sample leaving insufficient or no Ca^{2+} ions for gel formation. Thus, before LAL testing, additional amounts of Ca^{2+} ions should be added to samples of metal chelates to complex all unbound chelating agents. This will leave sufficient Ca^{2+} for gel formation in the test sample.

Toxicity

Before any radiopharmaceutical is approved for human use, as with any other drug, its toxic effect and safe dosage must be established. Toxic effects due to radiopharmaceutical administration include alterations in the histology or physiologic functions of different organs in the body or even death. These tests for acute or chronic toxicity can be carried out in various animals such as mice, rats, rabbits, and dogs. Typically they involve the administration of the radiopharmaceutical in certain dosage to animals for 2 to 6 weeks. The animals are sacrificed at various time intervals, and then a detailed autopsy examination of different organs is performed to observe any pathologic changes.

A quantity, called the $LD_{50/60}$, describes the toxic effect of a radiopharmaceutical; it is the dosage required to produce 50% mortality in 60 days in any species after administration of the radiopharmaceutical. For determination of the $LD_{50/60}$, the test substance is injected in increasing dosages into a large group of animals. The dosage at which 50% mortality of the animals is observed in 60 days following administration is established as the $LD_{50/60}$ for the material. The test must be carried out in at least two species of animals. From these studies, a safety factor is established, which should be as large as practicable for human use. It must be borne in mind that following the administration of drugs different animal species react differently from humans, and these species differences must be taken into consideration when the safety dosage of a radiopharmaceutical is determined for humans.

In most radiopharmaceuticals, toxicity arises from the pharmaceutical part of the radiopharmaceutical, not from the radionuclide part, because the latter in diagnostic dosages does not cause severe toxic effects. Since the quantity of radiopharmaceuticals used is usually small, the toxic effect is minimal. Because of strict regulations on the use of animals for research, nowadays toxicity is preferably studied using cell culture and computer modeling rather than in animals.

Record Keeping

In a radiopharmaceutical operation, record keeping is mandatory for legal reasons as well as for tracing any faulty preparation in the case of a poor-quality scan. These records help trace the history of a particular radiopharmaceutical should any untoward effect take place in a patient due to its administration. In some institutions, records are kept on separate sheets for each individual product, whereas in others a single log book is used in which a separate section is reserved for each individual product. Details of record keeping are given in Chapters 9 and 11.

Questions

1. What are quality control tests and why are they needed for a radiopharmaceutical?
2. Define radionuclidic purity and give some examples. Is ^{99}Mo in a ^{99m}Tc-labeled compound a radionuclidic or radiochemical impurity? Describe how the radionuclidic impurity can be estimated.

3. Define the radiochemical purity of a radiopharmaceutical. How do radiochemical impurities originate? Describe various methods of determining the radiochemical impurity in a radiopharmaceutical.
4. What are the three radioactive species in a ^{99m}Tc-radiopharmaceutical? Explain their origin.
5. For ^{99m}Tc-radiopharmaceuticals. ITLC methods are routinely used to detect radiochemical impurities. Which solvent and solid phase system is most common for this purpose and why?
6. An ITLC of a ^{99m}Tc-MDP sample was made with ITLC-SG paper and acetone. The strip was cut in the middle; the activity in the solvent front portion was found to be 3500 cpm and in the origin portion 38,000 cpm. Calculate the yield and impurity in percent. What is this impurity? Is the sample at origin after chromatography pure ^{99m}Tc-MDP?
7. If the experiment in Question 6 were performed with saline, what would be the results?
8. Describe the methods of sterilization and sterility testing.
9. What are pyrogens and their reaction symptoms? Describe the rabbit test and LAL test for pyrogens.
10. Define the $LD_{50/60}$ of a radiopharmaceutical. How can you determine this quantity?

Suggested Reading

Avis KE, Leuchuk JW. Parental Preparations. In: *Remington: The Science and Practice of Pharmacy*. 20th ed. Baltimore, MD: Lippincott, Williams and Wilkins; 2000:780.

Bobinet DD, Williams GC, Cohen MB. Comparison of commercial pyrogen testing laboratories. *Am J Hosp Pharm*. 1976; 33:801.

Dewanjee MK. The chemistry of ^{99m}Tc-labeled radiopharmaceuticals. *Semin Nucl Med* 1990; 20:5.

Eckelman WC, Levenson SM, Johnston GS. Radiochemical purity of ^{99m}Tc-radiopharmaceuticals. *Appl Radiol*. 1977; 6:211.

Guideline on validation of the Limulus Amebocyte Lysate test as an end-product endotoxin test for human and animal parenteral drugs, biological products, and medical devices. Rockville, MD; U.S. FDA; 1987.

Krogsgaard OW. Radiochemical purity of various ^{99m}Tc-labelled bone-scanning agents. *Eur J Nucl Med*. 1976; 1:15.

Pauwels EKJ, Feitsma RIJ. Radiochemical quality control of ^{99m}Tc-labeled radiopharmaceuticals. *Eur J Nucl Med*. 1977; 2:97.

Robbins PJ. Chromatography of technetium ^{99m}Tc-radiopharmaceuticals—a practical guide. New York: Society of Nuclear Medicine; 1984.

U.S. Pharmacopeia 26 & National Formulary 21 United States Pharmacopeial Convention, Rockville, MD: 2003.

9
Nuclear Pharmacy

Concept

We generally come across two terms in the literature: *nuclear pharmacy* and *radiopharmacy*. Is there any difference between the two? In my opinion, there is no difference between the two terms and they can be used interchangeably. The use of one term or the other is a matter of individual choice. The term *nuclear pharmacy* will be used in this chapter.

In a nuclear pharmacy radiopharmaceuticals are prepared, stored, and dispensed primarily for human use, just as regular drugs are in a pharmacy. The nuclear pharmacy is staffed with trained personnel such as radiopharmacists and radiochemists, that is, chemists or pharmacists with special training in radiopharmaceutical chemistry. The nuclear pharmacy may serve as a center for education and training of pharmacy and nuclear medicine technology students and engage in basic research in the design and development of new radiopharmaceuticals. Here the remedy for any adverse reaction in humans due to the administration of radiopharmaceuticals is sought and found. The nuclear pharmacists can provide education and consultation to the patients and health care personnel in this field.

Design of a Nuclear Pharmacy

Several common problems should be kept in mind when designing a nuclear pharmacy unit. Protection of personnel from radiation hazard, avoidance of contamination of work area and radiation-detection instruments, clean air circulation in the dispensing area, and disposal of radioactive waste are the common concerns. The design of a nuclear pharmacy should take into account daily operational protocols, proper utilization of available space, and provisions for future growth.

A nuclear pharmacy should be located within or near the nuclear medicine department because there is a close relationship between the two units. The nuclear pharmacy area can be as small as a 12×12 ft ($4\,\text{m} \times 4\,\text{m}$)

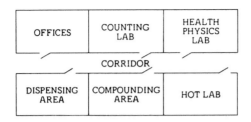

OFFICES	COUNTING LAB	HEALTH PHYSICS LAB
CORRIDOR		
DISPENSING AREA	COMPOUNDING AREA	HOT LAB

FIGURE 9.1. Conceptual design of a nuclear pharmacy unit.

room, depending on the volume of the operation. For a larger operation, the unit may consist of several rooms. Ideally, it should have enough space for accommodating offices, a counting room, and a health physics laboratory on one side of a corridor, and a high radiation (hot lab) laboratory, a compounding room, a storeroom, and a dispensing area on the other side. A conceptual design of a nuclear pharmacy unit is presented in Figure 9.1. The whole area should have minimal access to the public and the patient in order to avoid radiation hazard. Many institutions have a designated area for the storage and disposal of radioactive waste from all departments, and the nuclear pharmacy can share this facility for its own storage and waste disposal. The daily transfer of radioactive waste to a central area for storage and disposal eliminates high levels of radiation in the nuclear pharmacy.

The laboratory area where compounding and dispensing are done should be equipped with workbenches made of stainless steel or wood covered with laminated plastic. The floor should be made of removable tiles or be covered with rubber matting; in the event of spillage the contaminated tiles or rubber matting can be readily replaced with new ones. In each laboratory there should be an appropriate number of stainless steel sinks deep enough to prevent splashing and fitted with foot control. Each laboratory should have exhaust fumehoods fitted with filters to absorb gaseous and particulate radioactive materials, particularly radioiodine and radioxenon. A laminar flow hood should be installed in the dispensing area for a sterile environment. The storage area should be well built with thick concrete walls, and the walls of the storage safes should be lined with lead for radiation shielding. A safety shower and an eye-wash should be installed for use in the case of major body contamination.

Various pieces of equipment are essential for good operation of nuclear pharmacy. Examples are (1) a dose calibrator capable of measuring various types and levels of radioactivity, (2) chromatography equipment, (3) radiation survey meters, (4) an area monitor, (5) a pH meter, (6) a light microscope for particle size determination, (7) a NaI(Tl) or Ge(Li) detector coupled to a multichannel analyzer to identify contaminants in radiopharmaceuticals, (8) lead-lined refrigerators and freezers to store cold kits and radiopharmaceuticals under refrigeration, (9) a hot water bath, (10) a dry heat oven, and (11) a well-type NaI(Tl) counter equipped with an automatic sample changer for counting many samples. In addition, lead

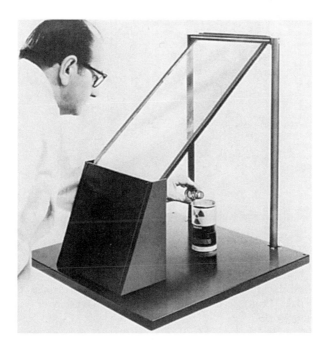

FIGURE 9.2. Lead barrier shield, behind which all formulations and manipulations of radioactive materials are carried out. (Courtesy of Nuclear Associates, Division of Victoreen, Inc., Carle Place, New York.)

barrier shields (Fig. 9.2) are essential for handling radioactive materials behind them. A sufficient number of lead containers of various designs to accommodate vials and syringes containing radioactivity are important for transporting radioactive materials (Fig. 9.3). Syringe shields are essential for injection for radiation protection unless contraindicated (Fig. 9.4). Lead-lined or leaded gloves, aprons, and eyeglasses are essential pieces of radiation safety equipment in any nuclear pharmacy operation. An autoclave is needed to sterilize certain materials in nuclear pharmacy, and a freeze-dryer would serve to lyophilize materials, if needed. An incubator is useful for incubation in sterility testing of radiopharmaceuticals. Certain basic equipment such as a balance, a centrifuge, pipetters, and a calculator should be available in nuclear pharmacy.

Various software packages that are used to manage the operation of nuclear pharmacies are available from several vendors. These programs are primarily used for record keeping of data related to nuclear pharmacy. Data such as logging of shipments, preparation of radiopharmaceuticals, dispensing of radiopharmaceuticals, and waste disposal can be stored in these programs. Survey and wipe test results and patient data also can be saved in these programs. All nuclear pharmacies should have these programs available for management of nuclear pharmacies.

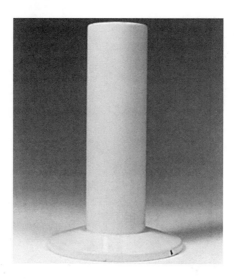

FIGURE 9.3. Lead-shield syringe holder for transporting the syringes containing radioactive material. (Courtesy of Nuclear Associates, Division of Victoreen, Inc., Carle Place, New York.)

Operation of a Nuclear Pharmacy

The daily operation of a nuclear pharmacy involves the following steps: (1) receiving of radioactive materials, (2) preparation of radiopharmaceuticals, (3) quality control tests of radiopharmaceuticals, (4) storage, (5) dispensing, (6) radioactive waste disposal, and (7) infectious waste disposal.

Before the day's operation is begun, the nuclear pharmacist must ensure that all equipment in the nuclear pharmacy such as the dose calibrator, survey meter, and NaI(Tl) well counter are in good operating condition.

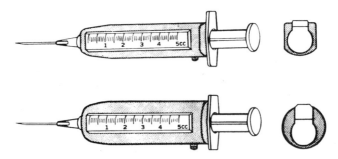

FIGURE 9.4. Syringe shields (Courtesy of Nuclear Associates, Division of Victoreen, Inc., Carle Place, New York.)

This is accomplished by proper calibration of each device with standard radioactive sources (e.g., ^{137}Cs, ^{226}Ra, ^{57}Co, etc.). If a malfunction is noted in any instrument, it must be remedied before any measurement is made. All personnel in the nuclear pharmacy must wear a laboratory coat and gloves while handling radioactive materials. A pair of long tongs should be used in the handling of high activity, preferably behind a lead barrier shield.

Receiving and Monitoring of Radioactive Packages

Individual users or institutions are authorized to possess and use radioactive materials upon issuance of a radioactive material license by the NRC or the Agreement State Agency (see Chapter 11). The suppliers require documentation of licensing of the user as to the types and limits of quantities of radioactive material before shipping. Normally, delivery of radioactive shipments is made directly to the nuclear medicine department or nuclear pharmacy because of the short half-lives of various radionuclides. In some institutions, radioactive shipments are delivered to the Radiation Safety Office, which then disburses to the respective user after the proper monitoring of the package for external exposure and contamination.

Monitoring of packages is required according to 10CFR20 if the packages are labeled as containing radioactive material, and is described in detail in Chapter 11. Briefly, the packages should be monitored within 3 hr if delivered during normal hours, or within 3 hr from the beginning of the next working day if delivered after working hours. The survey must be done on the surface of the package and at 1 m, using a GM survey meter and the readings should not exceed the limits of 200 mR/hr and 10 mR/hr, respectively. The wipe test of the package surface must be done according to 10CFR20 (see Chapter 11) and the limit for the test is 0.003 μCi (6600 dpm or 111 Bq) per 300 cm^2. All data must be entered in the receipt book (Fig. 9.5).

Preparation of Radiopharmaceuticals

All formulating should be carried out in a laminar flow hood and under aseptic conditions. Work should be done behind the lead barrier shields, and gloves should be worn for handling radioactivity.

Many radiopharmaceuticals, particularly ^{99m}Tc-labeled radiopharmaceuticals, are prepared daily for nuclear medicine tests. A few ^{123}I-labeled compounds such as ^{123}I-MIBG and fatty acids are labeled on site because they are not normally available from the commercial firm. For ^{99m}Tc-labeled radiopharmaceuticals, the ^{99m}Tc activity is eluted from the Moly generator daily early in the morning. After assaying in the dose calibrator and performing the tests for molybdenum breakthrough, aluminum breakthrough, pH, and radiochemical purity by chromatography, the ^{99m}Tc vial is identified with a label containing the information as to the total activity, concen-

RADIOISOTOPE RECEIPT FORM

Isotope-Chemical	Mfr.	Lot No.	No. of Vials	Total Vol. (ml)	Date Received	Date of Calib.	Activity Theoretical	Activity Measured	*Survey at Surface at 1 meter	Wipe Test ⊕ or ⊙	Received By

FIGURE 9.5. Typical radionuclide receipt form.

NUCLEAR PHARMACY/NUCLEAR MEDICINE
MOLY GENERATOR ELUTION FORM

Date of Calibration:

Activity:

Manuf. Lot No.:

DAY	DATE	TIME	ACTIVITY (mCi)	VOLUME (ml)	Mo-99 (μCi)	Mo-99/Tc-99m (μCi/mCi) A.L. $\geq$ 0.0425	Al $^{3+}$	Tc-99m LOT No.	TECH. NAME
MONDAY									
TUESDAY									
WEDNESDAY									
THURSDAY									
FRIDAY									
SATURDAY									
SUNDAY									

FIGURE 9.6. Typical log sheet for ^{99m}Tc-eluate.

tration, time of calibration, and a nuclear pharmacy control number. This information should be recorded on the generator control sheet (Fig. 9.6).

^{99m}Tc-labeled radiopharmaceuticals are prepared using kits from various manufacturers. The total ^{99m}Tc activity to be added to the kit vial depends on the number of patients and their scheduled time for the study. Sufficient activity must be added to allow for decay for the latter situations. Sometimes, the ^{99m}Tc eluate needs to be diluted because of the high concentration and it should be done with isotonic saline without preservative. Caution should be exercised not to introduce air in the vial. Most ^{99m}Tc-labeled preparations are made by simply mixing the kit contents with ^{99m}Tc activity. In some formulations, sequential addition of different ingredients are needed, and in others, heating of the contents is required. After reconstitution, a control number is assigned to the kit vial. A label with information such as control number, product name, concentration, date and time of calibration, and expiration is pasted on the lead container. A radiation label is also placed on the container. The above information as well as other items such as manufacturer's control number for the kits, saline if used for dilution, the volume of saline, and so forth are also recorded in a log book (Fig. 9.7).

Quality Control of Radiopharmaceuticals

Each radiopharmaceutical must pass several quality control tests before dispensing for human administration. Regular checks should be made for the sterility, apyrogenicity, and radiochemical purity of all labeled products. Commercial vendors often guarantee the quality and efficacy of labeled compounds and in those situations, rigorous quality control tests are not needed. However, ^{99m}Tc-labeled radiopharmaceuticals are prepared daily and the labeling efficiency must be determined by thin-layer or paper chromatography (see Chapter 8). Preparations with poor labeling should be discarded. Colloidal and macroaggregated preparations must be checked for particle size and preparations with inappropriate particle size must be discarded. New radiopharmaceuticals and investigational drugs require sterility and pyrogen testing besides radiochemical purity. For short-lived radionuclides, the sterility and pyrogen tests can be conducted on an "after-the-fact" basis. Such radiopharmaceuticals are administered to humans, while the biological tests are continued until the final results are obtained. If the results are positive, the subject is then followed up for any symptoms for which remedial medications are instituted.

Storage

All radiopharmaceuticals should be properly stored so that they are not degraded by light or temperature. For example, ^{99m}Tc-labeled macroaggregated albumin should be stored at 2° to 4 °C to prevent any bacterial growth and denaturation of proteins, whereas ^{99m}Tc-sulfur colloid can be stored at room temperature without any adverse effect.

Since radiation exposure is a serious problem in the nuclear pharmacy, the vials or syringes containing radiopharmaceuticals must be stored in lead containers or behind lead shields. In many institutions, lead safes are built into the walls of the room for storage of radioactive materials. To prevent

Tc-99m RADIOPHARMACEUTICAL RECORD

Date	Time	NP No	Tc-99m Pertechnetate				Kit Data						Saline			Total* Vol. (ml)	Conc. (mCi/ml)	Prep'd By
			Mfr.	Lot No	Activity (mCi)	Vol. (ml)	Type	Mfr.	Vol. (ml)	Lot No.	Mfr.	Lot No.	Vol. (ml)				

FIGURE 9.7. ^{99m}Tc-labeled radiopharmaceutical preparation record sheet.

the production of bremsstrahlung in high Z materials such as lead, ^{32}P-labeled compounds and ^{89}Sr-SrCl$_2$ are stored in low Z material containers such as plastic or lucite containers.

Dispensing

Dispensing starts with a prescription or a hospital requisition made by a written physician for a nuclear medicine study for a patient. In the case of a centralized nuclear pharmacy (see later), a verbal order by telephone can replace a written prescription. Each prescription or requisition should contain patient's name and identification number (clinic or hospital number), age, the date, the type of study, the type and dosage of radiopharmaceutical, and the signature of the authorized user physician.

In many institutions, the dosages for many routine nuclear medicine studies are standardized, such as 20 mCi (740 MBq) ^{99m}Tc-MDP for whole-body bone imaging, and 4 mCi (148 MBq) ^{99m}Tc-MAA for lung imaging and therefore, may be omitted in a prescription. A list of these standardized dosages should be readily available in the nuclear pharmacy. Before a dosage is drawn, the volume to be drawn is calculated from the knowledge of the concentration and the date and time of calibration by means of a decay table for the radionuclide in question. The required volume is then drawn in a syringe aseptically behind the lead barrier shield and the final dosage is assayed in the dose calibrator. Often, radiopharmaceutical dosages are drawn precalibrated. As a mater of policy, the dosages drawn should not deviate by more than $\pm 10\%$ from the calculated dosages. The syringe containing the dosage is labeled as to its content and quantity and then placed in a lead syringe holder. If the syringe label is not visible from outside, the holder must be labeled. If the dosage is to be transported to a distant institution, it should be recalibrated on arrival. Proper decay correction must be made for the time during the first and second calibrations.

Each time a radiopharmaceutical dosage is dispensed, the date and time of dispensing, the patient's name and identification number, the name, quantity, and control number of the radiopharmaceutical, and the name of the individual dispensing the dosage must be entered in the radiopharmaceutical dispensing record book (Fig. 9.8).

In a centralized nuclear pharmacy, the patient's name, the physician's name and a prescription number are given to each dosage of a radiopharmaceutical dispensed. The receiving institution must enter all pertinent information in the record book.

Pediatric Dosages

The metabolism, biodistribution, and excretion of drugs are different in children from those in adults and, therefore, radiopharmaceutical dosages for children must be adjusted. Several methods and formulas have been

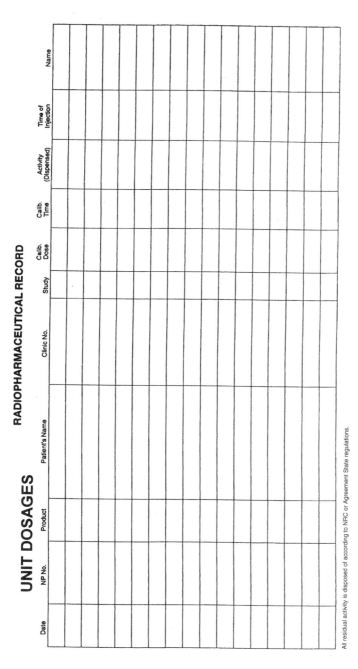

FIGURE 9.8. ^{99m}Tc-labeled radiopharmaceutical dispensing record sheet.

TABLE 9.1. Fraction of adult administered dosages for pediatric administration.

Weight in kg (lb)	Fraction	Weight in kg (lb)	Fraction
3 (6.6)	0.1	28 (61.6)	0.58
4 (8.8)	0.14	30 (66.0)	0.62
8 (17.6)	0.23	32 (70.4)	0.65
10 (22.0)	0.27	34 (74.8)	0.68
12 (26.4)	0.32	36 (79.2)	0.71
14 (30.8)	0.36	38 (83.6)	0.73
16 (35.2)	0.40	40 (88.0)	0.76
18 (39.6)	0.44	42 (92.4)	0.78
20 (44.0)	0.46	44 (96.8)	0.80
22 (48.4)	0.50	46 (101.2)	0.83
24 (52.8)	0.53	48 (105.6)	0.85
26 (57.2)	0.56	50 (110.0)	0.88

Adapted from Paediatric Task Group European Association Nuclear Medicine Members. A radiopharmaceuticals schedule for imaging in paediatrics. *Eur J Nucl Med.* 1990;17:127.

reported on pediatric dosage calculations based on body weight, body surface area, combination of weight and area, and simple ratios of adult dosages. The calculation based on body surface area is more accurate for pediatric dosages. The body surface area of an average adult is 1.73 m^2 and proportional to the 0.7 power of the body weight. Based on this information, the Paediatric Task Group European Association Nuclear Medicine Members published the fractions of the adult dosages needed for the children, which are tabulated in Table 9.1. However, for most nuclear studies, there is a minimum dosage required for a meaningful scan, which is primarily established in each institution based on experience.

Radioactive Waste Disposal

Radioactive waste generated in nuclear medicine and nuclear pharmacy (e.g., syringes, vials, needles, contaminated papers, tissues, etc.) is disposed of according to the methods outlined in 10CFR20 and 10CFR35 (see Chapter 11). These methods include decay-in-storage, release into sewerage system, incineration, and burial in a landfill. Because of the use of radionuclides with short half-lives, most of the radioactive waste in nuclear medicine is disposed of by the decay-in-storage method. In institutions where unit dosages are purchased from a central nuclear pharmacy, the syringes and vials with residual activities can be returned to the vendor who then disposes of them by following specific methods.

Although the columns of the ^{99}Mo–^{99m}Tc generators may be decayed to background for disposal to normal trash, a convenient method of disposing of these generators is to return them to the vendors who let them decay and later dispose of them. The out-of-use generators are packaged into the original shipping container, which is then properly labeled according to the instructions of the vendor. Normally, the generator is picked up by the authorized carrier when a new one is delivered.

Records must be maintained as to the date of storage,the amount stored and disposed, date of disposal, the meter used to monitor, and the name of the individual who is disposing.

Infectious Waste Disposal

In general, the states regulate the disposal of infectious waste containing body fluids, tissue, and other potentially infectious materials generated in health care institutions. Infectious waste may be incinerated, chemically treated, steam or dry sterilized, or sterilized with ionizing radiation. Blood, blood products, body fluids, and excreta can be discharged into the sanitary disposal system, if not otherwise prohibited. Infectious waste should be stored in puncture-resistant, leak-resistant bags or containers and conspicuously labeled with the international biohazard symbol. Local regulations may limit the amount of infectious waste that can be stored on-site and the storage time. If radioactive infectious waste is stored for a lengthy period, appropriate precautions such as spraying with disinfectants, freezing, and tightly sealing the container must be taken to prevent putrefaction.

Centralized Nuclear Pharmacy

Since radiopharmaceuticals play an important role in nuclear medicine, it is essential to evaluate the cost-effectiveness of the preparation, distribution, and dispensing of various radiopharmaceuticals. It is rather expensive to operate a separate nuclear pharmacy within a small nuclear medicine department. On the other hand, a large nuclear medicine department should be able to run a nuclear pharmacy unit of its own with some economic and operational benefit.

A centralized nuclear pharmacy in any region having reasonable transportation facilities can lead to significant savings of money and personnel time. It must be shared by many, if not all, hospitals in a given region; otherwise it may not be feasible to run it economically.

A centralized nuclear pharmacy would have the following advantages: Radiopharmaceuticals could be available in unit dosage form; the time the technologist spends in radiopharmaceutical preparation and dispensing could be used for clinical procedures; because a centralized nuclear pharmacy serves many institutions, the number of workers directly involved in the operation of the nuclear pharmacy is reduced and radiation exposure to the workers in general is minimized; and there is also less possibility of radioactive contamination of the nuclear medicine facilities than when radio-pharmaceuticals are prepared in individual institutions.

The primary advantage of a centralized nuclear pharmacy is an economic one. The preparation of radiopharmaceuticals from the basic ingredients in a centralized nuclear pharmacy would minimize the cost, if permissible by nuclear pharmacy guidelines approved by the FDA (see Chapter 11 as to when a registration is required in various situations of nuclear pharmacy practice). Even the kits purchased from the manufacturers could be better utilized with considerable economic benefits. Although the kits are guaranteed for sterility and apyrogenicity by the manufacturers, the in-house radiopharmaceutical preparation from basic ingredients require these tests and thus add to the total cost of manufacturing. In smaller institutions, where the patient load is not heavy, obviously the use of kits is not economical because relatively few studies are performed with the radiopharmaceutical from a kit and the bulk of it is wasted. A centralized nuclear pharmacy could provide an appreciable economic advantage to these institutions by dispensing unit dosages, as required by them.

Ideally, a centralized nuclear pharmacy should be located at the center of a geographic region and supply all radiopharmaceuticals in multidosages or unit dosages, as needed, to the participating hospitals. A nuclear pharmacist should be in charge of the unit. The nuclear pharmacist, or other personnel under his supervision, should prepare radiopharmaceuticals daily under aseptic conditions, test for radiochemical purity, sterility, and apyrogenicity, and finally dispense them, as required, to all institutions. The assay of the unit dosage or multidosage preparation should be doubly made by both the nuclear pharmacist in the central nuclear pharmacy and the technologist in the nuclear medicine department of the participating institution. The basic operation of a centralized nuclear pharmacy is similar to that of a regular nuclear pharmacy. The only difference lies in the organizational aspects of the operation. Since the centralized nuclear pharmacy serves a number of institutions in different locations, a precisely timed protocol is needed for procuring all the requisitions and then preparing and shipping radiopharmaceuticals to different customers at specified times. All requisitions from participating institutions should be received well before shipping. The shipping can be done via airplane, taxi, or car, depending on the distance and the transportation facilities available. If the shipping is to be done via an airline, the departure and arrival times should be chosen to match the time of examination requested by the ordering physician.

Nuclear pharmacists can be authorized by the NRC for their practice in nuclear pharmacy, provided they fulfill certain requirements of training and experience (10CFR35.980) (see Chapter 11). Such authorization allows nuclear pharmacists a wide latitude of freedom in their practice. Centralized nuclear pharmacies must be operated under an authorized nuclear pharmacist. Individuals who are not authorized by the NRC must practice in a nuclear pharmacy under the supervision of an authorized nuclear pharmacist or an authorized user.

Questions

1. Suppose you received a shipment of radiopharmaceuticals in your nuclear pharmacy. As a nuclear pharmacist, what are the steps you would take until it is dispensed?
2. What are the specific conditions of monitoring the radioactive shipments?
3. What are the limits of survey readings on radioactive shipments that require notifying the NRC or the Agreement State?
4. Give a general description of a nuclear pharmacy operation in a hospital.
5. How do you justify a centralized nuclear pharmacy in a large community having several hospitals? What are the salient advantages of a centralized nuclear pharmacy?

Suggested Reading

Callahan RJ. The role of commercial nuclear pharmacy in the future practice of nuclear medicine. *Semin Nucl Med.* 1996; 26:85.

Cox PH, Coenen HH, Deckart H, et al. Report and recommendations on the requirements of postgraduate training in radiopharmacy and radiopharmaceutical chemistry. 1989. *Eur J Nucl Med.* 1990; 17:203.

Elliot AT, Hilditch TE, Murray T, McNulty H. The design and construction of a central radiopharmacy. *Nucl Med Commun.* 1993; 14:328.

Gnau TR, Maynard CD. Reducing the cost of nuclear medicine. Sharing radiopharmaceuticals. *Radiology.* 1973; 103:641.

Guidelines for the preparation of radiopharmaceuticals in hospitals Special report no. 11. London: British Institute of Radiology; 1979.

Kawada TK, Tubis M, Ebenkamp T, Wolf W. Review of Nuclear pharmacy practice in hospitals. *Am J Hosp Pharm.* 1982; 39:266.

Rhodes BA, Hladik III WB, Norenberg JP. Chinical radiopharmacy: principles and practices. *Semin Nucl Med.* 1996; 26:77.

Saha GB. Nuclear pharmacy: a new discipline and its basis. *Pharm Int.* 1980; 1:137.

10
Internal Radiation Dosimetry

Radiation Units

There are three basic units related to radiation: the roentgen (R) for exposure, the rad (radiation absorbed dose) for absorbed dose, and the rem (roentgen equivalent man) for dose equivalent.

The *roentgen* is the amount of x or γ radiation that produces ionization of one electrostatic unit of either positive or negative charge per cubic centimeter of air at 0°C and 760 mmHg (STP). Since 1 cm^3 air weighs 0.001293 g at STP and a charge of either sign carries 1.6×10^{-19} Coulomb (C) or 4.8×10^{-10} electrostatic units, it can be shown that

$$1\,R = 2.58 \times 10^{-4}\,C/kg \tag{10.1}$$

It should be noted that the roentgen applies only to air and to x or γ radiations. Due to practical limitations of the measuring instruments, the R unit is applicable only to photons of less than 3 MeV energy.

The *rad* is a more universal unit. It is a measure of the energy deposited in unit mass of any material by any type of radiation. The rad is specifically defined as

$$1\,rad = 100\,ergs/g \text{ absorber} \tag{10.2}$$

Since 1 joule (J) $= 10^7$ ergs,

$$1\,rad = 10^{-2}\,J/kg \tag{10.3}$$

In SI units, the *gray* (Gy) is the unit of radiation absorbed dose and is given by

$$1\,gray\,(Gy) = 100\,rad \tag{10.4}$$

$$= 1\,J/kg \text{ absorber} \tag{10.5}$$

It can be shown that the energy absorbed per kilogram of air due to an exposure of 1 R is

$$1\,R = 86.9 \times 10^{-4}\,J/kg \text{ in air}$$

Therefore,

$$1\,R = 0.869 \text{ rad in air}$$

$$\text{or, } 1\,R = 0.00869 \text{ Gy in air}$$

This will be the absorbed dose to any matter or a person at the location of the exposure.

The rad is not restricted by the type of radiation or absorber nor by the intensity of the radiation. It should be understood that the rad is independent of the weight of a material. This means that a radiation dose of 1 rad (0.01 Gy) is always 1 rad (0.01 Gy) in 1, 2, or 10 g of the material. However, the integral absorbed dose is given in units of gram-rads (g·rad or g·Gy) and calculated by multiplying the rad (Gy) by the mass of material. For example, if the radiation dose to a mass of 45 g is 10 rad (0.1 Gy), then the integral radiation dose to the material is 450 g· rad (or 4.5 g·Gy); however, the radiation dose is still 10 rad (0.1 Gy).

The dose equivalent unit, H_r, in *rem*, has been developed to account for the differences in effectiveness of different radiations in causing biological damage. In radiobiology, the dose equivalent H_r for a particular radiation is defined as

$$H_r\,(\text{rem}) = \text{rad} \times (\text{RBE})_r \tag{10.6}$$

where $(\text{RBE})_r$ is the *relative biological effectiveness* of the radiation. It is defined as the ratio of the dose of a standard radiation to produce a particular biological response to the dose of the radiation in question to produce the same biological response. The standard radiation may be any suitable radiation such as 250-kV x-radiation or ^{60}Co radiations, and therefore the RBE of a radiation depends on the choice of the standard radiation.

In radiation protection, however, the H_r is defined as

$$H_r\,(\text{rem}) = \text{rad} \times W_r \tag{10.7}$$

where W_r is the radiation weighting factor for a given type of radiation. W_r is related to the linear energy transfer[a] of the radiation in a given medium and reflects the effectiveness of the radiation to cause biological or chemical damage. It is useful in the design of shielding and in the calculation of radiation dose to radiation workers. In the past, the W_r values were called *quality factors* (QFs), which are somewhat different, but still are adopted by the NRC. The QF values of various radiations are listed in Table 10.1.

---

[a] The linear energy transfer (LET) of a radiation is defined as the amount of energy deposited per unit length of the path by the radiation and is measured in kiloelectron volts per micrometer.

TABLE 10.1. Quality factors for different radiations.

Type of radiation	QF
X rays, γ rays, β particles	1.0
Neutrons and protons	10.0
α particles	20.0
Heavy ions	20.0

In SI units, the dose equivalent H_r is expressed in *sievert* (Sv), which is defined as

$$1 \text{ sievert (Sv)} = 100 \text{ rem} \tag{10.8}$$

In practical situations, all these radiation units are often expressed in milliroentgens (mR), millirads (mrad), and millirems (mrem), which are 10^{-3} times the units, roentgen, rad, and rem, respectively. In SI units, the equivalent quantities are milligrays (mGy) and millisieverts (mSv). A rad is also expressed as centigray (cGy).

Radiation Dosimetry

Radiation can cause deleterious effects in living systems. It is therefore essential to assess these effects in humans for a given nuclear medicine procedure involving the administration of a radiopharmaceutical. The damaging effects arise from the absorption of energy in tissues and depend on a number of factors: (1) the activity of the administered radiopharmaceutical, (2) the physical and biological half-lives of the radiopharmaceutical, (3) the distribution and metabolic fate of the radiopharmaceutical in the body, (4) the fraction of energy released per disintegration from a source region that is absorbed in the particular target volume, and (5) the shape, composition, and location of the source and target organs. The physical characteristics of a radiopharmaceutical are well established. Information concerning the biological handling of a radiopharmaceutical can be obtained from various experimental studies in humans and animals. Because there are variations from one individual to another in physiologic functions and in the shape, size, density, and relative location of different organs, the factors 3 to 5 listed above are approximated for a "reference" 70-kg man.

If the amount of energy in ergs absorbed in a mass of material is known, then the absorbed dose D in rad is obtained by dividing the absorbed energy by 100 and the mass of the material. However, D can be calculated from the radiation dose rate R and the duration of exposure from the source of radiation. The dose rate is defined as the amount of radiation energy absorbed per unit time per gram of material. The calculation of radiation dose due to internally absorbed radionuclides is detailed below.

Calculation of Radiation Absorbed Dose

Radiopharmaceuticals administered to patients are distributed in various regions of the body. These regions can be considered points, lines, surfaces, or volumes. In internal dosimetry calculations, a region of interest for which the absorbed dose is to be calculated is considered the "target," whereas all other regions contributing to the radiation dose to the target are considered "source" regions. The source and target regions become the same when the radiation dose due to radioactivity in the target itself is calculated. Suppose a source volume r contains A μCi of a radiopharmaceutical emitting several radiations. If the ith radiation has energy E_i and a fractional abundance N_i per disintegration, then the energy absorbed per hour by a target of mass m and volume v from the ith radiation emitted by the source volume r (dose rate) is given by

$$R_i(\text{rad/hr}) = A/m(\mu\text{Ci/g})N_iE_i(\text{MeV/disintegration})$$

$$\times \, [3.7 \times 10^4 \, \text{disintegrations/s} \cdot \mu\text{Ci})]$$

$$\times \, (1.6 \times 10^{-6} \, \text{erg/MeV})$$

$$\times \, (0.01 \, \text{g} \cdot \text{rad/erg})$$

$$\times \, (3600 \, \text{s/hr})$$

$$= 2.13(A/m)N_iE_i$$

If the target and the source are not the same, then a factor must be introduced to account for the partial absorption, if any, of the radiation energy. Thus,

$$R_i(\text{rad/hr}) = 2.13(A/m)N_iE_i\phi_i(v \leftarrow r) \tag{10.9}$$

Here $\phi_i(v \leftarrow r)$ is called the *absorbed fraction* and is defined as the ratio of the energy absorbed by the target volume v from the ith radiation to the energy emitted by the ith radiation from the source volume r. This is a very critical factor that is difficult to evaluate because the absorbed fraction ϕ_i depends on the type and energy of the radiation, the shape and size of the source volume, and the shape, composition, and distance of the target volume. However, in the case of β particles, conversion electrons, α particles, and x and γ rays of energies less than 11 keV, all of the energy emitted by a radionuclide is absorbed in the volume r larger than 1 cm. Then, ϕ_i becomes zero, unless v and r are the same, in which case $\phi_i = 1$. For x and γ rays with energies greater than 11 keV, the value of ϕ_i decreases with increasing energy and varies between 0 and 1, depending on the energy. The values of ϕ_i are calculated by statistical methods on the basis of fundamental mechanisms of interaction of radiations with matter and are available in many standard textbooks on radiation dosimetry, particularly the medical internal radiation dose (MIRD) pamphlets published by the Society of Nuclear Medicine.

The quantity $2.13 N_i E_i$ is a constant for the ith radiation and is often denoted by Δ_i. Thus,

$$\Delta_i = 2.13 \ N_i E_i \tag{10.10}$$

The quantity Δ_i is called the *equilibrium dose constant* and has the unit $g \cdot rad/(\mu Ci \cdot hr)$ based on the units chosen in Eq. (10.9). It should be pointed out that for γ-rays and α-particles, E_i is the maximum energy of these radiations. However, since β particles are emitted with a distribution of energy, the average energy $\bar{E}_\beta$ of β particles is used in the calculation of Δ_i. Now Eq. (10.9) becomes

$$R_i(\text{rad/hr}) = (A/m)\Delta_i \phi_i(v \leftarrow r) \tag{10.11}$$

The activity A will change due to the physical decay and biological elimination of the radiopharmaceutical, and therefore the dose rate will also change. Assuming an effective exponential change in A, Eq. (10.11) can be written

$$R_i(\text{rad/hr}) = (A_0/m)\Delta_i e^{-\lambda_e t}\phi_i(v \leftarrow r) \tag{10.12}$$

Here λ_e is the effective decay constant of the radiopharmaceutical and t is the time over which the original activity A_0 has decayed.

The cumulative radiation dose D_i due to the ith radiation during the period $t = 0$ to t can be obtained by integrating Eq. (10.12). Thus,

$$\begin{aligned}
D_i(\text{rad}) &= \frac{A_0}{m} \Delta_i \phi_i(v \leftarrow r) \int_0^t e^{-\lambda_e t} dt \\
&= \frac{A_0}{m} \Delta_i \phi_i(v \leftarrow r) \frac{1}{\lambda_e}(1 - e^{-\lambda_e t}) \\
&= 1.44 \frac{A_0}{m} \Delta_i T_e (1 - e^{-\lambda_e t})\phi_i(v \leftarrow r) \tag{10.13}
\end{aligned}$$

Here, T_e is the effective half-life of the radiopharmaceutical in hours (discussed in Chapter 6). If $t = \infty$, that is, the radiopharmaceutical is completely eliminated, then the exponential term $e^{-\lambda_e t}$ approaches zero and the absorbed dose in Eq. (10.13) may be written

$$D_i(\text{rad}) = 1.44(A_0/m)\Delta_i T_e \phi_i(v \leftarrow r) \tag{10.14}$$

If the radionuclide has n radiations with energies $E_1, E_2, \ldots, E_n$ and fractional abundances $N_1, N_2, \ldots, \cdot N_n$, per disintegration, then the total dose D

can be obtained by summing Eq. (10.14) over all radiations. Thus,

$$D(\text{rad}) = 1.44 \frac{A_0}{m} T_e \sum_{i=1}^{n} \Delta_i \phi_i (v \leftarrow r) \qquad (10.15)$$

This summation can also be applied to Eq. (10.12) for the dose rate R_i. The total dose to the target from other source regions can be calculated by summing Eq. (10.15) over all regions. Equation (10.15) assumes that the uptake in the organ is instantaneous and the radioactivity is eliminated by both physical decay and biological excretion. Modifications must be made if either physical decay or biological excretion only occurs, and if the uptake is not instantaneous. The reader is referred to standard radiobiology or physics textbooks for further details.

In the MIRD pamphlets, the values of Δ_i have been compiled on the basis of various nuclear characteristics of the radionuclide in question. The ϕ_i values have been calculated on the basis of different sizes and masses of the materials receiving the radiation dose and the radiation characteristics of the radionuclide. In MIRD pamphlet No. 11, $\tilde{A}$ has been substituted for the quantity $1.44 \times A_0 \times T_e$, and S for the quantity $(\sum_{i=1}^{n} \Delta_i \phi_i)/m$. $\tilde{A}$ is called the cumulated activity and S is called the mean absorbed dose per unit cumulated activity.

$$D = \tilde{A} \cdot S \qquad (10.16)$$

The values of S are tabulated in MIRD pamphlet No. 11. MIRD dose estimate reports are available for several radiopharmaceuticals and published periodically by the Society of Nuclear Medicine.

Problem 10.1
Calculate the absorbed dose to the liver of an adult patient who receives 3 mCi (111 MBq) ^{99m}Tc-sulfur colloid for a liver scan, assuming 85% liver uptake with no excretion.

Answer

$$\text{Mass of liver} = 1700 \, \text{g(for a standard man)}$$

$$A_0 \ \text{in the liver} = 3000 \times 0.85 = 2550 \, \mu\text{Ci}(86.7 \, \text{MBq})$$

$$T_e = 6 \, \text{hr [using Eq.(6.3)and assuming } T_b = \infty]$$

The major radiations of ^{99m}Tc are 140-keV photons, x rays, and Auger and conversion electrons. The Δ and ϕ values for these radiations are obtained from MIRD pamphlets (assuming uniform distribution) and given below.

Radiation	Δ_i	ϕ_i	$\Delta_i \phi_i$
140-keV photon	0.2640	0.160	0.0422
X rays (20 keV)	0.0031	0.784	0.0024
Electrons	0.0360	1.000	0.0360
Total			0.0806

From Eq. (10.15), the total dose to the liver is

$$D = 1.44 \times (2550/1700) \times 6 \times 0.0806 = 1.04 \text{ rad } (0.0104 \text{ Gy})$$

Radiation Dose in SI Units

The radiation dose in SI units due to the administration of a radiopharmaceutical can be calculated by assuming a source volume r containing A MBq of the radiopharmaceutical that emits several radiations. If the ith radiation has energy E_i and a fractional abundance N_i per disintegration, then the energy absorbed per hour by a target of mass m and volume v from the ith radiation emitted by the source volume r (dose rate) is given by

$$R_i(\text{Gy/hr}) = A/m(\text{MBq/g})N_iE_i(\text{MeV/disintegration})$$
$$\times 10^6 \text{ disintegrations}/(\text{s} \cdot \text{MBq})$$
$$\times (1.6 \times 10^{-6} \text{ erg/MeV})$$
$$\times (1 \times 10^{-4} \text{ g} \cdot \text{Gy/erg})$$
$$\times (3600 \text{ s/hr})$$
$$= 0.576(A/m)N_iE_i$$

When the target and the source are not the same, the absorbed fraction $\phi(v \leftarrow r)$ must be taken into account. Thus

$$R_i(\text{Gy/hr}) = 0.576(A/m)N_iE_i\phi_i(v \leftarrow r) \tag{10.17}$$

The quantity $0.576N_iE_i$ is a constant and can be denoted by Δ_i as in Eq. (10.10). Thus

$$\Delta_i = 0.576N_iE_i \tag{10.18}$$

With this value of Δ_i, Eqs. (10.11), (10.12), (10.13), (10.14), (10.15), and (10.16) are equally applicable to radiation doses in SI units. It should be understood that the equations in SI units contain a constant $\Delta_i = 0.576N_iE_i$ and activities expressed in MBq, whereas the equations in rad units contain the equilibrium constant $\Delta_i = 2.13N_iE_i$ and activities expressed in microcuries.

Table 10.2 presents radiation absorbed doses in different organs in adults from various radiopharmaceuticals. The doses have been obtained from package inserts of individual products, except ^{18}F-FDG.

Effective Dose

The concept of *effective dose* has been introduced by the ICRP because the stochastic effects of radiations vary in different tissues. While the *dose equivalent* is related to the variations of damage caused by different types of radiations, the effective dose relates to the radiosensitivity of different tis-

TABLE 10.2. Radiation absorbed doses in adults for various radiopharmaceuticals.

Radiopharmaceutical	Organ	Dose rad/mCi	Dose mGy/GBq
[99m]Tc-pertechnetate	Thyroid	0.130	35.1
	Upper large intestine	0.120	32.4
	Lower large intestine	0.110	30.0
	Stomach	0.051	13.8
	Ovaries	0.030	8.1
	Testes	0.009	2.4
[99m]Tc-sulfur colloid	Liver	3.375	912.2
	Spleen	2.125	574.3
	Marrow	0.275	74.3
	Ovaries	0.056	15.2
^{99m}Tc-DTPA	Bladder (2-hr void)	0.115	31.1
	Kidneys	0.090	24.3
	Gonads	0.011	3.0
[99m]Tc-gluceptate	Kidneys	0.170	45.9
	Bladder (2-hr void)	0.120	32.4
	Ovaries	0.080	21.6
[99m]Tc-tetrofosmin (Myoview) at rest	Gallbladder	0.180	48.7
	Upper large intestine	0.113	30.5
	Lower large intestine	0.082	22.2
	Heart (wall)	0.015	4.1
	Kidneys	0.046	12.4
	Ovaries	0.035	9.5
	Bladder (wall)	0.071	19.2
[99m]Tc-arcitumomab (CEA-scan)	Kidneys	0.371	100.3
	Bladder	0.061	16.6
	Spleen	0.059	15.9
	Liver	0.038	10.4
	Testes	0.017	4.5
	Red marrow	0.037	9.9
[99m]Tc-depreotide (NeoTect)	Kidneys	0.330	89.1
	Spleen	0.160	43.2
	Testes	0.110	29.7
	Bladder	0.033	8.9
	Thyroid	0.078	21.1
	Lungs	0.053	14.3
^{99m}Tc-MAA	Lungs	0.22	59.5
	Kidneys	0.011	3.0
	Liver	0.018	4.9
	Ovaries	0.008	2.2
	Testes	0.006	1.6
[99m]Tc-stannous pyrophosphate (blood pool imaging)	Bladder	0.034	9.2
	Red marrow	0.019	5.1
	Ovaries	0.023	6.2
	Testes	0.013	3.5
	Blood	0.051	13.8
^{99m}Tc-MDP	Bone	0.035	9.5
	Bladder wall (2-hr void)	0.130	35.1

TABLE 10.2 (*continued*)

Radiopharmaceutical	Organ	Dose	
		rad/mCi	mGy/GBq
	Kidneys	0.040	10.8
	Marrow	0.026	7.0
	Ovaries	0.012	3.2
	Testes	0.008	2.1
99mTc-mebrofenin (Choletec)	Liver	0.047	12.7
	Lower large intestine	0.474	128.1
	Upper large intestine	0.364	98.4
	Gallbladder	0.137	37.0
	Bladder	0.029	7.8
	Red marrow	0.034	9.1
	Ovaries	0.101	27.3
99mTc-MAG3	Bladder wall	0.480	129.7
	Gallbladder	0.016	4.3
	Kidneys	0.014	3.8
	Lower large intestine	0.033	8.9
	Ovaries	0.026	7.0
99mTc-HMPAO (Ceretec)	Brain	0.026	7.0
	Thyroid	0.100	27.0
	Kidneys	0.130	35.1
	Ovaries	0.023	6.2
	Gallbladder	0.190	51.4
	Lacrymal gland	0.258	69.7
99mTc-apcitide (AcuTect)	Bladder wall	0.22	60.0
	Kidneys	0.050	14.0
	Upper large intestine	0.038	10.0
	Uterus	0.034	9.2
	Lungs	0.016	4.3
	Red marrow	0.009	2.5
99mTc-DMSA	Bladder wall	0.070	18.9
	Kidneys	0.630	170.3
	Liver	0.031	8.56
	Bone marrow	0.022	5.86
	Ovaries	0.013	3.60
	Testes	0.007	1.80
99mTc-ECD (Neurolite)	Brain	0.020	5.4
	Gallbladder wall	0.092	24.9
	Upper large intestine	0.063	17.0
	Kidneys	0.027	7.3
	Liver	0.020	5.4
	Ovaries	0.030	8.1
	Bladder wall	0.270	72.9
99mTc-sestamibi (Cardiolite) at rest	Gallbladder	0.067	18.1
	Upper large intestine	0.180	48.6
	Lower large intestine	0.13	35.1
	Heart wall	0.017	4.6
	Kidneys	0.067	18.1
	Ovaries	0.050	13.5
	Bladder wall	0.067	18.1

TABLE 10.2 (*continued*)

Radiopharmaceutical	Organ	Dose	
		rad/mCi	mGy/GBq
[131]I-sodium iodide (25% uptake)	Thyroid	1300.00	3.50×10^5
	Ovaries	0.14	37.8
	Liver	0.48	129.7
[123]I-sodium iodide (25% uptake)	Thyroid	12.75	3445.9
	Bladder	0.30	81.1
	Ovaries	0.05	13.5
^{131}I-MIBG	Bladder (wall)	2.96	800.0
	Liver	2.92	789.2
	Spleen	2.18	589.2
	Heart (wall)	1.41	381.1
	Adrenal medulla	0.78	210.8
	Kidneys	0.33	89.2
	Ovaries	0.27	73.0
^{111}In-WBC	Spleen	26.00	7027.0
	Liver	38.00	10,270.0
	Red marrow	26.00	7027.0
	Skeleton	7.28	1967.6
	Ovaries	3.80	1027.0
[111]In-pentetreotide (OctreoScan)	Kidneys	1.807	488.4
	Liver	0.407	110.0
	Spleen	2.460	664.9
	Bladder wall	1.007	272.2
	Ovaries	0.163	44.1
[111]In-capromab pendetide (ProstaScint)	Liver	3.70	1000.0
	Spleen	3.26	881.1
	Kidneys	2.48	670.3
	Marrow	0.86	232.4
	Testes	1.12	339.0
	Prostate	1.64	443.2
^{18}F-FDG[a]	Brain	0.07	18.9
	Heart	0.22	59.5
	Bladder	0.70	189.2
	Spleen	0.14	37.8
	Ovaries	0.063	17.0
	Uterus	0.085	23.0
[82]Rb-rubidium chloride	Kidneys	0.032	8.6
	Heart (wall)	0.007	1.9
[201]Tl-thallous chloride	Heart	0.50	135.1
	Kidneys	1.20	324.3
	Liver	0.55	148.6
	Thyroid	0.65	175.7
	Testes	0.50	135.1
[67]Ga-gallium citrate	Liver	0.46	124.3
	Marrow	0.58	156.7
	Kidneys	0.41	110.8
	Spleen	0.53	143.2
	Upper large intestine	0.56	151.4
	Lower large intestine	0.90	243.2
	Gonads	0.26	70.0

TABLE 10.2 (*continued*)

Radiopharmaceutical	Organ	Dose	
		rad/mCi	mGy/GBq
[153]Sm-lexidronam (Quadramet)	Bone surfaces	25.000	6756.8
	Red marrow	5.700	1540.0
	Bladder wall	3.600	973.0
	Kidneys	0.065	17.6
	Ovaries	0.032	8.6
	Liver	0.019	5.1
[89]Sr-strontium chloride (Metastron)	Bone surfaces	63.0	17,000.0
	Red bone marrow	40.7	11,000.0
	Lower bowel	17.4	4700.0
	Bladder wall	4.8	1300.0
	Ovaries	2.9	800.0
	Kidneys	2.9	800.0
[90]Y-ibritumomab tiuxetan[b] (Zevalin)	Spleen	27.2	7350.0
	Liver	16.0	4320.0
	Lungs	7.6	2050.0
	Bladder wall	3.3	890.0
	Red marrow	2.2	590.0
	Kidneys	0.8	220.0
	Other organs	1.5	400.0
[133]Xe-xenon	Lungs	0.008	2.2

[a] From Stabin MG, Stubbs JB, Toohey RE. Radiation dose estimates for radiopharmaceuticals. Radiation Internal Dose Information Center, Oak Ridge Institute for Science and Foundation, 1996.
[b] From Wiseman GA, Kornmehl E, Leigh B, et al. Radiation dosimetry results and safety correlations from ^{90}Y-Ibritumomab tiuxetan radioimmunotherapy for relapsed or refractory non-Hodgkin's lymphoma: combined data from 4 clinical trials. *J Nucl Med.* 2003; 44:465.

sues. The effective dose H_E is the sum of weighted dose equivalents in different tissues and organs, and is calculated as

$$H_E = \sum_T W_T \times \sum_r H_{T,r} \qquad (10.19)$$

where W_T is the *tissue weighting factor* and $H_{T,r}$ is the absorbed dose in tissue T from radiation of type r. The values of W_T have been obtained from 10CFR20 and are listed in Table 10.3.

Table 10.4 lists the effective doses (H_E) from different radiopharmaceuticals for adults. The radiosensitivity of different organs is age-dependent, but only adult values are given. The effective doses give an estimate of possible risk of stochastic effects due to total body irradiation by external sources (e.g., diagnostic x-ray procedures) or internal sources (e.g., intravenous administration of radiopharmaceuticals).

TABLE 10.3. Tissue weighting factors, W_T.

Tissue	W_T [a]
Gonads	0.25
Breast	0.15
Red bone marrow	0.12
Lungs	0.12
Thyroid	0.03
Bone surfaces	0.03
Remainder	0.30
Total Body	1.00

[a] From 10CFR20.

TABLE 10.4. Effective doses from various radiopharmaceuticals in nuclear medicine.

Radiopharmaceuticals	Effective dose[a]	
	rem/mCi	mSv/MBq
[99m]Tc-pertechnetate	0.048	0.013
[99m]Tc-sestamibi (exercise)	0.030	0.008
^{99m}Tc-MAA	0.004	0.001
[99m]Tc-tetrofosmin (exercise)	0.026	0.007
^{99m}Tc-DTPA aerosol	0.022	0.006
^{99m}Tc-MDP	0.022	0.006
[99m]Tc-red blood cell (RBC)	0.026	0.007
[99m]Tc-iminodiacetic acid (IDA) derivatives	0.063	0.017
^{99m}Tc-DTPA	0.019	0.005
[99m]Tc-dimercaptosuccinic acid (DMSA)	0.033	0.009
[99m]Tc-sulfur colloid	0.033	0.009
[99m]Tc-white blood cell (WBC)	0.004	0.001
^{99m}Tc-HMPAO	0.033	0.009
[99m]Tc-gluceptate	0.019	0.005
^{99m}Tc-MAG3	0.026	0.007
[99m]Tc-depreotide[b]	0.084	0.023
[99m]Tc-apcitide[b]	0.003	0.009
^{111}In-WBC	0.133	0.036
^{111}In-DTPA	0.078	0.021
[111]In-pentetreotide	0.185	0.050
[123]I-NaI (35% uptake)	0.814	0.220
[131]I-NaI (35% uptake)	88.80	24.00
[201]Tl-TlCl	0.814	0.220
^{18}F-FDG	0.070	0.019
[67]Ga-citrate	0.370	0.100
^{131}I-MIBG	0.052	0.014
[82]Rb-RbCl	0.013	0.003

[a] Reproduced with permission from ICRP publication 80. New York: Elsevier, 1999.
[b] Adapted from package insert.

Questions

1. Define roentgen, rad, rem, gray, and sievert.
2. Calculate the absorbed dose to the lungs of an adult patient who received 3 mCi (111 MBq) ^{99m}Tc-MAA, assuming 99% uptake and uniform distribution of the radioactivity in the lungs. Pertinent data are: $T_b = 1.5\,hr$ and $S = 5.25 \times 10^{-5}\,rad/\mu Ci \cdot hr$ or $0.0142\,Gy/GBq \cdot hr$.
3. If the radiation dose to 1 g of an absorbing medium is 25 rad (0.25 Gy), what is the radiation dose to 2 g of the absorbing medium?
4. Calculate the dose in rem and sieverts to a tumor that received 20 rad (0.2 Gy) from neutron therapy ($\dot{Q}F = 10$ for neutrons).
5. What is the approximate average whole body dose from common ^{99m}Tc-radiopharmaceuticals?

Suggested Reading

Cloutier RJ, Edwards CL, Snyder WS, eds. Medical radionuclides: radiation dose and effects. CONF-691212. US Atomic Energy Commission, Oak Ridge; 1970.

Fourth International Radiopharmaceutical Dosimetry Symposium, Oak Ridge, November, 1985, CONF-851113.

Howell RW, Wessels BW, Loevinger R. The MIRD perspective. *J Nucl Med.* 1999; 40:3S–10S.

International Commission on Radiation Protection. Radiation dose to patients from radiopharmaceuticals (ICRP 80) ICRP Publications; 1999.

Loevinger R, Budinger T, Watson E. MIRD primer for absorbed dose calculations. Society of Nuclear Medicine, New York, 1991.

National Council on Radiation Protection and Measurements. General concepts for the dosimetry of internally deposited radionuclides (NCRP 84). Bethesda: NCRP Publications; 1985.

Reports of Medical Internal Radiation Dose (MIRD) Committee. Pamphlet Nos. 1–11. Society of Nuclear Medicine, New York; 1968–1977.

U.S. Food and Drug Administration. Radioactive drugs and radioactive biological products. *Fed Register.* 1975; 40:144.

Zanzonico PB. Internal radiation dosimetry: a review of basic concepts and recent developments. *J Nucl Med.* 2000; 41:297.

11
Radiation Regulations, Protection, and Uses

The use of radiations and radiolabeled products for any purpose is governed by regulatory agencies in different countries all over the world. This chapter focuses on regulations that pertain only to the United States, and only a brief summary of European regulations is given at the end.

The use of radiopharmaceuticals in humans was almost unregulated until the late 1950s. Since then, a progression of regulations has been imposed on the use of radiations in humans. Until 1963, all reactor-derived radiopharmaceuticals were under the control of the Atomic Energy Commission (AEC, now the Nuclear Regulatory Commission, (NRC)) only for their radiation hazards. The therapeutic or diagnostic efficacy and the pharmaceutical quality of radiopharmaceuticals were not regulated by the AEC or by the U.S. Food and Drug Administration (FDA) until the early 1960s. In 1963 the FDA introduced rules stating that the clinical efficacy of all radiopharmaceuticals, for that matter, all drugs, must be reported. However, under an agreement between the AEC and the FDA, all investigational new radioactive drugs were exempted from these regulations. In July 1975, the exemption of all new drugs was revoked by the FDA and all radiopharmaceuticals came under its regulations. Thus, the FDA regulates the safety and efficacy of radiopharmaceuticals in humans, whereas the NRC controls the radiation safety of the worker, the patient, and the public. For approved radiopharmaceuticals, the state boards of pharmacies regulate the pharmacy aspect of nuclear pharmacy operations. Also, state agencies regulate the cyclotron-produced radionuclides and man-made radiations, such as x-rays.

Food and Drug Administration (FDA)

Use of all drugs in humans is regulated by the FDA in two ways—either by submission of Notice of Claimed Investigational Exemption for a New Drug (IND) by an investigator or by submission of a New Drug Application (NDA) by a manufacturer.

Investigational New Drug (IND)

Approval for the use of investigational radiopharmaceuticals in humans must be obtained from the FDA by submitting an IND on Forms FDA 1571 and 1572. The IND must include the names and credentials of the investigators, purpose of the project, manufacturing and toxicologic data of the radiopharmaceutical, the technical details of the project, and the clinical protocol.

In all human investigations, the FDA requires that investigators obtain written consent from patients or their relatives for the proposed study. In the consent form, details of the safety and hazard of the radiopharmaceutical, the benefit from the study, financial compensation, if any, and a brief outline of the procedure are given.

In almost all institutions, an institutional review board (IRB) is established to supervise and regulate the use of radiopharmaceuticals in humans. This committee is approved by the FDA. The IRB is composed of scientists, laymen, lawyers, clergymen, and others, and is responsible for the close monitoring of clinical protocols in humans in the institution. This committee approves the contents of the consent form to be presented to the patient.

An IND is sponsored by a physician or a drug company. The drug company sponsors a group of investigators who conduct the clinical protocol of a new drug on behalf of the company. In contrast, the physician-sponsored IND is carried out under his own protocol only for a specific radiopharmaceutical. The IND is run for a limited period and a specific number of patients are undertaken in the protocol. An annual report must be submitted stating the progress and various findings of the study. Any serious adverse reactions must be reported to the FDA immediately. Identical INDs may be submitted by several individual sponsors for the same product. The FDA collects all data on the safety and efficacy of the product to be shared among individual sponsors.

The clinical investigation of a new drug is carried out in three phases:

Phase I: In this phase, only a limited number of patients are included to determine the pharmacologic distribution, metabolism, excretion, toxicity, optimum dosage, and any adverse reactions.

Phase II: In this phase, studies are conducted in a limited number of patients for a specific disease.

Phase III: A large number of patients with the specific disease are involved in Phase III clinical trial to assess the drug's safety, efficacy, and dosage necessary in diagnosing or treating the disease. This phase of the study is normally conducted by several investigators for better statistical data.

New Drug Application (NDA)

Usually the drug companies apply to the FDA for approval of an NDA for marketing a new radiopharmaceutical for one or more clinical uses. As already mentioned, the drug company submits an IND to the FDA for the new radiopharmaceutical and collects data through a group of investigators whose names are filed with the FDA by the company for conducting the study.

When all of the studies are completed as required by the FDA, the sponsor (normally a drug company) submits all pertinent supporting data from all investigators in an NDA to the FDA for approval prior to marketing the product for clinical use. When the FDA is convinced of the efficacy and safety of the radiopharmaceutical supported by the data, it approves an NDA to the sponsor for the marketing of the product. In its approval, the FDA specifies the indications and contraindications of the radiopharmaceutical, its dosimetry, clinical pharmacological information, method of formulation route of administration, and any precaution to be taken. All the information must be included in the package insert.

In 1997, the U.S. Congress passed the Food and Drug Administration Modernization Act (FDAMA) to improve the regulation of food, drugs, devices, and biologic products and for other purposes. Section 121 of the FDAMA required the FDA to come up with a new rule for the approval of radiopharmaceuticals used for diagnosis or monitoring of human diseases. Accordingly, the FDA introduced the final rule for requirements of in vivo diagnostic radiopharmaceutical approval under title 21 of the Code of Federal Regulations (21CFR315). The section describes various issues related to the pharmacologic and toxicologic effects, clinical effectiveness, proposed indications for use, and the estimated absorbed dose of the diagnostic radiopharmaceutical. These data are needed for an NDA approval of a diagnostic radiopharmaceutical.

Radioactive Drug Research Committee

To expedite investigations of new radiopharmaceuticals, the FDA allows institutions to form the so-called Radioactive Drug Research Committee (RDRC), which functions like a mini-FDA. The committee is composed of a nuclear physician, a radiochemist or radiopharmacist, a radiation safety officer (RSO), and at least two more individuals of other disciplines, and is primarily charged with the approving and monitoring of protocols involving the investigational use of radiopharmaceuticals in humans. Under this category, the study cannot be used for diagnostic and therapeutic purposes; only pharmacokinetic data (biodistribution, absorption, metabolism, and excretion) can be obtained; the radiation dose to the critical organ cannot be more than 3 rem (0.03 Sv) in a single dose, and a total of greater than 5 rem (0.05 Sv) per year during the entire study; and only 30 patients can be studied.

The RDRCs are approved by the FDA, and annual progress reports on all active protocols must be submitted to the FDA.

PET Radiopharmaceuticals

Section 121 of FDAMA directs the FDA to establish appropriate approval procedures and current good manufacturing practice (CGMP) requirements for positron emission tomography (PET) radiopharmaceuticals. Accordingly, the FDA has published a preliminary draft guidance on CGMP that addresses the issues of meticulous validation, calibration, and documentation for the production of PET radiopharmaceuticals. However, final rules have not been published yet. The guidance outlines the standards to adopt in manufacturing PET radiopharmaceuticals to meet the requirements of safety, identity, strength, quality, and purity of the product. All of these activities must be accomplished through validation and documentation. The FDA also requires a PET center to employ a sufficient number of personnel with essential training and experience to perform the required CGMP.

The FDAMA requires the FDA to set regulations for the approval of PET radiopharmaceuticals pursuant to Section 505 of Federal Food, Drug, and Cosmetic Act (FFDCA). Since methods of production of PET radiopharmaceuticals vary considerably among centers, the FDA considers PET radiopharmaceuticals as new drugs, and therefore each facility is required to have an NDA or abbreviated NDA (ANDA) approved by the FDA, based on the safety and effectiveness data. The FDA has approved ^{18}F-fluorodeoxyglucose (FDG), ^{13}N-ammonia, and ^{18}F-sodium fluoride for clinical use in humans based on literature review and input from the medical community. One can apply for an NDA for these products referring to an already approved NDA, provided their ingredients, route of administration, dosage form, and strength are identical. However, the FDA considers an ANDA to be a more appropriate application, rather than a full NDA, for an already approved drug for a particular indication. The FDA has not yet addressed the issues of future potential PET radiopharmaceuticals, but it expects to apply standards similar to those of approved PET radiopharmaceuticals.

FDA Regulations for Nuclear Pharmacies

Section 503A of the FDAMA specifies the criteria and requirements for pharmacy compounding. Under this section, drug products that are compounded by a licensed pharmacist or physician on a customized basis for an individual patient on the basis of a valid prescription may be entitled to exemptions from three provisions of the Act: (1) the adulteration provision of Section 501(a)(2)(B) (concerning the good manufacturing practice requirements); (2) the misbranding provision of Section 502(f)(1) (concerning the labeling of drugs with adequate directions for use; and (3) the new drug provision of Section 505 (concerning the approval of drugs under NDA or ANDA).

For this exemption, the drug compounded in bulk or small quantities must meet the requirements of the United States Pharmacopoeia (USP) or National Formulary (NF) monograph and has components approved by the FDA and manufactured by a registered manufacturer. The compounded drug cannot be a product that has been withdrawn from the market because of the unsafe and ineffective characteristics or a copy of the commercial drug in inordinate amounts or routinely produced.

However, Section 503A does not apply to PET drugs and other radio-pharmaceuticals, even though the radiopharmaceuticals are compounded by a nuclear pharmacist or physician under a valid prescription. Thus, these drug products are not exempted from the requirements of Sections 501(a)(2)(B), 502(f)(1), and 505. Although compounding of radiopharmaceuticals is identical to that of conventional drugs, radiopharmaceutical handling is distinctly different because of radiation. In 1984 the FDA set guidelines for nuclear pharmacy practice and for requirements for registering as a manufacturer. The FDA is considering various guidelines and corresponding compliance guides to be implemented in the future. In 2001 the American Pharmaceutical Association (APhA) published a treatise on nuclear pharmacy guidelines based on the principles of the 1984 Nuclear Pharmacy Guideline. It is hoped that the forthcoming FDA guidelines and compliance guides will follow those of the APhA.

There are centralized nuclear pharmacies that supply radiopharmaceuticals to many local and distant hospitals. Nuclear pharmacies may operate as stand-alone units or within a pharmacy or nuclear medicine department and supply all radiopharmaceuticals to the department of nuclear medicine in different hospitals. All these organizations must possess licenses from the NRC or the Agreement State agency (see later) for the use of radioactive materials. The state boards of pharmacy in the U.S. have set specific guidelines regarding the practice of nuclear pharmacies, but the guidelines vary from state to state. Nuclear pharmacies at times may perform some activities that are considered "manufacturing." In 1984 the FDA set guidelines for nuclear pharmacies as to when they are required to register with the FDA as a manufacturer. Here are some examples:

Source of drug	Activities of the nuclear pharmacy	Registration required
Radioactive drug is supplied by a manufacturer (product is subject to an approved NDA or IND).	Dispenses the drug under a prescription in the manufacturer's original container.	No
	After storing the drug, ships the drug in the manufacturer's original container to another nuclear pharmacy or to a physician with or without having received a prescription.	No
	Fills the drug into single- or multiple-dosage containers in anticipation of a future need and its subsequent dispensing under a prescription.	No

Source of drug	Activities of the nuclear pharmacy	Registration required
	Dispenses a drug that was diluted or filled into single- or multiple-dosage containers upon receipt of a prescription.	No
	Dilutes or fills the drug into single- or multiple-dosage containers and dispenses the drugs without a prescription but upon receipt of an appropriate order, for use within the same institution.	No
	Dilutes or fills the drug into single- or multiple-dosage containers and ships it without a prescription to another nuclear pharmacy or institution that, irrespective of its location or ownership, is recognized as a separate entity by the State Board of Pharmacy.	Yes
	Upon a request from a physician, routinely dilutes or fills the drug into single- or multiple-dosage containers and ships the drug to the physician for his/her own professional use.	Yes
Radioactive drug (not involving use of a nonradioactive kit) prepared by the nuclear pharmacy.	Upon receipt of a prescription, prepares a radioactive drug and dispenses it.	No
	Prepares a radioactive drug in anticipation of a future need and its subsequent dispensing under a prescription.	No
	Prepares a radioactive drug and dispenses it without a prescription but upon receipt of an appropriate order for use within the same institution.	No
	Prepares a radioactive drug and ships it without a prescription to another pharmacy or institution that, irrespective of its location or ownership, is recognized as a separate entity by the State Board of Pharmacy.	Yes
	Operates an accelerator or nuclear reactor to produce radionuclides and radiochemicals to manufacture radioactive drugs to be dispensed under a prescription.	No
	Prepares radiochemicals and ships them to other nuclear pharmacies or institutions as drug components.	Yes
	Upon a request from a physician, routinely prepares a drug in single- or multiple-dosage containers and ships the drug to the physician for his/her own professional use.	Yes
A reagent kit and generator are supplied by a manufacturer (the kit and generator are subject to an approved NDA and IND).	Radiolabels the reagent kit according to the manufacturer's directions and dispenses the drug under a prescription.	No
	Radiolabels the reagent kit according to instructions in a prescription and dispenses the drug.	No

Source of drug	Activities of the nuclear pharmacy	Registration required
	Radiolabels a reagent kit in anticipation of a future need and its subsequent dispensing under a prescription.	No
	Radiolabels a reagent kit and ships it without a prescription to another pharmacy that, irrespective of its location or ownership, is recognized as a separate entity by the State Board of Pharmacy.	Yes
	Upon request from a physician, routinely radiolabels a reagent kit for the physician's own use in his/her professional practice.	Yes
A reagent kit is prepared by the nuclear pharmacy.	Upon receipt of a prescription, prepares and radiolabels the reagent kit and dispenses it.	No
	Prepares a reagent kit in anticipation of a future need; upon receipt of a prescription, radio-labels and dispenses it.	No
	Prepares a reagent kit and ships it without a prescription, either before or after radiolabeling, to another pharmacy that, irrespective of its location or ownership, is recognized as a separate entity by the State Board of Pharmacy.	Yes
	Prepares a reagent kit and ships it without a prescription, either before or after radiolabeling, to another institution.	Yes
	Upon a request from a physician, routinely prepares reagent kits and ships them either before or after radiolabeling, to the physician (or his/her own professional use).	Yes
Radioactive drug or reagent kit obtained from another nuclear pharmacy, institution, or practitioner.	Uses the radioactive drug or reagent kit to perform one or more steps in the manufacture of a radioactive drug as a service for the nuclear pharmacy or institution that supplied the radioactive drug or kit, i.e., custom manufacturing.	Yes

State Boards of Pharmacy

The practice of nuclear pharmacy is regulated by a board of pharmacy in each state. More than two thirds of the states have specific regulations for nuclear pharmacy, while the remaining states regulate nuclear pharmacy under other forms of pharmacy, such as retail pharmacy, etc. However, strict implementation of specific regulations in nuclear pharmacy is lacking in many states, although basic pharmacy practice regulations are applied equally to nuclear pharmacy.

The National Association of Nuclear Pharmacies (NANP) has introduced Model Nuclear Pharmacy Regulations that are available to state boards of pharmacies for implementation. These regulations include training requirements, requirements for space, equipment quality control, and other related aspects of pharmacy practice.

Nuclear Regulatory Commission

The Nuclear Regulatory Commission (NRC) regulates all reactor-produced byproduct materials with regard to their use and disposal and the radiation safety of all personnel using them as well as the public. The NRC does not regulate naturally occurring and accelerator-produced radionuclides, which are regulated by the individual states. The details of these topics are given below.

State Agencies and Agreement States

The cyclotron- or accelerator-produced radionuclides are regulated by one of the state agencies in each state. These state agencies include a health department, an environmental protection section, and similar divisions. They operate in the same vein as the NRC regarding radiation protection and the use of radionuclides. Licenses are issued to applicants upon submission of an application with details of the intended use of the radionuclide. Adoption of strict radiation protection principles is required of all authorized users.

At present, for convenience of operation, 33 states have entered into an agreement with the NRC, which authorizes each state to regulate the reactor-produced byproduct materials, in addition to the naturally occurring and accelerator-produced materials. These states are called the Agreement States. The rules and regulations of the states must be at least as strict as, if not stricter than, those of the NRC.

Licenses

Authorization for the use of byproduct material is granted by issuance of a license by the NRC or the Agreement state. There are two categories of licenses:

1. *General domestic license*: Although the general domestic license is given for the use of byproduct material in various devices according to 10CFR31, only the provisions of 10CFR31.11 are applicable for general license for the use of byproduct material in certain in vitro clinical laboratory tests. Such general licenses are given to physicians, veterinarians, clinical laboratories, and hospitals only for in vitro tests, not for the use of byproduct material in humans or animals. An application must be filed with the NRC using the

Form NRC-483 "Registration Certificate—In vitro Testing with Byproduct Material under General License" and a validated copy must be obtained prior to the use of byproduct material. The total amount to be possessed at any one time should not exceed 200 μCi (7.4 MBq) of ^{125}I, ^{131}I, ^{75}Se, and/or ^{59}Fe. The amount of ^{14}C and ^{3}H can be obtained in units of 10 μCi (370 kBq) and 20 μCi (740 kBq), respectively. The products must be supplied in prepackaged units.

2. *Specific licenses*: The specific licenses are given in two categories: one to manufacture or transfer for commercial distribution certain items containing byproduct material (10CFR32), and the other to possess, use, and transfer byproduct material in any chemical or physical form with the limitations of the maximum activity specified (10CFR33). The former types of specific licenses are typically given to commercial manufacturers. The latter type is called the specific license of broad scope or "broad license" and has three categories based on the maximum activity allowed for the receipt, acquisition, ownership, possession, use, and transfer of any chemical or physical form of byproduct material (10CFR33.11). The Type A broad license allows specified quantities of activities, usually in multicuries; the Type B broad license allows maximum activities of byproduct material specified in 10CFR33.100, Schedule A, Column I; and the Type C license permits maximum activities of byproduct material specified in 10CFR33.100, Schedule A, Column II, which are two orders of magnitude less than those in the Type B license.

The Type A licenses are mainly issued to large medical institutions with previous experience that are engaged in medical research, and in diagnostic and therapeutic uses of byproduct material. Individual users in the institution are authorized by licensee's management to conduct specific protocols using byproduct materials. The Type B licenses are normally issued to physicians in private practice or group practice and smaller medical institutions where use of byproduct material is limited and the names of all authorized users are indicated on the license. The Type C licenses are issued to physicians in practice using only a limited quantity of byproduct material. The licensee provides a statement that the byproduct material will be used by him, or persons under his supervision who satisfy the training requirement in 10CFR33.15.

In all cases of specific licenses, an application must be signed by the licensee's management and filed with the NRC using the NRC Form 313. All information related to the possession, use, and disposal of byproduct material must be provided on the application.

Radiation Protection

Because radiation can cause damage in living systems, international and national organizations have been established to set guidelines for the safe handling of radioactive materials. The International Committee on Radiological Protection (ICRP) and the National Council on Radiation Protection and Measurement (NCRP) are two such organizations. They set guidelines for all radiation workers to follow in handling radiations. The NRC adopts these recommendations into regulations for implementing radiation protection programs in the U.S. At present, the 10CFR20 contains all major radiation protection regulations applicable in the U.S. Since it is beyond the scope of this book to include the entire 10CFR20, only the relevant highlights of it are presented here.

Definitions

Several terms relate to absorbed doses and radiation areas as defined in the revised 10CFR20:

Committed dose equivalent ($H_{T,50}$) is the dose equivalent to organs or tissues of reference (T) that will be received from an intake of radioactive material by an individual during the 50-year period following the intake. It is given by Eq. (10.19) in Chapter 10.

Deep-dose equivalent (H_d), which applies to the external whole-body exposure, is the dose equivalent at a tissue depth of 1 cm (1000 mg/cm^2). It is given by Eq. (10.19).

Shallow-dose equivalent (H_S), which applies to the external exposure of the skin or an extremity, is the dose equivalent at a tissue depth of 0.007 cm (7 mg/cm^2) averaged over an area of 1 cm^2. It is given by Eq. (10.19).

Effective dose equivalent (H_E) is the sum of the products of the weighting factors applicable to each of the body organs or tissues that are irradiated and the dose equivalent to the corresponding organ or tissue ($H_E = \Sigma W_T \times H_{T,r}$). The values of W_T are given in Table 10.3. Note that this is due to committed dose equivalent from internal uptake of radiation. This quantity is termed simply effective dose.

Annual limit on intake (ALI) is the derived limit on the amount of radioactive material taken into the body of an adult worker by inhalation or ingestion in a year. These values are given in Table 1, Appendix B, in 10CFR20.

Derived air concentration (DAC) is the concentration of a given radionuclide in air that, if breathed by the reference man for a working year of 2000 hours under conditions of light work, results in an intake of ALI. DAC values are given in Table 1, column 3 of Appendix B in 10CFR20.

Total effective dose equivalent (TEDE) is the sum of the deep-dose equivalent (for external exposure) and the committed effective dose equivalent (for internal exposure).

Radiation area is an area in which an individual could receive from a radiation source a dose equivalent in excess of 5 mrem (0.05 mSv) in 1 hr at 30 cm from the source.

High radiation area is an area in which an individual could receive from a

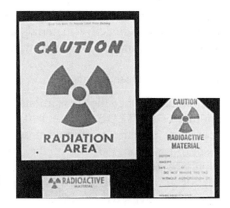

FIGURE 11.1. Radiation caution signs and labels.

radiation source a dose equivalent in excess of 100 mrem (1 mSv) in 1 hr at 30 cm from the source.

Very high radiation area is an area in which an individual could receive from radiation sources an absorbed dose in excess of 500 rad (5 Gy) in 1 hr at 1 m from the source.

Restricted area is an area of limited access that the licensee establishes for the purpose of protecting individuals against undue risks from exposure to radiation and radioactive materials.

Unrestricted area is an area in which an individual could receive from an external source a maximum dose of 2 mrem (20 μSv)/hr, and access to the area is neither limited nor controlled by the licensee.

Caution Signs and Labels

The NRC requires that specific signs, symbols, and labels be used to warn people of possible danger from the presence of radiations. These signs use magenta, purple, and black colors on a yellow background, and some typical signs are shown in Fig. 11.1.

Caution: Radiation Area: This sign must be posted in radiation areas.

Caution: High Radiation Area or Danger: High Radiation Area: This sign must be posted in high radiation areas.

Caution: Radioactive Material or Danger: Radioactive Material: This sign is posted in areas or rooms in which 10 times the quantity or more of any licensed material specified in Appendix C of 10CFR20 are used or stored. All containers with quantities of licensed materials exceeding those specified in Appendix C of 10CFR20 should be labeled with this sign. These labels must be removed or defaced prior to disposal of the container in the unrestricted areas.

Caution signs are not required in rooms storing the sealed sources, provided the radiation exposure at 1 foot (30 cm) from the surface of the source reads less than 5 mrem (0.05 mSv) per hr. Caution signs are not needed in rooms where radioactive materials are handled for less than 8 hr, during which time the materials are constantly attended.

Occupational Dose Limits

The annual limit of the occupational dose to an individual adult is the more limiting of (a) TEDE of 5 rem (0.05 Sv) or (b) the sum of the deep-dose equivalent and the committed dose equivalent to any individual organ or tissue other than the lens of the eye being equal to 50 rem (0.5 Sv). It should be noted that there is no lifetime cumulative dose limit in the revised 10CFR20, although the NCRP recommends a lifetime cumulative dose of 1 rem (0.01 Sv) × age in years.

The annual limit on the occupational dose to the lens of the eye is 15 rem (0.15 Sv).

The annual limit on the occupational dose to the skin and other extremities is the shallow-dose equivalent of 50 rem (0.5 Sv).

Depending on the license conditions, both internal and external doses have to be summed to comply with the limits. A licensee may authorize under *planned special procedures* an adult worker to receive additional dose in excess of the prescribed annual limits, provided no alternative procedure is available. The total dose from all planned procedures plus all doses in excess of the limits must not exceed the dose limit (5 rem or 0.05 Sv) in a given year, nor must it exceed five times the annual dose limits in the individual's lifetime.

The annual occupational dose limits for minors are 10% of the annual dose limits for the adults. The dose limit to the fetus/embryo during the entire pregnancy (gestation period) due to occupational exposure of a declared pregnant woman is 0.5 rem (0.005 Sv).

The total effective dose equivalent to individual members of the public is 0.1 rem (0.001 Sv) per year. However, this limit can be increased to 0.5 rem (0.005 Sv) provided the need for such a higher limit is demonstrated.

The dose in an unrestricted area from an external source is 2 mrem (0.02 mSv) in an hour.

ALARA Program

The dose limits are the upper limits for radiation exposure to individuals. The NRC has instituted the ALARA (as low as reasonably achievable) concept to reduce radiation exposure to individuals. The ALARA concept calls for a reasonable effort to maintain individual and collective doses as low as possible. Under this concept, techniques, equipment, and procedures are all critically evaluated. According to Regulatory Guide NUREG-1556, volume 9, Appendix L, under the ALARA concept, when the exposure to a radiation worker exceeds 10% of the occupational exposure in a quarter (Action level I), an investigation by the RSO takes place and the report is reviewed by the radiation safety committee (RSC). When the occupational exposure exceeds 30% of the occupational exposure (Action level II), corrective actions are taken or the institution must justify a higher dose level for ALARA in that particular situation.

Principles of Radiation Protection

Of the various types of radiation, the α particle is most damaging due to its great charge and mass, followed by the β particle and the γ rays. Heavier particles have shorter ranges and therefore deposit more energy per *unit* path length in the absorber, causing more damage. These are called *nonpenetrating* radiations. On the other hand, γ and x rays have no charge and mass and therefore have a much longer range in matter. These electromagnetic radiations are called *penetrating* radiations. Knowledge of the type and energy of radiations is essential in understanding the principles of radiation protection.

The cardinal principles of radiation protection from external sources are based on four factors: time, distance, shielding, and activity.

Time

The total radiation exposure to an individual is directly proportional to the time the person is exposed to the radiation source. The longer the exposure, the higher the radiation dose. Therefore, it is wise to spend no more time than necessary near radiation sources.

Distance

The intensity of a radiation source, and hence the radiation exposure, varies inversely as the square of the distance. It is recommended that an individual remains as far away as possible from the radiation source. Procedures and radiation areas should be designed such that only minimum exposure takes place to individuals doing the procedures or staying in or near the radiation areas.

The radiation exposure level from γ- and x-ray emitters can be estimated from the *exposure rate constant*, Γ, which is defined as the exposure due to γ and x rays in R/hr from 1 mCi (37 MBq) of a radionuclide at a distance of 1 cm. Each γ- and x-ray emitter has a specific value for Γ^a and it has the unit of R-cm^2/mCi-hr at 1 cm or, in SI units, μGy-m^2/GBq-hr at 1 m. Since γ or x rays below some 10 or 20 keV are absorbed by the container and thus do not contribute to radiation exposure, often γ and x rays above these energies only are included in the calculation of Γ. In these instances, they

---

[a] The Γ value of photon-emitting radionuclides can be calculated from the expression $\Gamma = 199\Sigma N_i E_i \mu_i$ where N_i is the fractional abundance of photons of energy E_i in MeV and μ_i is the mass absorption coefficient (cm^2/g) of air for photons of energy E_i.

TABLE 11.1. Exposure rate constants and half-value layer values in lead of commonly used radionuclides.[a]

Radionuclides	Γ^{20} (R-cm²/mCi-hr at 1 cm)	Γ^{20} (μGy-m²/GBq-hr at 1 m)[b]	HVL, Pb (cm)
^{137}Cs	3.26	88.11	0.65
^{99m}Tc	0.59	15.95	0.03
^{201}Tl	0.45	12.16	0.02
^{99}Mo	1.46	39.46	0.70
^{67}Ga	0.76	20.54	0.10
^{123}I	1.55	41.89	0.04
^{111}In	2.05	55.41	0.10
^{125}I	1.37	37.03	0.003
^{57}Co	0.56	15.16	0.02
^{131}I	2.17	58.65	0.30
^{18}F[c]	5.7	154.05	0.39

[a] Adapted from Goodwin PN. Radiation safety for patients and personnel In: *Freeman and Johnson's Clinical Radionuclide Imaging.* 3rd ed. Philadelphia: WB Saunders; 1984:320.
[b] R-cm²/mCi-hr is equal to 27.027 μGy-m²/GBq-hr.
[c] Personal communication with Dr. M. Stabin, Oak Ridge Associated Universities, Inc., Oak Ridge, Tennessee.

are denoted by Γ^{10} or Γ^{20}. The values of Γ^{20} for different radionuclides are given in Table 11.1.

The exposure rate X from an n (mCi) radionuclide source at a distance d (cm) is given by

$$X = \frac{n\Gamma}{d^2} \tag{11.1}$$

where Γ is the exposure rate constant of the radionuclide.

Problem 11.1
What is the exposure rate at 30 cm from a vial containing 20 mCi (740 MBq) of ^{131}I?

Answer
The exposure rate constant Γ^{20} for ^{131}I is 2.17 R-cm²/mCi-hr at 1 cm from Table 11.1. Therefore, using Eq. (11.1), at 30 cm

$$X = \frac{20 \times 2.17}{30^2} = 0.048 \text{ R/hr}$$

Since Γ^{20} for ^{131}I in SI units is 58.65 μGy-m²/GBq-hr at 1 m, X for 740 MBq ^{131}I at 30 cm is

$$X = \frac{0.74 \times 58.65}{(0.3)^2} = 482.2 \text{ } \mu\text{Gy/hr}$$

Shielding

Various high atomic number (Z) materials that absorb radiations can be used to provide radiation protection. Since the ranges of α and β particles are short in matter, the containers themselves act as shields for these radiations. However, γ radiations are highly penetrating, and therefore highly absorbing material must be used for shielding of γ-emitting sources. For economic reasons, lead is most commonly used for this purpose. The concept of half-value layer (HVL) of an absorbing material for penetrating radiations is important in the design of shielding for radiation protection. It is defined as the thickness of shielding that reduces the exposure from a radiation source by one half. Thus, an HVL of an absorber placed around a source of radiation with an exposure rate of 100 mR/hr will reduce the exposure rate to 50 mR/hr. The HVL is dependent on both the energy of the radiation and the atomic number of the absorbing material. The HVL value is greater for high-energy radiations and smaller for high Z materials. The greater the HVL of any material for a radiation, the larger the amount of material necessary to shield the radiation. The HVLs in lead of different radionuclides are given in Table 11.1.

Obviously, shielding is an important means of protection from radiation. Radionuclides should be stored in a shielded area. The dosages for patients should be transported in lead containers, and injected using syringe shield. Radionuclides emitting β particles should be stored in containers of low Z material such as aluminum and plastic because in high Z material such as lead they produce highly penetrating bremsstrahlung radiation. For example, ^{32}P should be stored in plastic containers instead of lead containers.

Activity

It should be obvious that the radiation hazard increases with the intensity of the radioactive source. The greater the source strength, the more the radiation exposure. Therefore, one should not work unnecessarily with high quantities of radioactivity.

Receiving and Monitoring of Radioactive Packages

According to 10CFR20, all packages carrying radioactive labels must be monitored for radioactive contamination. Monitoring should be done within 3 hr after delivery if the package is delivered during the normal working hours or no later than 3 hr from the beginning of the next working day if it is received after working hours. Two types of monitoring are performed: survey for external exposure, and wipe test for removable contamination on the surface of the package due to leakage of the radioactive material. The external survey is made by using a GM survey meter at the surface and at 1 m from the package. The wipe test for removable contamination is carried out by swabbing 300 cm^2 areas on the package surface using absorbent paper and counting the swab in a NaI(Tl) scintillation counter. The NRC limits of these measurements are:

Tests	Limits
Survey at the surface	<200 mR/hr
Survey at 1 m	<10 mR/hr
Wipe test	6600 dpm/300 cm^2

If any of the readings exceeds the limit, the NRC and the final delivery carrier must be notified by telephone and telegram, mailgram, or facsimile.

After the completion of the survey, all information as to the date of the receipt, the manufacturer, the lot number, name and quantity of the product, date and time of calibration, the survey readings, and the name of the individual performing the tests should be entered into a record book.

Radioactive Waste Disposal

Radioactive waste generated in nuclear medicine or pharmacy (e.g., syringes, needles, vials containing residual activities, liquid waste, gas, and contaminated papers, tissues, and liners) is disposed of by the following methods according to the guidelines set forth in 10CFR20:

1. Decay-in-storage
2. Release into a sewerage system
3. Transfer to an authorized recipient (commercial land disposal facilities)
4. Other disposal methods approved by the NRC (e.g., incineration and atmospheric release of radioactive gases).

The following is a brief description of the different methods of radioactive waste disposal, but one should consult 10CFR20 and 10CFR35 for further details.

Decay-in-Storage

Although 10CFR20 does not spell out the conditions of the decay-in-storage method, 10CFR35.92 describes this method in detail. Radionuclides with half-lives less than 120 days usually are disposed of by this method. The waste is allowed to decay for a period of time and then surveyed. If the radioactivity of the waste cannot be distinguished from background, it can be disposed of in the normal trash after removal of all radiation labels. In the previous 10CFR35.92, a decay for 10 half-lives of the radionuclide was required, but this requirement has been omitted in the new regulation. This method is most appropriate for short-lived radionuclides such as ^{99m}Tc, ^{123}I, ^{201}Tl, ^{111}In, and ^{67}Ga, and therefore it is routinely employed in nuclear medicine. Radioactive waste should be stored separately according to the similar half-lives of radionuclides for convenience of timely disposal of each radionuclide.

Release into a Sewerage System

The NRC permits radioactive waste disposal into a sewerage system provided the radioactive material is soluble (or dispersible biological material) in water and the quantity disposed of monthly does not exceed the limits of the maximum permissible concentrations (MPCs) set in 10CFR20. When more than one radionuclide is released, the fraction of each radionuclide is calculated from the limit given in 10CFR20, and the sum of the fractions of all radionuclides should not exceed unity. Disposal depends on the flow rate of water but is limited to 1 Ci (37 GBq) of ^{14}C, 5 Ci (185 GBq) of ^{3}H, and 1 Ci (37 GBq) for all other radionuclides annually. Excreta from humans undergoing medical diagnosis or treatment with radioactive material are exempted from these limitations. However, items contaminated with excreta (such as linens and diapers contaminated with urine or feces) are not exempted from these limitations. To follow this method of radioactive disposal in an institution, one has to determine the average daily flow of sewer water in the institution from the water usage bill, and the number of users of a radionuclide, so that for each individual user a limit can be set for sewer disposal of the radionuclide in question.

Transfer to an Authorized Recipient

A transfer to an authorized recipient method is adopted for long-lived radionuclides and usually involves transfer of radioactive waste to authorized commercial firms that bury or incinerate at approved sites or facilities.

Each shipment of radioactive waste must be accompanied by a shipment manifest that contains the names, addresses, and telephone numbers of the waste generator and waste collector, and identity, volume, and total radioactivity of the radionuclide. The manifest shall include a certification that the shipment is properly classified, packaged, marked, and labeled according to the regulations of the Department of Transportation.

Other Disposal Methods

A licensee may adopt separate methods of radioactive waste disposal other than those mentioned above, provided approval is obtained from the regulatory agency. The impact of such disposal methods on the environment, nearby facilities, and the population is heavily weighed before approval is granted. Incineration of carcasses of research animals containing radioactive materials is allowed by this method up to the limit of MPCs. Radioactive gas such as ^{133}Xe is also released by this method as long as the radioactive effluent into the atmosphere does not exceed the NRC limits of MPCs. Radioactive waste containing 0.05 μCi (1.85 kBq) or less of ^{3}H or ^{14}C per gram of medium used for liquid scintillation counting or of animal tissue may be disposed of in the regular nonradioactive trash. The disposed tissue must not be used for human or animal consumption.

Records must be maintained of the date of storage and the amount and kind of activity in a waste disposal log book. The stored packages must be labeled with pertinent information. The date of disposal, the amount of disposed activity, and the name of the individual who is disposing must also be recorded in the logbook.

Radioactive Spill

Accidental spillage of radioactivity can cause unnecessary radiation exposure to personnel and must be treated cautiously and expeditiously. There are two types of spills: major and minor. No definitive distinction exists between a major and a minor spill. A major spill usually occurs when the spilled activity cannot be contained in a normal way and can cause undue exposure to personnel around. In the case of a major spill, the radiation safety office should be notified immediately. In either case, the access to the area should be restricted. Appropriate procedures must be established for decontamination. Areas, personnel, and equipment have to be decontaminated, keeping in mind the principle of containment of radioactivity. Survey and wipe test have to be done after decontamination. The RSO investigates the accident and recommends corrective action if a major spill occurs.

Personnel Monitoring

Personnel monitoring is required under the following conditions:

1. Occupational workers including minors and pregnant women likely to receive in 1 year a dose in excess of 10% of the annual limit from the external radiation source
2. Individuals entering high or very high radiation areas.

Monitoring for occupational intake of radioactive material is also required if the annual intake by an individual is likely to exceed 10% of the ALIs in Table 1, Appendix B of 10CFR20, and if the minors and pregnant women are likely to receive a committed effective dose equivalent in excess of 0.05 rem (0.5 mSv) in 1 year.

   Three devices are used to measure the exposure of ionizing radiations received by an individual: the pocket dosimeter, the film badge, and the thermoluminescent dosimeter. The pocket dosimeter works on the principle of a charged electroscope (Fig. 11.2) provided with a scale inside. The scale is so designed that when the dosimeter is fully charged it reads zero, and as the charge is reduced by radiation, the reading on the viewable scale increases. The dosimeter is initially charged to read zero. Ionizing radiation discharges the dosimeter by ionization in the sensitive volume of the chamber and the amount of exposure can be read from the scale. The dosimeter has the advantage of giving an immediate reading, but it requires frequent charging for reuse. Because the charge leaks over time, the cumulative reading over a long period of time can be erroneous. These dosimeters are available in full-scale readings of 200 mR, 500 mR, and 1 R.

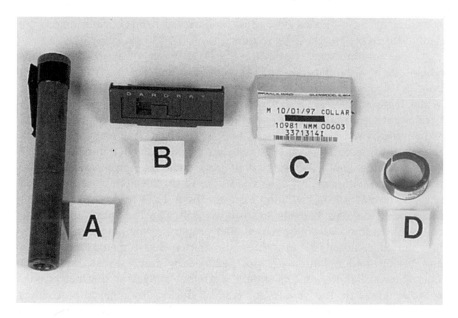

FIGURE 11.2. Devices to measure personnel radiation exposure. A: Pocket dosimeter. (Courtesy of Nuclear Associates, Division of Victoreen, Inc., 100 Voice Rd, Carle Place, New York.) B: Film badge holder. C: Film badge. D: Thermoluminescent chip in finger badge.

The film badge is most popular and cost-effective for personnel monitoring and gives reasonably accurate readings of exposures from β, γ, and x radiations. The film badge consists of a radiation-sensitive film held in a plastic holder (Fig. 11.2). Filters of different materials (aluminum, copper, and cadmium) are attached to the holder in front of the film to differentiate exposures from radiations of different types and energies. The optical density of the developed film after exposure is measured by a densitometer and compared with that of a calibrated film exposed to known radiations. Film badges are usually changed by radiation workers on a monthly basis and give an integrated dose for each individual for a month. The main disadvantage of the film badge is the long waiting period before the exposed personnel know about their exposure. The film badge also tends to develop fog due to heat and humidity, particularly when in storage for a long time, and this may obscure the actual exposure reading.

In many institutions the film badges of all workers are sent to a commercial firm approved by National Voluntary Laboratory Accreditation Program (NVLAP) of the National Institute of Standards and Technology that develops and reads the density of the films and sends the report of exposure to the institution. When an individual is employed at a radiation facility, a record of his accumulated dose must be retrieved from previous employers and added to his present dose account.

A thermoluminescent dosimeter (TLD) consists of inorganic crystals (chips) such as lithium fluoride (LiF) and manganese-activated calcium fluoride (CaF_2:Mn) held in holders like the film badges or finger rings. When these crystals are exposed to radiations, electrons from the valence band are excited and trapped by the impurities in the forbidden band. If the radiation-exposed crystal is heated to 300° to 400°C, the trapped electrons are raised to the conduction band, wherefrom they fall back into the valence band, emitting light. The amount of light emitted is proportional to the amount of radiation energy absorbed in the TLD. The light is measured and read as the amount of radiation exposure by a TLD reader, a device that heats the crystal and reads the exposure as well. The TLD gives an accurate exposure reading and can be reused after proper heating (annealing).

It should be noted that exposures to radiation due to medical procedures and background radiation are not included in occupational dose limits. Therefore, radiation workers should wear film badges or dosimeters only at work. These devices should be taken off during any medical procedures involving radiation such as radiographic procedures and dental examinations, and also when leaving after the day's work.

Dos and Don'ts in Radiation Protection Practice

Do post radiation signs in radiation areas.
Do wear laboratory coats and gloves when working with radioactive materials.
Do work in a ventilated fumehood when working with radioactive gases.
Do cover the trays and workbench with absorbent paper.
Do store and transport radioactive material in lead containers.
Do wear a film badge while working in the radiation laboratory.
Do identify all radionuclides and dates of assay on the containers.
Do survey work areas for any contamination as frequently as possible.
Do clean up spills promptly, and survey the area after cleaning.
Do not eat, drink, or smoke in the radiation laboratory.
Do not pipette any radioactive material by mouth.
Do monitor hands and feet after the day's work.
Do notify the RSO in case of any major spill or other emergencies related to radiation.

Medical Uses of Radioactive Materials

The NRC regulates the medical use of byproduct materials by enforcing 10CFR35; similar regulations are implemented by the states for naturally occurring and accelerator-produced radionuclides. However, the Agreement States regulate both categories of radionuclides. The revised 10CFR part 35 has been in effect as of October 24, 2002 when all NRC-regulated states must adopt all new regulations. However, the Agreement States have been given a 2-year grace period to adopt these regulations, after which time 10CFR35 will be effective for medical use of byproduct material equally for all states.

There are six categories of medical uses of radioactive materials according to 10CFR35: (1) radiopharmaceuticals for uptake, dilution, and excretion (10CFR35.100); (2) radiopharmaceuticals for imaging and localization including generators and kits (10CFR35.200); (3) radiopharmaceuticals for therapy (10CFR35.300); (4) sealed sources for brachytherapy (10CFR35.400); (5) sealed sources for diagnosis such as sources of ^{125}I and ^{153}Gd for bone mineral analysis (10CFR35.500); and (6) sealed sources for teletherapy such as sources of ^{60}Co and ^{137}Cs in teletherapy units (10CFR35.600).

The regulations for the medical use of all radioactive materials are given in 10CFR35, but radiopharmaceuticals under categories 1, 2, and 3 only are relevant in nuclear medicine. These radiopharmaceuticals must be approved for human clinical use by the FDA under an IND or NDA. The ^{99m}Tc activity is eluted from the ^{99}Mo-^{99m}Tc generator and reagent kits are used to prepare ^{99m}Tc-labeled radiopharmaceuticals according to instructions given in the package inserts. Only reagent kits that are approved by the FDA under an IND or NDA may be used for radiopharmaceutical preparation.

Applications, Amendments, and Notifications

As already mentioned, applications for a license and its renewals must be made by the licensee's management for the medical uses of byproduct materials. Amendments to the license must be made by the licensee's management for the following:

1. Appointment or discontinuation of an authorized user, radiation safety officer, authorized medical physicist, or authorized nuclear pharmacist
2. Change of name or address of the licensee
3. Change or addition of the use areas
4. Use of excess or new byproduct materials not permitted before in the license.

Notification of the above must be made within 30 days of occurrence. Change or addition of areas of use for uptake and dilution (10CFR35.100) and for localization and imaging (10CFR35.200) need not be amended. The Type A specific licenses of broad scope are exempted from these requirements.

Authority and Responsibilities of the License

According to 10CFR35.24, the licensee's management is responsible for the overall implementation of a radiation safety program in the medical uses of byproduct material. The licensee's management shall approve in writing all new authorized users, an RSO, or a nuclear pharmacist, and ministerial changes in the radiation safety program that do not require license amendment (10CFR35.26).

The licensee's management shall appoint an RSO, who accepts in writing responsibilities to implement a radiation protection program. Management may appoint one or more temporary RSOs for 60 days in a year, if all conditions of an RSO are met.

The licensee's management also must appoint an RSC, if the licensee is authorized for two or more different types of uses of byproduct material. Examples are the use of therapeutic quantities of unsealed byproduct material (10CFR35.300) and manual brachytherapy (10CFR35.400), or manual brachytherapy and low-dose-rate therapy units (10CFR35.600), or teletherapy units (10CFR35.600) and gamma knife units (10CFR35.600). Use of byproduct materials for both uptake and dilution (10CFR35.100) and imaging and localization (10CFR35.200) does not require an RSC. The RSC must include as a minimum an authorized user of each type of use permitted in the license, the RSO, a representative of the nursing service, a representative of management, and other members, if appropriate. The NRC does not prescribe any definite frequencies of the RSC meetings nor record keeping of the minutes.

Supervision

According to 10CFR35.27, a licensee that permits an individual to work under an authorized user or authorized nuclear pharmacist using byproduct material must instruct the supervised individual to strictly follow all regulations and conditions of the license and all procedures involving byproduct material. There is no requirement for periodic review of the supervised individual's work and records. The licensee is responsible for the acts and omissions of the supervised individuals.

Mobile Nuclear Medicine Service

According to 10CFR35.80, a licensee providing mobile nuclear medicine service to a client must

1. have a letter signed by the licensee and the management of each client spelling out the details of the responsibility and authority of the client and the licensee,
2. calibrate and daily check the instruments for measuring dosages and surveying,
3. measure dosages and perform surveys of the area of uses at the client address, and
4. the client must have a license for receiving and using byproduct material.

Written Directives

According to 10CFR35.40, a written directive is required when a dosage greater than 30 μCi (1.11 MBq) of ^{131}I-NaI or a therapeutic dosage of an unsealed byproduct material other than ^{131}I-NaI is administered to a patient or human research subject. The written directive must be dated and signed by an authorized user and must contain the patient's name, the dosage, the name of the drug and route of administration. A revision of the written directive can be made, if necessary, provided it is signed and dated by the authorized user before the administration. In case of an emergency, an oral revision to an existing written directive is acceptable, which must be followed by a written directive within 48 hr.

According to 10CFR35.41, the licensee shall develop and maintain a copy of the written procedures for the written directive that include specific verifications of the identity of the patient before each administration, and that the administration is in accordance with the written directive. The identity of the patient may be verified by the name, driver's license, birthday, any hospital's I.D. number, etc.

Measurement of Dosages

According to 10CFR35.63, all dosages for patient administration must be measured in an instrument (dose calibrator) that is calibrated with nationally recognized standards or the manufacturer's instructions (10CFR35.60). Although the methods of calibration are not specifically prescribed in 10CFR35, the constancy, accuracy, linearity, and geometry of the dose calibrator must be checked as described in Chapter 8.

For unit dosages, the activity can be determined by direct measurement or by the decay correction of the activity provided by the licensed manufacturer. For dosages other than unit dosages, the activity must be determined by direct measurement, a combination of measurement of radioactivity and mathematical calculations, or a combination of volumetric measurements and mathematical calculations based on the activity provided by the manufacturer.

Unless otherwise directed by the authorized user, the licensee may not use a dosage if it does not fall within the prescribed dosage range, or if it differs from the prescribed dosage by more than 20%. The licensees who use only unit dosages supplied by the manufacturer may not need to have a dose calibrator.

Calibration, Transmission, and Reference Sources

The following sources of byproduct material are permitted for check, calibration, transmission, and reference use (10CFR35.65):

1. Sealed sources not exceeding 30 mCi (1.11 GBq) manufactured and supplied by a licensed manufacturer, or a licensee authorized to redistribute such sources

2. Any byproduct material with a half-life not longer than 120 days in individual amounts not exceeding 15 mCi (0.56 GBq)
3. Any byproduct material with a half-life longer than 120 days in individual amounts not to exceed the smaller of 200 μCi (7.4 MBq) or 1000 times the quantities in Appendix B of 10CFR30
4. ^{99m}Tc in amounts needed.

A licensee may only use sealed sources for medical use, manufactured by a licensed manufacturer (10CFR.49).

Requirement for Possession of Sealed Sources

According to 10CFR35.67, sealed sources of radionuclides with a half-life greater than 30 days and containing more than 100 μCi (3.7 MBq) of γ-emitting material or more than 10 μCi (370 kBq) α-emitting material must be leak tested and inventoried semiannually. If a source shows a leak of 0.005 μCi (185 Bq) or more of removable contamination, it must be immediately removed from use and stored, disposed of, or repaired according to regulations, and a report must be filed with the NRC within 5 days of the leak test describing the source involved, the test results, and the action taken.

Labeling of Vials and Syringes

Each syringe and vial containing radioactivity must be labeled to identify the radioactive drug (10CFR35.69). Each syringe or vial shield also must be labeled, unless the label on the syringe or vial is visible through the shield. Although syringe shields are not required by the NRC regulations for administration of radiopharmaceuticals, they should be used to maintain ALARA exposures.

Surveys of Ambient Radiation Exposure Rate

According to 10CFR35.70, the NRC requires that the licensee shall survey all areas where unsealed byproduct material requiring a written directive is prepared for use or administered. The survey must be performed at the end of each day of use with a radiation detection instrument.

According to 10CFR35.61, the survey meter must be calibrated before its first use, annually, and after repairs that affect calibration. Calibration must be made in all scales with readings up to 1000 mrem (10 mSv) per hour with a radiation source, and two separated readings must be calibrated on each scale or decade (digital) that is used to show compliance. The date of calibration must be noted on the instrument. The licensee may not use the survey instruments if the difference between the indicated exposure rate and the calculated exposure rate is more than 20%. Requirement for wipe testing of various areas of use for removable contamination has been eliminated in the new 10CFR35 regulations. However, it is advisable to adopt wipe testing for removable contamination for better radiation protection.

Training and Experience Requirements for Medical Uses
of Byproduct Materials

Authorized users, RSOs, and nuclear pharmacists are required to have appropriate training and experience for medical uses of byproduct materials. Normally there are two methods of approval: (1) certification by a specific medical specialty board, and (2) training and work experience in radionuclide handling techniques applicable to specific medical use of byproduct material.

The specialty boards are not listed in 10CFR35; however, each board must meet all requirements of the training and work experience in a specific category described below and be approved by the NRC.

The training part includes a specified period of classroom and laboratory instruction in the areas of (1) radiation physics and instrumentation, (2) radiation protection, (3) mathematics pertinent to radioactivity, (4) chemistry of byproduct material, and (5) radiation biology and radiation dosimetry (for RSO).

The work experience must be under an authorized user, RSO, or nuclear pharmacist and must include (1) ordering, receiving, and unpacking radioactive materials, and surveying; (2) calibration of dose calibrators and survey meters; (3) calculating, measuring, and preparing dosages for patients; (4) procedures for spill management; (5) safely administering dosages to patients (for authorized users only); and (6) elution of radioactive generators (for localization and imaging studies).

In addition, approval by training and experience method requires a written certification by a preceptor that the individual has acquired competence in the techniques to function independently for a specified use of byproduct material.

The required hours of training and experience vary for different types of uses of radioactive material:

Radiation safety officer	200 hr of training plus 1 year of work experience under a radiation safety officer
Nuclear pharmacist	700 hr of combined training and work experience
Authorized user (uptake, dilution, and excretion)	60 hr of combined training and work experience
Authorized user (localization and imaging)	700 hr of combined training and work experience
Authorized user (therapeutic use)	700 hr of combined training and work experience, plus three cases in each therapeutic use of byproduct material
Authorized user (hyperthyroidism using less than 33 mCi [1.22 GBq] ^{131}I-NaI)	80 hr of combined training and work experience, plus three cases of hyperthyroid treatments
Authorized user (thyroid cancer using greater than 33 mCi [1.22 GBq] ^{131}I-NaI)	80 hr of combined training and experience, plus three cases of thyroid cancer treatments

Report and Notification of a Medical Event

The term *medical event* has been substituted for *misadministration* and *recordable event* under the revised 10CFR35. A medical event occurs when a dose exceeds 5 rem (0.05 Sv) effective dose equivalent, or 50 rem (0.5 Sv) to an organ or tissue or skin from any of the following situations:

1. the total dosage delivered differs from the prescribed dosage by 20% or more, or falls outside the prescribed dosage range; or ·
2. administration of a wrong radioactive drug containing byproduct material; or
3. administration by a wrong route; or
4. administration to a wrong individual.

The licensee must notify a medical event by telephone to the NRC Operation Center no later than one calendar day after discovery of the event, followed by a written report to the NRC Regional Office within 15 days. The report must include the licensee's name; prescribing physician's name; brief description of the event; cause of the event; effect of the event, if any, on the individual; corrective action taken, if any; and whether the affected individual or his or her relative or guardian has been notified. The individual's name or identification number shall not be included in the report.

The licensee shall notify the individual and the referring physician of the event no later than 24 hours after the discovery, unless the referring physician personally takes the responsibility of informing or not informing the individual based on medical judgment. If a verbal notification is made, the licensee shall inform the individual of the availability of a written description of the event, which the licensee will provide upon request.

In addition, the licensee shall annotate a copy of the report filed with the NRC with the name and social security number or other identification number of the affected individual and provide a copy of the annotated report to the referring physician, if other than the licensee, within 15 days of occurrence of the event. Record keeping of medical events is not required since the reports are provided to the NRC.

Report and Notification of a Dose to an Embryo/Fetus or a Nursing Child

The licensee shall report to the NRC an event in which an embryo/fetus receives more than 5 rem (50 mSv) dose equivalent due to the administration of byproduct material to a pregnant individual, unless such a dose was specifically approved in advance by the authorized user. Also, a report must be made to the NRC if the dose to a nursing child, from the administration of byproduct material to a breast-feeding individual, exceeds total effective dose equivalent 5 rem (50 mSv) or has resulted in unintended permanent functional damage to an organ or a physiological system of the child.

The conditions, timing, and descriptions of the report are identical to those of the medical events described above.

Bioassay

Regulatory guide 8.20 gives the details of bioassay requirements for ^{131}I and ^{125}I radionuclides. Bioassays are required when the level of radioiodine activity handled (volatile or dispersible) exceeds the following values:

Open bench: 1 mCi (37 MBq)
Fumehood: 10 mCi (370 MBq)
Glovebox: 100 mCi (3.7 GBq)

When the radioiodinated material is nonvolatile, the limits of activity are higher by a factor of 10. ^{131}I-capsules (e.g., diagnostic capsules) may be considered with iodine in nonvolatile form, and bioassay may not be necessary unless they are inadvertently opened (e.g., dropped or crushed).

For iodine radionuclides, bioassay is performed by the thyroid uptake test within 72 hr to 14 days, depending on the frequency of handling radioiodine but at least 6 hr after the exposure or intake. Sometimes urine analysis may also be required. Bioassays may be required for other radionuclides depending on the amount and type of the radionuclide.

Release of Patients Administered with Radiopharmaceuticals

According to 10CFR35.75, a licensee can release a patient administered with a radiopharmaceutical or a permanent radioactive implant, provided the TEDE to any other individual from exposure to the released patient is not likely to exceed 500 mrem (5 mSv). Practically in nuclear medicine, patients treated with ^{131}I-NaI are commonly considered under these regulations. In these cases, when the activity in the patient is less than 33 mCi (1.2 GBq) or the measured exposure rate is less than 7 mrem/hr (0.07 mSv/hr) at 1 m, then the patient can be released. However, patients administered with higher ^{131}I-activities, as high as 200 mCi (7.4 GBq), may be released provided the dose calculations using patient-specific parameters show that the potential TEDE to any individual would be no greater than 0.5 rem (5 mSv) (NRC Regulatory Guide 8.39). The patient-specific calculations depend on the choice of the occupancy factor and the physical or effective half-life. An occupancy factor of 0.75 is chosen for $t_{1/2}$ of less than 1 day and a value of 0.25 for $t_{1/2}$ greater than 1 day. A value of 0.25 for the occupancy factor would be valid if the patient follows the instructions, such as for the first 2 days: (1) maintain the distances from others; (2) sleep alone or, better yet, live alone; (3) do not travel by airplane or mass transportation; (4) do not travel in automobiles with others; (5) have the sole use of the bathroom; (6) drink plenty of water; and (7) limit visits by others. These instructions must be given in writing to the patient to follow after release.

The released patient must be given instructions, including written instructions, to maintain the dose as low as reasonably achievable if the TEDE to any other individual is likely to exceed 100 mrem (1 mSv). In the case of ^{131}I treatment, instructions must be given to the patient when the activity in the

TABLE 11.2. Limits of activities that require instructions to breast-feeding patients and record keeping.[a]

Radiopharmaceutical	Activity above which instructions are needed [mCi (MBq)]	Activity above which record is needed [mCi (MBq)]	Recommended duration of cessation of breast-feeding
[131]I-NaI	0.004 (0.01)	0.002 (0.07)	Complete cessation
[123]I-NaI	0.5 (20)	3 (100)	
^{123}I-MIBG	2 (70)	10 (400)	12 hr (4 mCi/150 MBq)
^{99m}Tc-DTPA	30 (1000)	150 (6000)	
^{99m}Tc-MAA	1.3 (50)	6.5 (200)	12.6 hr (4 mCi/ 150 MBq)
[99m]Tc-pertechnetate	3 (100)	15 (600)	12 hr (12 mCi/440 MBq)
^{99m}Tc-DISIDA	30 (1000)	150 (6000)	
[99m]Tc-glucoheptonate	30 (1000)	170 (6000)	
[99m]Tc-sestamibi	30 (1000)	150 (6000)	
^{99m}Tc-MDP	30 (1000)	150 (6000)	
^{99m}Tc-PYP	25 (900)	120 (4000)	
^{99m}Tc-RBC in vivo	10 (400)	50 (2000)	6 hr (20 mCi/740 MBq)
^{99m}Tc-RBC in vitro	30 (1000)	150 (6000)	
[99m]Tc-sulfur colloid	7 (300)	35 (1000)	6 hr (12 mCi/440 MBq)
^{99m}Tc-MAG3	30 (1000)	150 (6000)	
^{99m}Tc-WBC	4 (100)	15 (600)	12 hr (12 mCi/440 MBq)
[67]Ga-citrate	0.04 (1)	0.2 (7)	1 mo (4 mCi/150 MBq)
^{111}In-WBC	0.2 (10)	1 (40)	1 wk (0.5 mCi/20 MBq)
[201]Tl	1 (40)	5 (200)	2 wk (3 mCi/110 MBq)

[a] NRC Regulatory Guide 8.39.

patient is more than 7 mCi (259 MBq) or when the measured exposure rate exceeds 2 mrem/hr (0.02 mSv/hr) at 1 m. If the dose to a breast-fed infant or child could exceed 100 mrem (1 mSv) assuming continuous breast-feeding by a patient administered with radiopharmaceutical, then instructions on discontinuation of breast-feeding and consequences of failure to follow the guidance must also be given. Table 11.2 lists the activity limits for giving instructions to the breast-feeding patients and activity limits for cessation of breast-feeding.

Records of release of patients are required if the TEDE is calculated by using the retained activity rather than the administered activity, using an occupancy factor less than 0.25 at 1 m, using a biological or effective $t_{1/2}$, or considering the shielding by tissue. Records are also required if instructions are given to a breast-feeding woman who may give a TEDE exceeding 500 mrem (5 mSv) to the infant from continuous breast-feeding (10CFR35.2075). Table 11.2 gives the activity limits that require record keeping in case of breast-feeding.

Record Keeping

Records must be maintained for the receipt, storage, and disposal of radioactive materials, and for various activities performed in the radiation laboratories. According to the NRC regulations, these records must contain specific information and be kept for certain period of time. Table 11.3 lists the records that are required by the NRC and the period of time to be kept.

Department of Transportation

The transportation of radioactive materials is governed by the U.S. Department of Transportation (DOT), which sets the guidelines for packaging, types of packaging material, limits of radioactivity in a package, and exposure limits. Title 49 of the Code of Federal Regulations (49CFR) contains all these regulations related to packaging and transportation of radioactive materials.

There are two types of packaging:

Type A: This type of packaging is primarily used for most radiopharmaceuticals. Packaging is sufficient to prevent loss of radioactive material with proper shielding to maintain the prescribed exposure during normal transportation. The limits of radioactivities of various radionuclides under this category are specified in 49CFR.

Type B: When the radioactivity exceeds the limits specified in Type A, Type B packaging must be utilized. Such packaging is considerably more accident-resistant and is required for very large quantities of radioactive material.

The packages must pass certain tests such as the drop test, corner drop test, compression test, and 30-min water spray test.

The radioactive packages must be labeled properly prior to transportation. There are three types of labels (Fig. 11.3) according to the exposure reading at 1 m (transport index, TI). The TI criteria for three labels are given in Table 11.4. The TI must be indicated on the label, and the sign "RADIOACTIVE" must be placed on the package. The maximum permissible TI value is 10, although it is limited to 3 for passenger-carrying aircrafts. For liquids, the label "THIS SIDE UP" must be placed on the package. Each package must be labeled on opposite sides with the appropriate warning label (one of the labels in Fig. 11.3). The label must identify

TABLE 11.3. Record keeping of various activities related to radioactive materials.

Type of operation	Information needed	Time to maintain the records
Written directives (10CFR35.2040)	Copy of the written directives	3 years
Procedures requiring written directives (10CFR35.2041)	Copy of the procedures	Duration of the license
Dosage of radiopharmaceuticals dispensed (10CFR35.2063)	Name, lot number, expiration date, patient's name or identification number, prescribed dosage and dispensed dosage, date and time of administration, and name of the individual	3 years
Calibration of dose calibrator (10CFR35.2060)	Model, serial number of the dose calibrator, date and results of test, and name of the individual	3 years
Calibration of survey meters (10CFR35.2061)	Model and serial number of the instrument, date and results of calibration, and name of the individual	3 years
Semiannual leak tests and inventory of sealed sources (10CFR35.2067)	Model and serial number of each source and its radionuclide, estimated activity, measured activity in μCi (Bq), date of test, location of source (inventory) and name of the individual	3 years
Molybdenum breakthrough (10CFR35.2204)	μCi (MBq) of ^{99}Mo per mCi (MBq) of ^{99m}Tc, date and time of measurement, name of the individual	3 years
Thyroid bioassay and whole body counting (10CFR20.2106)	Name of the individual having the bioassay, date of reading and the individual taking the measurement	Until the NRC terminates the license
Personnel exposure monitoring records (10CFR20.2106)	Must be on Form NRC-5 according to items described in the form	Until the NRC terminates the license
Radioactive waste disposal by decay-in-storage (10CFR35.2092)	Date of disposal, instrument used, background reading and surface reading of the waste container and the name of the individual	3 years
Planned special procedures (10CFR20.2105)	Circumstances, name of authorizing individual, doses expected	Until the NRC terminates the license

TABLE 11.3 (*continued*)

Type of operation	Information needed	Time to maintain the records
Surveys (10CFR35.2070)	Date, area, trigger level (mR/hr), survey data, instrument used, and name of the individual	3 years
Release of patients with unsealed byproduct material (10CFR35.2075)	Basis of calculation to release the patient, such as retained activity, occupancy factor less than 0.25 at 1 m, using T_p or T_e or considering shielding by tissue	3 years
Instruction given to breast-feeding female (10CFR35.2075)	Instruction given if dose to the infant exceeds 0.5 rem (5 mSv)	3 years

the contents and amounts of radionuclide in curies or becquerels. The package must contain shipping document inside bearing the identity, amount, and chemical form of the radioactive material and the TI (Table 11.4).

Placards are necessary on the transport vehicles carrying yellow-III labeled packages and must be put on all four sides of the vehicle.

According to 49CFR173.421, radionuclides are exempted from the packaging and labeling requirements if only a limited quantity is shipped. The surface exposure readings should not exceed 0.5 mR/hr at all points of the package surface, and the wipe test indicates no removable contamination in excess of 6600 dpm/300 cm^2. A notice or a label indicating "Radioactive—Limited Quantity" must be enclosed inside or pasted outside or forwarded with the package. The notice must include the name of the shipper and the consignee, and the following statement must be in or on the package: "This package conforms to the conditions and limitations specified in

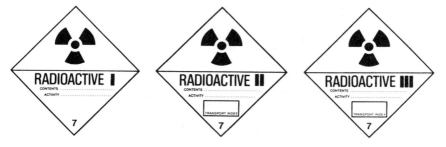

FIGURE 11.3. Three types of Department of Transportation (DOT) labels required for transportation of radioactive materials.

TABLE 11.4. Labeling categories for packages containing radioactive materials.

	Exposure (mR/hr)	
Type of label	At surface	At 1 m
White—I	<0.5	—
Yellow—II	>0.5 ≤50	<1
Yellow—III	>50 ≤200	>1 ≤10

Note: No package shall exceed 200 mR/hr at the surface of the package or 10 mR/hr at 1 m. Transport index is the reading in mR/hr at 1 m from the package surface.

TABLE 11.5. Limited quantities of several radionuclides that are exempted from shipping and labeling requirements, according to 49CFR 173.425.

Radionuclide	Quantity (mCi)	Quantity (MBq)	Radionuclide	Quantity (mCi)	Quantity (MBq)
^{57}Co	22	800	^{111}In	5	200
^{67}Ga	16	600	^{32}P	0.8	30
^{123}I	16	600	^{99m}Tc	22	800
^{125}I	5.4	200	^{201}Tl	27	1000
^{131}I	1.4	50	^{133}Xe gas	541	20,000

49CFR173.421 for radioactive material, excepted package—limited quantity of material, UN2910." The limited quantities for some important radionuclides are given in Table 11.5, based on $10^{-4}A_2$ as stated in 49CFR173.425. The values of A_2 are obtained from 49CFR173.435.

Employees who ship hazardous material (hazmat) including radioactive material must have hazmat training to be able to recognize and identify hazardous material, to conduct their specific function, and to enforce safety procedures in shipping to protect the public. The training must be given to new employees within 90 days of employment and then repeated every 3 years. The training is provided by the hazmat employer or other public or private sources, and a record of training must be made.

European Regulations Governing Radiopharmaceuticals

Regulations governing the use of radioactive drugs in humans varied in European countries until 1989 when the European Union (EU, a union of 15 European countries) adopted the EU Directives involving radiopharmaceuticals. As implied in the charter of the EU, medical products, among others, are transported and distributed free of regulatory constraints of individual countries. The European Regulatory Organizations have three main instruments: Directives, Guidelines, and Regulations. Directives are mandatory rules to be translated into national legislation and implemented in each member country. Guidelines are recommendations (not mandatory) for effective implementation of Directives by the member countries. Regulations are mandatory for all member countries without adoption into national legislation.

Directive 65/65 EEC, amended by 83/570 EEC, 87/21 EEC, and 98/431 EEC, defines medicinal products and details the requirements for registration for commercialization of the medicinal products by each member state. Directive 75/319 EEC establishes the requirements for an application for registration with all pharmaceutical data, pharmacological and toxicological data, and clinical effectiveness of the medicinal product. Directive 89/341 EEC exempts certain drugs from the registration requirements, which include primarily drugs compounded by the pharmacy for patients and those for research and clinical trials. Until 1989, radiopharmaceuticals were exempt from these requirements, but then Directive 89/343 EEC was introduced requiring the registration of all radiopharmaceuticals in all EU member states for human use.

A drug can be registered for commercialization by a centralized or decentralized registration procedure. In the centralized procedure, which is governed by the European Medicines Evaluation Agency (EMEA), an application for a drug is reviewed and approved by one member state nominated by the EU, and the approved drug is valid in all member states. In the decentralized procedure, an application is made to one member state that approves/disapproves it after review. The applicant state can then present the authorization to other member states for registration. The centralized registration procedure is mandatory for certain drugs, such as monoclonal antibodies or radionuclides.

Directive 91/356 EEC provides the principles of good manufacturing practice (GMP), which apply to drug manufacturing at the industrial levels as well as to compounding in hospitals. For an approved radiopharmaceutical for marketing, a summary of the product characteristics (SPC), equivalent to package inserts in the U.S., must be included, which lists relevant information, such as chemical form, approved clinical indication, internal dosimetry, instructions for labeling kits, method to verify radiochemical purity, shelf life, storage temperature, etc. For a change or a new clinical indication, new authorization must be obtained.

The European Pharmacopoeia specifies characteristics of all radiopharmaceuticals in monograph forms, regarding radionuclidic and radiochemical purity, pH, sterility, pyrogenicity, etc. It is mandatory in drug product manufacturing in the entire EU and equivalent to the USP in the U.S.

Within the EU, it is the responsibility of the radiopharmacist to ensure the quality, safety, and efficacy of a radiopharmaceutical if it is intended for human administration. Similarly, the nuclear physician is responsible for administration of the radiopharmaceutical to the patient and the clinical care of the patient for any adverse reactions thereof. Claims may be made against any adverse reaction for up to 10 years after the event; therefore, the patient's and preparation's records must be maintained for this length of time.

Clinical trials are conducted by qualified clinicians based on protocols approved by an Ethics Committee in each institution. Data are collected on pharmacokinetic characteristics, clinical efficacy, safety, etc., for a particular indication of a disease, which are then submitted for marketing authorization. Any modification in a product or its administration requires a new clinical trial.

The radiation aspect of the radiopharmaceuticals is regulated by Directives from the European Atomic Energy Community (EURATOM) (84/466 EURATOM and 84/467 EURATOM). These directives mandate regulations for radiation protection for patients, workers, and the public. These regulations mostly follow the ICRP regulations. Much of these regulations are similar to those of the NRC. The dose limits set by the ICRP are accepted for regulations by the EURATOM. The optimization principle (similar to the ALARA principle of the NRC) for dose reduction applies to all radiation workers in the EU. Similar to the RSO in the U.S., a radiation protection advisor (RPA) is an expert in radiation protection principles who implements and supervises radiation safety regulations in an institution. Personnel monitoring is mandatory for all radiation workers using specific monitoring devices. The use of radiation is approved by the issuance of a license to a qualified person with experience in handling radiation. All activities in the radiation area must be recorded and maintained.

Although all EU regulations and Directives are equally applicable to all member states, the actual situation is very different from country to country because of the lack of effective implementation in many states. So in some member states, these Directives are effectively applied, while in others they are loosely applied, and in some cases there may be a breach of the community law.

Questions

1. What are the occupational dose limits for the following parts of the body of a radiation worker: (a) whole body, gonads, and eye lens; (b) hands; and (c) skin? How many rem can a radiation worker receive per week?

2. What is the occupational dose limit for pregnant women during the gestation period?

3. What are the features of planned special procedures?

4. What are the cardinal rules of protection from external sources of radiation?

5. If a source of radioactivity shows an exposure rate of 50 mR/hr at 4 m from the source, calculate the exposure rate at (a) 3 m from the source and (b) 6 m from the source.

6. What will be the exposure rate in percent of a radioactive sample surrounded by an HVL of absorbing material? Calculate the exposure rate if the source exposure rate is 75 mR/hr.

7. Describe the principles of personnel monitoring by film badges and thermoluminescent dosimeters. What are the merits and disadvantages of these two methods?

8. What are the steps you would take in the event of a spill of a liquid radioactive sample on the floor of a radioisotope laboratory?

9. What are the dose limits to (a) individual members of the public and (b) an unrestricted area?

10. A patient has been treated with 200 mCi (7.4 GBq) ^{131}I for thyroid cancer. What are the factors you would take into consideration for the release of the patient from the hospital?

11. At what limits of activity and exposure would you give instructions to the patients and breast-feeding women who are released after treatment with ^{131}I?

12. What is the maximum value of transport index that is allowed for transportation of radioactive material?

13. When do you need a bioassay if handling ^{131}I-NaI?

14. Describe the situations in which a medical event will occur.

15. What are the requirements for a physician to become authorized?

Suggested Reading

Cox PH. European legislation and its effects on the production of radiopharmaceuticals. In: Sampson CB, ed. *Textbook of Radiopharmacy*. Amsterdam: Gordon and Breach Science Publishers; 1999.

Gollnick DA. *Basic Radiation Protection Technology*. 2nd ed. Altadena, CA: Pacific Radiation Corporation; 1988.

International Commission on Radiological Protection. General principles for the radiation protection of workers. ICRP 75. New York: Elsevier; 1997.

International Commission on Radiological Protection. 1990 recommendations of the ICRP. ICRP 60. New York: Elsevier; 1990.

National Council on Radiation Protection and Measurements. Limitation of exposure to ionizing radiation (NCRP 116). Bethesda, MD: NCRP Publications; 1993.

National Council on Radiation Protection and Measurements. Maintaining radiation protection records (NCRP 114). Bethesda, MD: NCRP Publications; 1992.

National Council on Radiation Protection and Measurements. Nuclear medicine factors influencing the choice and use of radionuclides in diagnosis and therapy (NCRP 70). Bethesda, MD: NCRP Publications; 1982.

National Council on Radiation Protection and Measurements. Radiation protection and allied health personnel (NCRP 105). Bethesda, MD: NCRP Publications; 1989.

Nuclear Regulatory Commission. Consolidated guidance about material licenses: program specific guidance about medical license. NUREA-1556, Vol 9. Washington DC; 1998.

Nuclear Regulatory Commission. Medical Use of Byproduct Material. 10CFR Part 35. Washington, DC; 2002.

Nuclear Regulatory Commission. Standards for protection against radiation. 10CFR Part 20. Washington, DC; 1995.

Shapiro J. *Radiation Protection*. 4th ed. Cambridge, MA: Harvard University Press; 2002.

U.S. Food and Drug Administration. Food and Drug Administration Modernization Act of 1997. Rockville, MD: 1997.

U.S. Food and Drug Administration. Nuclear pharmacy guideline: criteria for determining when to register as a drug establishment. Washington, DC: 1984.

U.S. Food and Drug Administration. Radioactive drugs and radioactive biological products. *Fed Register*. 1975; 40:144.

U.S. Food and Drug Administration. Regulations for in vivo radiopharmaceuticals for diagnosing and monitoring. 21CFR Part 315. Rockville, MD: 1999.

12
In Vitro and In Vivo Nonimaging Tests

Radioimmunoassay

The radioimmunoassay (RIA) method was first developed by S.A. Berson and R.S. Yalow in the late 1950s for the determination of insulin in human serum. The method is employed to determine numerous hormones, enzymes, antigens, and drugs in minute quantities (10^{-9}–$10^{-12}M$) in human plasma in order to assess various disease conditions.

Principle

The RIA method is based on the formation of an antigen–antibody complex and utilizes the principles of the isotope dilution technique. An antigen (Ag) is a substance (e.g., protein) that is able to induce the production of an antibody in the body and binds to that antibody very specifically. Conversely, an antibody (Ab) is usually a protein that is produced in immunologic response to an antigen and forms a specific complex with the antigen. In an RIA method, a mixture of radiolabeled antigen (Ag*) and unlabeled antigen is added to a quantity of its antibody that is *insufficient* to form the antigen–antibody complex with all antigen (both labeled and unlabeled). In the formation of this complex, both types of antigen will be competing for the limited binding sites on the antibody, and both labeled and unlabeled complexes will be formed in proportion to the amounts of respective antigen. Thus, in an RIA mixture, the following reactions take place:

$$Ab + Ag \rightleftharpoons Ab - Ag + Ag$$

$$Ab + Ag^* \rightleftharpoons Ab - Ag^* + Ag^*$$

Here the antibody is present in an *insufficient* amount to bind all the labeled and unlabeled antigen. Most often, in an RIA mixture the unreacted labeled antigen is referred to as free antigen and its concentration is denoted F, and labeled antigen–antibody complex (Ab–Ag*) is referred to as bound antigen and its concentration is denoted by B. For constant amounts of antibody and labeled antigen (with antibody insufficient to form complexes with all of the labeled and unlabeled antigen), the amount of bound antigen will be inversely proportional to the quantity of unlabeled antigen; that is, if the amount of unlabeled antigen is increased, the amount of bound antigen will decrease with a concomitant increase in the amount of free antigen left in the mixture and vice versa. Thus, the ratio of bound to free antigen (B/F) is a function of the concentration of unlabeled antigen in the RIA mixture, and can be used in the determination of an unknown concentration of antigen in a sample by using the so-called standard or dose-response curve as described below.

Methodology

A series of standard samples are prepared with increasing but known concentrations of unlabeled antigen, including one sample without any unlabeled antigen; the latter is referred to as the zero standard. To each of these samples, a known amount of labeled antigen and a constant quantity of antibody (remember, insufficient antibody to bind to all labeled and unlabeled antigen) are added and the mixture is incubated. The period of incubation and the temperature vary with the type of antigen to be assayed.

After incubation, the bound and free antigens of each sample are separated by an appropriate chemical method. Some of the common methods of separation are (1) precipitation with reagents such as ethanol, polyethylene glycol, and ammonium sulfate; (2) adsorption of antigen on a solid surface such as talc, charcoal, cellulose, and silica; (3) adsorption of antibody on a solid phase such as glass or plastic; (4) gel filtration using Sephadex and Bio-Rad Gel; and (5) a double antibody method in which a second antibody is added to the RIA mixture to precipitate bound antigen. The reader is referred to any standard book on RIA for details of these methods.

After separation, the amounts of bound and free antigens are determined by measuring the activity in a counter, and the B/F ratio or percent bound is calculated for each sample. These values are then plotted against the logarithms of the unlabeled antigen concentration of each sample. The plot is the standard curve for the RIA of the antigen in question. A typical standard curve for digoxin RIA is shown in Fig. 12.1. For a sample with an unknown amount of antigen, an identical procedure is followed, B/F or percent bound calculated, and the corresponding level of antigen is read from the standard curve.

Instead of B/F, sometimes F/B and B/B_0 are plotted in constructing the standard curve. Here B_0 is the concentration of bound antigen in the zero standard sample. These curves are not linear as seen in Fig. 12.1. However, a linear standard curve can be obtained by using the logit function, which is defined as

$$logit(Y) = \log_e\left(\frac{Y}{1-Y}\right) \qquad (12.1)$$

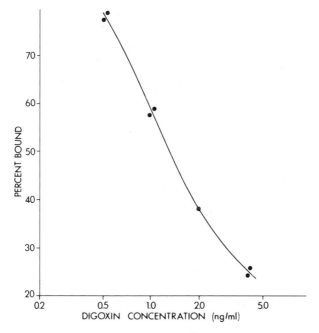

FIGURE 12.1. Typical standard curve for digoxin RIA.

where $Y = B/B_0$. A plot of logit (Y) against log [Ag] gives a linear standard curve on which it is easier to read the data for an unknown sample.

Sensitivity and Specificity

The RIA method is highly sensitive due to the presence of radioactivity that can be detected in tracer quantities. In RIA, the immunologic reaction between the antigen and the antibody is highly specific, and hence the method has high specificity. Peptides, hormones, drugs, and so on can be detected in the range of 10^{-9} to 10^{-12} M. The accuracy of the method depends on various experimental factors and the specificity of the antigen–antibody reaction. The precision of RIA is affected by experimental errors in pipetting of reagents, chemical separation of the complex, and counting.

Application

The RIA method is useful in the assay of various hormones, enzymes, steroids, and peptides in plasma. These measurements yield information on the normal and abnormal states of patients. Some examples of substances that are assayed by RIA are T_3, gastrin, angiotensin, and aldosterone.

Another area of application of RIA is in the determination of the serum level of a drug that has been administered to a patient.

Kits are marketed by commercial manufacturers for the RIA of the above-mentioned substances. In a given kit, the following materials are included: (1) a series of standard samples containing increasing amounts of unlabeled antigen, (2) a vial of labeled antigen, and (3) a vial of antibody solution. Depending on the type of the RIA method, other supplementary materials may be provided. Mostly ^{125}I-antigens are used.

At present, the use of RIA has been curtailed considerably, because of the applications of the other nonradioactive methods such as enzyme-linked immunosorbent assay (ELISA), chemoluminiscence immunoassay, enzyme immunoassay, and immunofluorescence assay.

Schilling Test

The Schilling test indicates normal or abnormal absorption of vitamin B_{12} (cyanocobalamin), as in pernicious anemia. Vitamin B_{12} labeled with ^{57}Co is administered to fasting patients and the 24-hr urinary excretion of the tracer is measured and used as an index of the disease state.

In the actual procedure, the patient is asked to fast overnight; 0.5 μg ^{57}Co–vitamin B_{12} containing 0.5 μCi (18.5 kBq) radioactivity is then given orally, followed by intramuscular administration of a large dosage ($\sim 1000\,\mu$g) of cold vitamin B_{12}. The latter is given to promote urinary excretion of vitamin B_{12} and to saturate the liver and other tissues. A radioactive standard is prepared with an aliquot or identical amount of the administered dosage. Urine is collected over a period of 24 hr. The activities in the 24-hr urine and the standard are measured, and the percent excreted in 24 hr is calculated. The normal values of urinary excretion of vitamin B_{12} are in the range of 10% to 40% (mean 18%). Values lower than this limit indicate malabsorption of vitamin B_{12}.

If the values are lower than normal ($<7\%$), pernicious anemia may be suspected and can be distinguished from other related diseases. The procedure is repeated several days later with 30 mg intrinsic factor given orally along with radioactive vitamin B_{12}. In the case of pernicious anemia or total gastrectomy, the 24-hr urinary excretion becomes normal (10–40%). In syndromes not affected by intrinsic factor, the value still remains low.

Alternatively, a dual-isotope method may be applied, and repetition of the Schilling test in the case of pernicious anemia is avoided. In this method, a capsule containing both ^{57}Co–vitamin B_{12} and intrinsic factor, and another capsule containing only ^{58}Co–vitamin B_{12} are administered orally simultaneously. Both isotopes in the 24-hr urine sample are counted in a well counter on two energy windows. In the case of pernicious anemia, the 24-hr urinary excretion should be normal for ^{57}Co and low for ^{58}Co.

Blood Volume

The two common methods of measuring blood volume are the ^{125}I-labeled serum albumin method and the ^{51}Cr-labeled red blood cell method.

[125]I-Serum Albumin Method

The principle of the ^{125}I-serum albumin method is that after ^{125}I-RISA is administered, it is thoroughly mixed with the circulating blood, and therefore blood volume can be determined from the activity of a blood sample and the total administered activity.

In this procedure, 10 μCi (0.37 MBq) ^{125}I-RISA is injected intravenously and a 5- to 10-ml blood sample is collected in a tube containing heparin 10 to 20 min after injection. A standard is prepared using the same amount as the injected dosage. If a fraction of the injected dosage is used for the standard, a correction factor must be considered in the final calculation. The hematocrit is determined and the plasma is separated by centrifugation of the remaining blood. Then 1 ml plasma and 1 ml standard are counted in a NaI(Tl) well counter. From the measured activities, the blood volume is calculated as follows:

$$\text{Plasma volume} = \frac{C_s \times V_s}{C_p} \tag{12.2}$$

where

C_s = radioactivity (cpm) in 1 ml of the standard

V_s = volume (ml) of the standard corrected for
      fraction of the injected dosage.

C_p = radioactivity (cpm) in 1 ml plasma

$$\text{Blood volume} = \frac{\text{Plasma volume}}{1 - (\text{Hematocrit} \times 0.92)} \tag{12.3}$$

where 0.92 is the correction factor for the trapped plasma in the red blood cells and for the difference between the venous and whole-body hematocrits.

[51]Cr-Labeled Red Blood Cell Method

The blood volume can be measured with ^{51}Cr-labeled red blood cells using the same principle as in the ^{125}I-RISA method.

About 50 to 100 μCi (1.85–3.7 MBq) ^{51}Cr-labeled red blood cell suspension is injected intravenously into the patient, and a separate aliquot of the suspension is used as a standard. A blood sample is collected 15 to 20 min after the injection and a hematocrit is determined. The plasma sample, the whole blood sample, and the standard are counted in a NaI(Tl) well counter, and the blood volume is calculated from the measured counts.

Application

The normal blood volume for humans is 4000 to 5500 ml. Determination of blood volume is most useful in pre- and postoperative patient care. From both these methods, the red cell volume can be easily calculated as

$$\text{Red cell volume} = \text{Blood volume} \times \text{Hematocrit} \times 0.92 \qquad (12.4)$$

Determination of red cell volume is particularly useful in patients with polycythemia vera, specifically in the evaluation of their response to treatment.

Red Blood Cell Survival

The lifetime of a red blood cell is 120 days. However, red cells of different ages are present in blood, and one can measure only the average survival half-time of these cells, which is done by means of ^{51}Cr-labeled red cells. About 50 μCi (1.85 MBq) of labeled red blood cells is injected into the patient, and a 24-hr blood sample is collected and considered as the 100% sample. Serial blood samples of 6 to 10 ml are then obtained every 48 hr until the activity in the last sample is less than half of the 100% sample. An

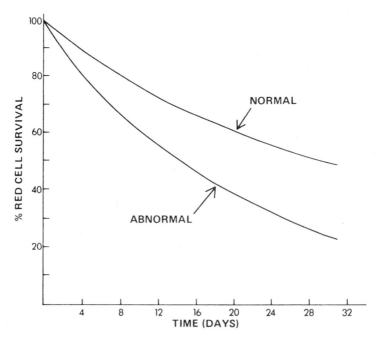

FIGURE 12.2. Normal and abnormal red blood cell survival curves with ^{51}Cr-labeled red blood cells.

aliquot of each blood sample is taken and hemolyzed. All samples are counted in a well counter on the same day to avoid decay correction. The activities are then plotted against time after injection and the red cell survival half-time is determined from the curve. The normal values range between 25 and 33 days with a mean value of 28 days (Fig. 12.2). In hemolytic anemia patients, the red cell survival half-time is much shorter (Fig. 12.2).

Questions

1. Describe the general principles of the RIA method.
2. Why is the RIA method so highly sensitive and specific? What is a logit function?
3. What is a standard curve in RIA? How do you construct it?
4. In the Schilling test, why is a large dosage of nonradioactive vitamin B_{12} injected intramuscularly following the oral administration of ^{57}Co–vitamin B_{12}? What are the normal values of urinary excretion of ^{57}Co–vitamin B_{12}? What additional test do you do in cases of suspected pernicious anemia?
5. In a blood volume measurement, 2 ml plasma and 1 ml of the standard measured 6020 cpm and 13,590 cpm, respectively. If the volume of the standard was 500 ml, calculate the blood volume of the patient whose hematocrit was 45%.
6. In a red blood cell survival study, the following data were obtained after injection of ^{51}Cr-labeled red blood cells:

Time (day)	Blood (cpm/ml)
1	3010
2	2810
3	2683
6	2235
8	2001
10	1789
12	1601
14	1412

Plot these activities versus time and find the red cell survival half-time. Is it normal or abnormal?

Suggested Reading

Chase GC, Rabinowitz JL. *Principles of Radioisotope Methodology*. 3rd ed. Minneapolis: Burgess; 1970.

Moss AJ Jr, Dalrymple GV, Boyd CM, eds. *Practical Radioimmunoassay*. St Louis: Mosby; 1976.

Odell WD, Daughaday WH, eds. *Principles of Competitive Protein-Binding Assays*. Philadelphia: Lippincott; 1974.

Rothfeld B, ed. *Nuclear Medicine In Vitro*. Philadelphia: Lippincott; 1974.

Thorell JI, Larson SM. *Radioimmunoassay and Related Techniques*. St Louis: Mosby; 1978.

13
Diagnostic Uses of Radiopharmaceuticals in Nuclear Medicine

In previous chapters, we described various characteristics and production of radionuclides, preparation of different radiopharmaceuticals using various radionuclides, and their quality control. In the present chapter we shall describe clinical applications of these radiopharmaceuticals in the diagnosis of various diseases in humans. The discussion is primarily divided into sections on different organs. In each section the anatomic structure and physiologic function of the organ are briefly described and appropriate nuclear medicine tests are discussed along with their clinical usefulness, particularly with respect to the radiopharmaceuticals used, their pharmacologic aspect, the mechanism of their localization, and diagnosis of various diseases.

Central Nervous System

Anatomy and Physiology

The central nervous system (CNS) consists of two parts—the brain in the skull and the spinal cord in the vertebral column. The brain consists of two symmetric cerebral hemispheres (left and right) separated by longitudinal fissures. Each hemisphere has four lobes—the frontal, parietal, temporal, and occipital—and these lobes are separated by fissures (Fig. 13.1). Both the cerebellum and the pons are dorsally located behind the cerebral hemispheres in the posterior fossa of the skull. The cerebellum is responsible for motor coordination and space orientation of the body, while the pons forms the bridge between the connecting links. The medulla oblongata is a region of passage for nerve fiber tracts that extend between the spinal cord and the higher regions of the brain, and it contains reflex centers and cranial nerves. The thalamus and hypothalamus are situated inside the interbrain and their function involves general sensations (pain, temperature, pleasant feelings, and feeding reflexes). The pituitary gland is suspended underneath the hypothalamus. Between the left and right halves of the interbrain lies the third ventricle as a continuation of the cerebral aqueduct. The third ventricle communicates with the first and second lateral ventricles via an interven-

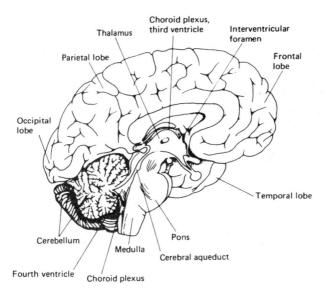

FIGURE 13.1. Sagittal section of a normal brain.

tricular foramen. The fourth ventricle exists as an expansion of the neural canal above the medulla. The ventricles are fluid-filled spaces within the brain. The choroid plexus is a mass of blood vessels lying in the lateral ventricles.

The outer layer of the cerebral hemispheres is composed of gray matter and is known as the cerebral cortex. Beneath this lie tracts of fiber comprising the white matter along with clumps of gray matter. It has been estimated that the human cortex contains about 10 to 14 billion neurons, which are nerve cells with afferent and efferent nerve fibers. All of these cells are formed before birth and none of them, if injured, is ever replaced. The brain and spinal cord are covered with meninges, through which the cerebrospinal fluid (CSF) circulates. The CSF is a colorless liquid containing a few lymphocytes and is similar in composition to plasma. Most of the components of CSF are secreted by vascular plexuses (e.g., choroid plexus) lining the ventricles. The CSF is secreted at a rate of 50 to 400 ml/day into the cisterns and the subarachnoid space (a space between two layers of meninges in the CNS) and is finally reabsorbed into the venous blood leaving the cranium. This fluid acts as a shock absorber for the brain.

Nerve cells need a constant supply of oxygen for survival; this supply is maintained by the blood vessels. The brain receives nearly 20% of the total cardiac output and consumes about 20% of total oxygen used by the whole body at rest. The two internal carotid and the two vertebral arteries supply blood to the brain, and a single anterior and two spinal arteries supply blood to the spinal cord. All of the venous blood from the CNS eventually drains into the superior vena cava.

Radiopharmaceuticals and Imaging Techniques

Brain Imaging

The principle of brain imaging is governed by a mechanism called the blood–brain barrier (BBB), which excludes many substances from entering the brain from the blood. The BBB is probably a functional mixture of anatomic, physiologic, and metabolic phenomena, and which of these are effective in a particular instance depends on the physicochemical properties of the substance in question. The barrier perhaps results from a tight intracellular junction of endothelial cells in the brain capillaries, lack of extracellular fluid space, lack of pinocytosis, and limited transport mechanism. The barrier is selective: some substances such as water, glucose, sodium chloride, and so on enter the brain readily, whereas compounds such as sodium nitrite, sodium iodide, sucrose, bile pigments, and many commonly used radiopharmaceuticals do so with difficulty or not at all. The breakdown of the BBB, as in the case of tumors or other diseases, results in the penetration of the latter compounds into the brain.

Based on the principle of BBB, radiopharmaceuticals for brain imaging can be broadly grouped into two categories: diffusible and nondiffusible. Diffusible tracers are typically lipophilic and readily cross the BBB. Examples are ^{99m}Tc-HMPAO, ^{99m}Tc-ECD, and ^{18}F-FDG. Nondiffusible tracers are hydrophilic and polar and cannot cross the BBB except in abnormal tissues where the BBB is broken. Examples are ^{99m}TcO$_4^-$ and ^{99m}Tc-DTPA.

In earlier years, in the absence of diffusible radiopharmaceuticals, nondiffusible tracers were the agents of choice for brain imaging. However, with the introduction of diffusible tracers, nondiffusible tracers such as ^{99m}TcO$_4^-$ and ^{99m}Tc-DTPA are no longer used for brain imaging. Among the diffusible tracers, ^{99m}Tc-HMPAO, ^{99m}Tc-ECD, and ^{18}F-FDG are most commonly used for brain imaging. ^{18}F-fluorodopa is used for brain imaging to detect cerebral diseases related to dopamine receptors. The characteristics of the commonly used radiopharmaceuticals for brain imaging are summarized in Table 13.1.

TABLE 13.1. Radiopharmaceuticals for brain imaging.

Characteristics	^{99m}Tc-HMPAO	^{99m}Tc-ECD	^{18}F-FDG	^{18}F-Fluorodopa
$t_{1/2}$ (physical)	6 hr	6 hr	110 min	110 min
Photon energy (keV)	140	140	511	511
Usual dosage (mCi)	10–20	10–20	10–15	5–10
Usual dosage(MBq)	370–740	370–740	370–555	185–370
Usual time for imaging (hr)	0.3–2	0.5–1	0.6	0.3–0.5

^{99m}Tc-Hexamethylpropylene Amine Oxime (HMPAO; Ceretec)

As stated in Chapter 7, the primary complex d, l isomer of ^{99m}Tc-HMPAO, not the meso isomer, is a lipophilic moiety which diffuses into the brain by crossing the BBB. In the brain, it is converted to a secondary complex, most likely due to a reaction with glutathione which is hydrophilic and is unable to back out of the brain. The blood clearance is rapid after intravenous injection resulting in a blood level of 12% of the injected dosage at 1 hr after injection (Sharp et al., 1986). The maximum brain uptake of $\sim$4% occurs within 1 min of injection. Only 15% of the brain activity washes out within 2 min postinjection, after which the brain activity remains at a plateau over a period of 24 hr. The urinary excretion is about 35% in 24 hr after injection. The soft tissue, liver, and gastrointestinal uptakes are high ($\sim$10%).

Approximately 10 to 20 mCi (370–740 MBq) ^{99m}Tc-HMPAO is administered intravenously to patients with altered cerebral perfusion as in stroke. SPECT images are obtained 20 to 250 min after injection at 3° to 10° intervals over 180° or 360° using a rotating camera equipped with a low-energy parallel hole collimator. Some nuclear medicine departments use special collimators such as "fan beam" collimators that focus in the brain giving better spatial resolution (6–7 mm, compared to $\sim$15 mm for low-energy parallel hole collimator) of the images. Data are acquired in a 64×64 matrix and later used to reconstruct the transverse (short axis), sagittal (vertical long axis), and coronal (horizontal long axis) images. Perfusion abnormalities due to infarction, stroke, tumor, and so forth show decreased uptake of ^{99m}Tc-HMPAO. A typical SPECT image obtained with ^{99m}Tc-HMPAO is shown in Figure 13.2.

^{99m}Tc-Ethyl Cysteinate Dimer (ECD; Neurolite)

^{99m}Tc-ECD is a neutral lipophilic complex that localizes in the brain by crossing the BBB via passive diffusion and is used as a brain perfusion

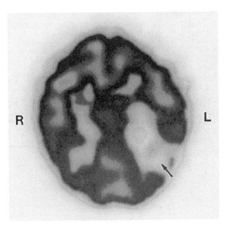

R   L

FIGURE 13.2. A SPECT image (mid-transverse slice) obtained with 20 mCi (740 MBq) ^{99m}Tc-HMPAO demonstrating decreased uptake in the left hemisphere in a patient with stroke.

FIGURE 13.3. A SPECT image (transverse) of the brain obtained with ^{99m}Tc-ECD indicating an acute stroke in the right hemisphere in a patient.

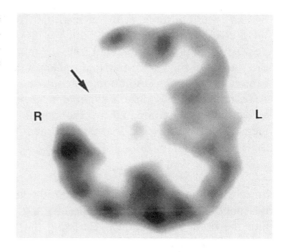

agent. However, in the brain, an enzyme-catalyzed hydrolysis of one of the ester groups to carboxylic acid results in the formation of an anionic complex, which cannot diffuse across the BBB, thus preventing the washout from the brain. After intravenous administration, the blood clearance of ^{99m}Tc-ECD is very rapid and the blood activity is less than 10% after 5 min. The brain uptake is very rapid and amounts to 5% to 6% of the injected dosage with very slow washout. The ratio of gray to white matter uptake is greater than 2:1. The lung uptake is negligible and the hepatobiliary excretion is about 11%. The urinary excretion is $55 \pm 10\%$ in 2 hr and about $78 \pm 14\%$ in 24 hr after injection (Leveille et al., 1989; Vallabhajosula et al., 1989).

Approximately 10 to 20 mCi (370–740 MBq) ^{99m}Tc-ECD is injected intravenously into the patient. Both planar and SPECT images can be obtained using an appropriate camera and suitable collimators. Imaging can start immediately for dynamic flow studies, or static images can be obtained at 30 to 60 min later. SPECT images are obtained by collecting data at 3° to 10° intervals over 180° or 360° using a rotating camera equipped with a low-energy parallel hole collimator. Perfusion abnormalities in the brain are seen as cold defects on the images (Fig 13.3). ^{99m}Tc-ECD has also been used to detect the epileptic foci in epilepsy patients.

Interventional Studies

Interventional studies using acetazolamide (ACZ, Diamox) are performed to assess the cerebrovascular reserve capacity of the brain because ACZ causes vasodilation of cerebrovascular arteries to the extent of 20% to 40%, causing increased blood flow. The action of ACZ begins within 10 min of injection, reaches maximum at 25 min, and fades within 1 hr.

In a typical interventional study, the patient is injected with 15 mCi (555 MBq) ^{99m}Tc-ECD, and pre-ACZ scan is started 15 min after injection and SPECT images taken for about 30 min. Fifteen minutes into the scan, the patient is administered with reconstituted ACZ containing 1 g. Soon after the pre-ACZ scan is finished, 25 mCi (850 MBq) ^{99m}Tc-ECD is injected and post-ACZ images are obtained after 15 min postinjection. Similar protocol can be used for ^{99m}Tc-HMPAO. Data are collected with a triple-head camera using a high-resolution collimator. Comparison of the pre- and post-ACZ images shows only a slightly increased blood flow in the abnormal areas (ischemic) compared to the normal areas that show significantly increased blood flow. This technique identifies the areas at highest risk of ischemia and lateralization of the severity of the disease in the brain.

^{18}F-Fluorodeoxyglucose (FDG)

Since the brain derives its energy from the metabolism of glucose, ^{18}F-FDG is a good candidate for metabolic imaging of the brain. ^{18}F-FDG diffuses into the brain from blood by crossing the BBB and is metabolized in the brain cells wherein FDG is phosphorylated to FDG-6-phosphate mediated by hexokinase. Since FDG lacks a hydroxyl group at the 2-position, its first metabolite, FDG-6-phosphate is not a substrate for glycolysis and does not undergo further metabolism. Because of its negative charge, FDG-6-phosphate remains trapped in the brain for several hours, thus facilitating imaging of the brain at convenience. However, over the past decade several studies have been reported suggesting that a significant fraction of ^{14}C-DG-6-phosphate undergoes further metabolism and is incorporated into glycogen (Virkamaki et al, 1997). Also, evidence has been found that almost 20% of ^{14}C-deoxyglucose-6-phosphate is further metabolized in the brain, which diffuses into the blood pool (Dienel et al, 1993). It is expected that ^{18}F-FDG-6-phosphate would metabolize similar to ^{14}C-DG-6-phosphate, and failure to account for further metabolism would underestimate the rate of tissue uptake of ^{18}F-FDG.

The brain uptake in humans is 6.9% at 2 hr postinjection. The uptake values for other organs at 1 hr postinjection are as follows (Mejia et al, 1991): heart, 3.3%; kidneys, 1.3%; liver, 4.4%; red marrow, 1.7%; and bladder content, 6.3%. The urinary excretion is 19.6 ± 10.9% at 1 hr and 21.2 ± 5.0% at 2 hr.

Before ^{18}F-FDG administration, data for attenuation correction is acquired. This is achieved either by a theoretical calculation using a computer program or by actual measurements using a rotating ^{68}Ge source around the brain of the subject. After collecting the attenuation correction data, approximately 10 to 15 mCi (370–555 MBq) ^{18}F-FDG is injected intravenously. Imaging is performed using a PET camera or a coincidence gamma camera about 40 min after injection. Data are collected in a 64×64 matrix for sufficient time to give statistical accuracy, and then corrected for attenuation with the information mentioned above. The corrected data are then applied to reconstruct the images in short axis (transverse), vertical long axis (sagittal), and horizontal long axis (coronal).

During focal seizures (ictal state) in epileptic patients, brain metabolism and blood flow are increased at the focus and therefore increased ^{18}F-FDG

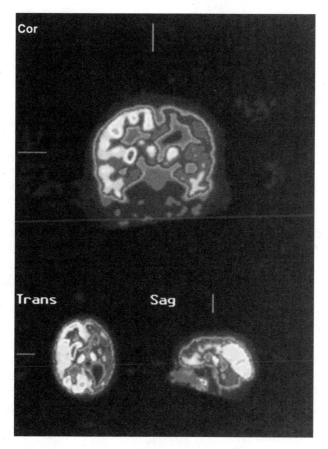

FIGURE 13.4. ^{18}F-FDG PET image (coronal, transverse, and sagittal) of the brain indicating hypometabolism in the left lobe including frontal, parietal, temporal, and occipital lobes extending up to basal ganglia and thalamus in the interictal state in an epilepsy patient.

uptake is seen. In the periods between seizures (the interictal state), both metabolism and blood flow are reduced at the focus and hence the decreased ^{18}F-FDG uptake. However, ^{18}F-FDG PET imaging during the interictal state is more useful than in the ictal state in localizing the epileptogenic focus in epilepsy patients for surgical ablation. An ^{18}F-FDG PET image indicating the hypometabolism in the brain is shown in Figure 13.4. The study of presurgical evaluation of epilepsy by ^{18}F-FDG-PET has been approved for reimbursement by the Center for Medicare and Medicaid Survices (CMS) in the U.S.

^{18}F-FDG PET imaging is useful in differentiating the recurrent brain tumors from necrotic brain tissue such as in radiation necrosis. Recurrent brain tumors exhibit high glucose metabolism, whereas necrotic brain tissue does not metabolize glucose. Thus, ^{18}F-FDG PET shows increased uptake in brain tumors, whereas decreased uptake is seen in necrotic brain tissue.

Brain tumor imaging with ^{18}F-FDG is discussed in detail under tumor imaging in this chapter.

^{18}F-FDG has also been used in the metabolic study of the brain in demented patients and Alzheimer's patients.

^{18}F-Fluorodopa

As a neurotransmitting agent, ^{18}F-fluorodopa crosses the BBB and accumulates in the brain with the highest uptake in the striatum (caudate nucleus and putamen) and lowest in the cerebellum. After intravenous administration, the plasma concentration of ^{18}F-fluorodopa peaks quickly and then decreases to approximately 10% of the injected dosage at 5 min after injection. The maximum brain uptake occurs in 20 min postinjection (Barrio et al., 1990). It is largely metabolized in circulation by dopa decarboxylase (DDC) to ^{18}F-fluorodopamine and by catechol-O-methyl-transferase to ^{18}F-3-O-methylfluorodopa (3-OMFD) before crossing the BBB. This complicates the uptake of ^{18}F-fluorodopa. Inhibitors of DDC such as carbidopa and nitecapone are injected prior to administration of ^{18}F-fluorodopa to improve brain uptake of the tracer. Since ^{18}F-3-OMFD also enters the brain along with ^{18}F-fluorodopa, L-phenylalanine has been used to prevent the entry of ^{18}F-OMFD.

Approximately 5 to 10 mCi (185–370 MBq) ^{18}F-fluorodopa is administered intravenously to patients with Parkinson's disease or other neurodegenerative diseases. Sequential images are obtained after injection using a PET scanner. Attenuation correction is made using either a theoretical program or a rotating ^{68}Ge rod. In the Parkinson's disease, the accumulation of the tracer is markedly reduced in the striatum of the brain.

Other Radiopharmaceuticals

^{123}I-isopropyl-p-iodoamphetamine (IMP) is a lipid-soluble tracer that crosses the BBB easily to localize in the brain. After injection, its blood clearance is rapid and only a small faction remains in the blood 6 to 10 min after administration. The brain uptake is about 5% compared to the lung uptake of 33% and the liver uptake of 44% at 3 hr postinjection (Kuhl et al, 1982). Urinary excretion is about 23% in 24 hr and 40% in 48 hr. Imaging immediately and 3 hr after administration of 3 mCi (111 MBq) ^{123}I-IMP shows only slight uptake in ischemic regions on immediate images that are filled on delayed images. However, infracted areas show decreased uptake in both sets of images. This agent is useful for the evaluation of cerebral stroke. This product is not available commerically in the United States.

^{15}O–O$_2$ has been used to measure the oxygen consumption by the brain tissue, which measures the metabolic status of the brain. ^{15}O–H$_2$O, n-^{15}O-butanol and ^{133}Xe have been used to measure the blood flow in the brain. ^{11}C-labeled ligands such as ^{11}C-N-methylspiperone have been used to image the D2 dopamine receptor density in schizophrenic patients in whom D2 dopamine receptors increase in number in the caudate nucleus and putamen.

The highly mu-selective opiate agonist ^{11}C-carfentanil has been used to quantify mu opiate receptors in patients with idiopathic unilateral temporal lobe epilepsy. In other instances, benzodiazepine receptors are imaged with ^{11}C-flumazenil and ^{123}I-iomazenil to detect areas of seizure foci in epilepsy patients.

Cisternography

Cisternography is employed in the investigation of the rate of formation, flow, and resorption of CSF. Any obstruction in the cerebral ventricular system results in abnormal circulation of CSF. These abnormalities are manifested in hydrocephalus, CSF leakage, and other similar conditions.

^{111}In-DTPA

The radiopharmaceutical most commonly used in cisternography is ^{111}In-DTPA, although ^{99m}Tc-DTPA also can be used. Approximately 0.5 mCi (18.5 MBq) ^{111}In-DTPA is injected into the patient by lumbar puncture. Imaging with a gamma camera fitted with a medium-energy collimator is performed 4 hr and 24 to 48 hr after injection, and anterior, posterior, and lateral views are obtained. Under normal conditions, at 24 hr, the radioactivity appears in the basal cisterns, convexities, and parasagittal locations. In the case of normal pressure hydrocephalus (NPH), the radioactivity is refluxed into the lateral ventricles and is still seen in them at 24 to 48 hr with no activity found in the convexities.

In patients with CSF leakage, cotton pledgets are placed in the nostrils for a period of 24 hr after lumbar puncture administration of ^{111}In-DTPA, and then removed at the end of the study. The activities in the pledgets and the blood are measured in a well counter, and compared. If the pledget activity is greater than the blood activity by a factor of 1.5 or more, CSF leakage (rhinorrhea) is suspected. If the patient is actively leaking, the actual site of CSF leakage can be detected by gamma camera scintigraphy using a larger dosage of ^{111}In-DTPA (2–3 mCi or 74–111 MBq).

^{111}In-DTPA is also used to assess the shunt patency in patients with obstructive hydrocephalus who have been implanted with ventriculoatrial or ventriculoperitoneal shunts. The radiotracer (0.5 mCi or 18.5 MBq) is usually injected into the reservoir or the tubing under aseptic condition, and the passage of the tracer is observed by gamma camera scintigraphy. In the case of shunt patency, the rapid passage of radioactivity through the shunt should be seen within 30 min to 1 hr after administration.

Diagnosis

Various diseases of the brain diagnosed by radionuclidic procedures are primary tumors such as gliomas and meningiomas, metastatic tumors, cerebrovascular infarcts, intracranial abscess, subdural hematoma, metabolic defects, epileptogenic focus, blood flow abnormalities as in stroke, alterations in the receptor density distribution as in schizophrenia, and various other related diseases. Normal pressure hydrocephalus (communicating and noncommunicating), CSF rhinorrhea (leakage), and CSF shunt patency can be detected by cisternography.

Thyroid

Anatomy and Physiology

The thyroid gland is composed of two lobes situated below the larynx, one on either side of the trachea (Fig. 13.5). The two lobes are connected by an isthmus lying near the surface of the neck. The normal weight of a thyroid gland is approximately 15 to 30 g. The thyroid gland is primarily composed of numerous spherical acini, each of which contains a variable amount of a homogeneous colloid material. These acini cells are responsible for the formation of thyroid hormones utilizing iodine obtained from dietary sources.

The primary function of the thyroid gland is to regulate the basal metabolic rate by controlling the synthesis and secretion of two important thyroid hormones, triiodothyronine (T3) and thyroxine (T4). These hormones act as stimulants to all metabolic processes, which are reflected by increased oxygen consumption and heat production. These hormones are essential for growth and sexual maturation.

There are five major steps in the synthesis of thyroid hormones:

1. trapping of iodide from blood by the thyroid gland
2. oxidation of iodide to $I°$ or I^+ by peroxidase enzyme
3. organification, whereby monoiodotyrosine (MIT) and diiodotyrosine (DIT) are formed by iodination of tyrosine with iodine produced in step 2; tyrosine molecules are bound by peptide linkage in thyroglobulin, which is stored in the lumen of the acinus

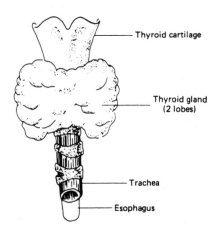

Thyroid cartilage

Thyroid gland (2 lobes)

Trachea

Esophagus

FIGURE 13.5. Position of the thyroid gland.

4. condensation or coupling in which one DIT molecule combines with either an MIT molecule or another DIT molecule to form T3 or T4, respectively

5. release of T3 and T4 into the circulation by enzymatic hydrolysis of thyroglobulin; in the blood approximately 90% of T4 is bound to T4-binding globulin (TBG) (the biological $t_{1/2}$ of T3 and T4 are 2 days and 7 days, respectively).

Control of the synthesis and secretion of thyroid hormones is maintained by a feedback mechanism with the thyrotropin or thyroid-stimulating hormone (TSH) secreted by the pituitary gland. TSH acts on the thyroid to increase trapping, organification, and release of thyroid hormones, primarily by stimulating the activity of the proteolytic enzyme responsible for the breakdown of thyroglobulin. Excessive amounts of T3 and T4 in the blood inhibit the release of TSH from the pituitary gland, thus maintaining thyroid function at an optimum level. TSH is in turn regulated by the action of TSH-releasing hormone (TRH) produced in the hypothalamus.

Thyroid diseases are primarily associated with the iodine uptake and functional status of the thyroid glands. When the thyroid produces excessive amounts of T4, the condition is called hyperthyroidism, which is manifested by symptoms such as increased appetite, restlessness, and hyperactivity. Endemic goiter results from an iodine-deficient diet, particularly in areas where the dietary intake of iodine is very low. This condition can be rectified by the addition of an adequate amount of iodide to the food. Severe hyperfunctioning of the thyroid is called thyrotoxicosis, Graves' disease, or exophthalmic goiter.

Underfunctioning of the thyroid gland leads to the condition called hypothyroidism, which is manifested by lethargy, a tendency to gain weight, and cold intolerance. The level of circulating thyroid hormones remains low. Severe hypothyroidism is called myxedema, which is manifested by infiltration of the skin.

Radiopharmaceuticals and Imaging Techniques

^{131}I- or ^{123}I-Sodium Iodide

Since iodine is an essential element for the function of the thyroid gland, ^{131}I- or ^{123}I-NaI has been the agent of choice for assessing its functional and structural status.

After oral administration of ^{131}I-NaI or ^{123}I-NaI, iodide is absorbed through the intestine and its level in the blood reaches a maximum within 3 hr. Up to 90% of the administered dosage is excreted by the kidneys and only a small fraction is excreted in feces and sweat. Urinary excretion is almost 50% in 24 hr after administration. Two tests are performed—the radioiodide uptake and the imaging of the thyroid glands.

In the iodide uptake test, approximately 10 to 15 μCi (0.37–0.56 MBq) ^{131}I-NaI or 100 μCi (3.7 MBq) ^{123}I-NaI in capsule form is placed in a thyroid phantom, and the activity in counts is measured with a thyroid probe of NaI(Tl) crystal fitted with a long-bore collimator of lead, placed at the same distance as the patient would be seated for the uptake measurement. A room background count is taken and subtracted from the phantom counts, which gives the net standard count. The capsule or capsules are then administered orally to the patient and the uptake is normally determined at 6 hr and 24 hr after administration. The patient is seated at the same distance as the phantom and the thyroid count is obtained using the thyroid probe. A thigh count is taken and subtracted from the thyroid count to correct for extrathyroidal activity. The thyroid uptake as a percentage of the administered dosage is calculated as follows:

$$\% \text{ Uptake} = \frac{A - B}{C - D} \times 100 \tag{13.1}$$

where

A = total cpm of the thyroid
B = total cpm of the thigh
C = total cpm of the thyroid phantom corrected for decay
D = total cpm of the room background corrected for decay.

The normal values for thyroid uptake of ^{131}I-NaI or ^{123}I-NaI are 10% to 35% for 24 hr and 7% to 20% for 6 hr, but the values vary from institution to institution.

Thyroid scans are obtained at 24 hr after oral administration of 100 μCi (3.7 MBq) ^{131}I-NaI or 300 μCi (11.1 MBq) ^{123}I-NaI. A gamma camera equipped with a pinhole collimator is used to image the thyroid glands. Some laboratories use a parallel-hole collimator instead of a pinhole collimator. Imaging is useful in the assessment of the thyroidal structure, position, and function in cases of thyroid carcinoma and hyperthyroid. A normal image with ^{131}I at 24 hr is shown in Fig. 13.6.

Various drugs and chemicals in blood influence the thyroid uptake of iodine and are listed in Table 13.2. Iodine uptake should not be performed during the period of the effects of these drugs and chemicals.

[99m]Tc-Sodium Pertechnetate

Due to their common ionic characteristics, iodide and $^{99m}TcO_4^-$ behave similarly following intravenous administration. Like iodide, $^{99m}TcO_4^-$ localizes in the thyroid, salivary glands, gastric mucosa, and choroid plexus of the brain. Following intravenous administration, $^{99m}TcO_4^-$ partly becomes protein-bound in plasma. The plasma clearance is rapid and it is secreted by gastric mucosa in the stomach and the intestine. It is trapped but not organified in the thyroid gland and is primarily used for assessing the structure of the thyroid gland. Approximately 30% of the injected activity is

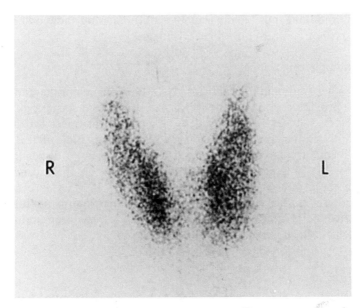

FIGURE 13.6. Normal thyroid image obtained with ^{131}I-iodide 24 hr after administration of the dosage showing uniform distribution of activity in both lobes.

excreted in the urine in the first 24 hr; fecal excretion becomes important after 24 hr. The total urinary and fecal excretion of ^{99m}Tc is about 50% in 3 days and nearly 70% in 8 days. In contrast, reduced ^{99m}Tc and ^{99m}Tc-chelates are promptly cleared by the kidneys and do not accumulate in the thyroid and the choroid plexus.

Approximately 10 mCi (370 MBq) ^{99m}TcO$_4^-$ is administered intravenously and images are taken 10 to 30 min after injection using a gamma camera equipped with a pinhole collimator or a parallel-hole collimator. The images demonstrate the trapping phenomenon indicating the structure

TABLE 13.2. Inhibitory effect of drugs or chemicals on thyroid uptake of iodine

Drugs or chemicals	Duration of effect
T3, thiouracil (PTU, etc.), sulfonamides, cobaltous ions, penicillin, adrenocorticotropic hormone (ACTH), isoniazid, steroids, bromides, perchlorate, pentothal, nitrates, butozolidine, thiocyanate	1 week
Iodides, some vitamin mixtures, some cough medicine, seaweed, dinitrophenol	2–3 weeks
Thyroid extract, T4	4–6 weeks
Radiographic contrast media (e.g., Conray), oral contrast media (e.g., Cholografin)	8 weeks
Contrast media used in bronchography, myelography and arthography (e.g., Lipiodol)	>1 year

of the thyroid, and thus, at times cold nodules seen on radioiodine images may appear hot or warm on $^{99m}TcO_4^-$ images.

Other Radiopharmaceuticals

Among other radiopharmaceuticals, ^{201}Tl-thallous chloride and ^{99m}Tc-sestamibi provide a good sensitivity in detecting the metastasis of thyroid cancer. $^{99m}Tc^{5+}$-DMSA has proved to be an excellent tracer for the detection of both primary and metastatic medullary carcinoma of the thyroid. Thyroid medullary carcinoma is also detected by using ^{111}In-pentetreotide, because of the presence of somatostatin receptors on these cancer cells. Although these radiopharmaceuticals (except Tc^{5+}-DMSA) are approved for clinical use in other indications by the FDA, their routine use for thyroid cancer detection is limited. Recently ^{18}F-FDG PET has been approved for reimbursement in staging thyroid follicular cancer.

Diagnosis

Common diseases that are diagnosed by the thyroid iodine-uptake test include hypothyroidism and hyperthyroidism. Thyroid imaging is useful in detecting any palpable mass (nodule). Clinically, thyroid nodules can be classified into various categories—solitary or multiple, firm or soft, tender or nontender, and benign or malignant. Hyperfunctioning nodules accumu-

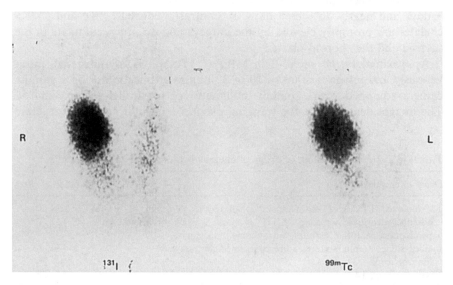

FIGURE 13.7. Thyroid images obtained with ^{131}I (24 hr after oral administration) and ^{99m}Tc (1 hr after injection) and showing a "hot" nodule in the upper right lobe. Both images are similar in the distribution of radioactivity except that there is slightly more uptake of ^{131}I in the left lobe.

late relatively higher amounts of radioactivity and are termed "toxic," "hot," or "autonomous" nodules. Hypofunctioning nodules behave in an opposite manner. Thyroid carcinoma does not concentrate radioiodine well and therefore is seen as a cold spot on the image. Figure 13.7 shows thyroid images with ^{99m}Tc and ^{131}I indicating a hot nodule in the upper right lobe.

Lung

Anatomy and Physiology

The airway of the respiratory tract starts at the nostrils and passes through the pharynx and then through the trachea in the neck. The upper end of the trachea is the larynx. The trachea branches at the lower end into two main bronchi, one going to each of the two lungs. The bronchi branch into bronchioles that in turn terminate into alveolar sacs. There are approximately 700 million alveoli in an adult man, providing a surface area of almost 80 m^2. A schematic diagram of the respiratory system is shown in Figure 13.8.

The lungs are covered by a connecting tissue membrane called the visceral pleura. The pleural cavity between the visceral pleura and the thoracic lining (parietal pleura) is filled with serous fluid which lubricates the two surfaces as they slide over one another during breathing.

Blood circulation is maintained by the pulmonary artery carrying deoxygenated blood from the right ventricle of the heart to the lungs, and the pulmonary veins returning oxygenated blood from the lungs to the left atrium of the heart. The pulmonary arterial distribution is similar to airway segmental distribution. The pulmonary artery branches into distribution arteries ranging in diameter from 60 to 100 μm. These arteries branch into precapillary arterioles with diameters of 25 to 35 μm, which in turn terminate in capillary units whose average diameter is approximately 8 μm. The capillaries are just large enough for the 7-μm red cells to pass through without any deformation. There are about 280 billion arterial capillaries that connect to venules at the other end and ultimately to the veins. About 500 to 1000 capillaries surround each alveolus.

Deoxygenated blood carried by arterial capillaries comes in contact with the inhaled air in the alveolus, where oxygen almost instantaneously diffuses into the blood; venous carbon dioxide is released into the alveolus, wherefrom it is exhaled. Blood flow through the pulmonary arterial system is called pulmonary perfusion and air flow through the bronchial system is called ventilation. Both proper ventilation and perfusion are essential for normal respiration. Overall, the lungs receive 106% of the cardiac output, 100% through the pulmonary artery and about 5% to 6% through the bronchial artery.

In the lungs there is a network of lymphatic vessels lined mainly by phagocytic cells, called macrophages. Dust particles on the walls of the

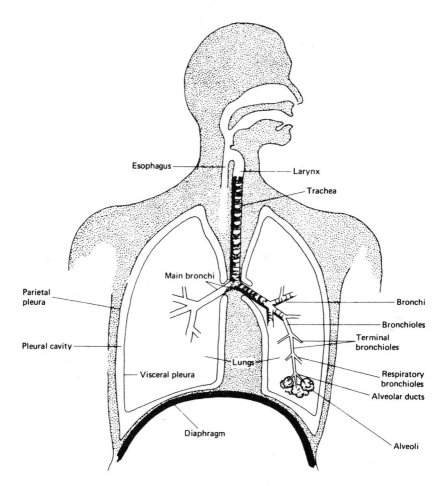

FIGURE 13.8. Structure of the respiratory tract.

alveoli are phagocytosed by these macrophages. Particles that are not removed by the macrophages enter the lymphatics and are deposited at the roots of the lung; for example, the deposits of coal dust in coal miners are seen as " black lung."

Radiopharmaceuticals and Imaging Techniques

The characteristics of the radiopharmaceuticals used in lung imaging are listed in Table 13.3.

Perfusion Imaging

Lung perfusion imaging is based on the trapping of large particles in the capillary bed of the lungs. Particles larger than 10 μm are lodged in the

TABLE 13.3. Radiopharmaceuticals for lung imaging.

Characteristics	^{99m}Tc-MAA	^{133}Xe	^{99m}Tc-aerosol
$t_{1/2}$ (physical)	6 hr	5.3 day	6 hr
$t_{1/2}$ (effective)	2–3 hr	—	0.67
Photon energy (keV)	140	80	140
Usual dosage (mCi)	2–4	10–15	30
Usual dosage (MBq)	74–148	370–555	1110
Usual time to start imaging	Immediately	Immediately	Immediately
Uses	Perfusion study	Ventilation study	Ventilation study

capillaries in the first pass of circulation through the pulmonary artery following intravenous administration.

^{99m}Tc-Labeled Macroaggregated Albumin

Approximately 2 to 4 mCi (74–148 MBq) ^{99m}Tc-MAA (10–90 μm) is injected intravenously into patients lying in a supine position. Approximately 100,000 to 400,000 particles of MAA are administered per injection to adults and a lesser number to children. The number of capillaries occluded (compared to a total of 280 billion) is almost negligible, whereas less than 1% of the precapillary arterioles and distribution arteries may be occluded. Larger particles ($>150\,\mu$m) may occlude the larger arteries, thus causing regional pulmonary embolism. Almost 95% of the administered activity is trapped in the lungs. The effective half-life of the macroaggregates in the lung is approximately 2 to 3 hr. The particles are broken down into smaller ones by mechanical movement of the lungs and some enzymatic action (proteolysis) and then released into the circulation; these particles are then removed by phagocytes in the reticuloendothelial system.

Since occluded particles can cause a rise in pulmonary arterial pressure, not more than 100,000 particles are recommended in patients with pulmonary hypertension. In patients with right-to-left cardiac shunt, MAA particles may induce cerebral microembolization and, therefore, the number of particles should be reduced in these patients.

Images of the lungs are obtained immediately after injection by means of a large-field-of-view gamma camera fitted with a low-energy, all-purpose, parallel hole collimator and placed over the lung field. The position of the patient must be supine for there to be a uniform distribution of particles throughout the lung field; in a sitting position a greater fraction of particles localize in the lower part of the lungs due to gravity, resulting in an uneven distribution of radioactivity in the lung field. A lung image obtained with ^{99m}Tc-MAA showing normal perfusion is shown in Figure 13.9 and another demonstrating pulmonary embolism is presented in Figure 13.10. Detection of lung tumors is discussed under Tumor Imaging, later.

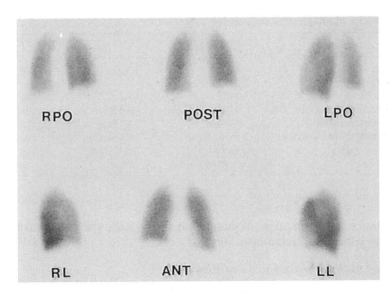

FIGURE 13.9. Normal lung images obtained with ^{99m}Tc-MAA in different projections. The distribution of radioactivity is uniform in both lungs. RL, right lateral; LPO, Left posterior oblique; RPO, right posterior oblique; LL, left lateral; ANT, anterior; POST, posterior.

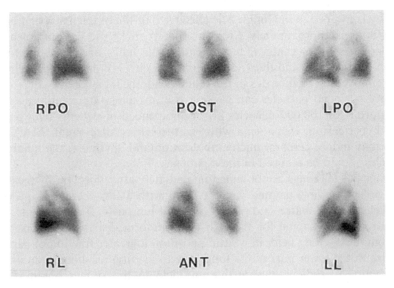

FIGURE 13.10. Lung images obtained with ^{99m}Tc-MAA in different projections indicating multiple pulmonary emboli in both lobes of the lungs (see Fig. 13.9 for abbreviations).

Ventilation Studies

In addition to perfusion, the lung has another physiologic parameter, that is, ventilation, to maintain the respiratory function. Radionuclidic ventilation studies of the lung indicate the presence of any obstruction in its airways.

^{133}Xe Gas

The radionuclide ^{133}Xe, available in gas form, is used for ventilation studies. In ^{133}Xe ventilation studies, the patient is asked to inhale ^{133}Xe (10–15 mCi or 370–555 MBq) gas mixed with air in a closed system in a xenon machine and to hold breath for 15 to 35 s, at which time all parts of the lungs are maximally ventilated and a image is obtained with a gamma camera fitted with a low energy parallel hole collimator. The patient is then asked to breathe while equilibrium is reached and images are taken. The patient then inhales fresh air and exhales ^{133}Xe into a collecting bag or a xenon machine containing a charcoal trap. This period is called the "washout" period, during which all radioactivity should clear out of the lungs in about 3 to 5 min in normal men. Any obstruction in the airways should appear as a hot spot on the images obtained during the washout period. The relatively low-energy photons (80 keV) of ^{133}Xe are not suitable for good resolution with a scintillation camera and ^{99m}Tc-DTPA aersols have replaced it for lung ventilation studies.

^{99m}Tc-Labeled Aerosol

^{99m}Tc-labeled aerosols, 0.5 to 3 μm in size, are used routinely for lung ventilation studies. Radiolabeled aerosols are produced by nebulizing ^{99m}Tc-DTPA (or other appropriate ^{99m}Tc-products) in commercially available nebulizers. These commercial aerosol units are disposable. Approximately 30 mCi (1.11 GBq) ^{99m}Tc-DTPA in 3 ml is placed in the nebulizer. Air or oxygen is forced through the nebulizer at 30 to 50 psi to produce aerosol droplets that are then inhaled by the patient through a mouthpiece. Exhaled air from the patient is trapped in the filter attached to the aerosol unit, thus preventing any contamination of the surrounding area. About 10% of the activity is deposited in the lungs of a normal patient and the remainder remains airborne and is exhaled. This deposition depends on size, shape, density, and electrical charge of the aerosol particles. The larger particles tend to settle in the central area, while the smaller particles deposit in the peripheral areas. The biological $t_{1/2}$ of ^{99m}Tc-DTPA aerosol is about 0.75 hr in normal subjects and is much shorter in smokers due to increased alveolar permeability.

After 5 to 10 min of inhalation by the patient, the aerosol unit is disconnected and stored for decay prior to disposal. The patient is then imaged in different projections with a gamma camera equipped with a low-energy, parallel hole collimator. Images show the distribution of the aerosol in

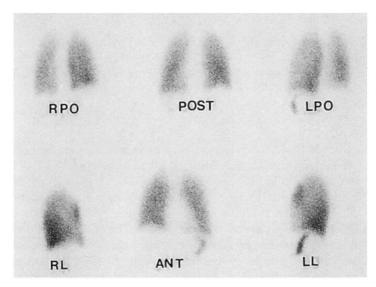

FIGURE 13.11. Normal lung ventilation images obtained with ^{99m}Tc-DTPA aerosol (see Fig. 13.9 for abbreviations).

bronchial spaces. Images are comparable to those obtained with ^{133}Xe. Normal and abnormal lung ventilation images obtained with ^{99m}Tc-aerosol are shown in Figures 13.11 and 13.12 respectively.

^{99m}Tc-Technegas

Although ^{99m}Tc-technegas is not approved for clinical use in the U.S., it is used clinically in other countries for the ventilation studies. The preparation of ^{99m}Tc-technegas has been described in Chapter 7. The technegas is administered to the patient through closed, single-use circuit breathing tubes until a counting rate of 2000 counts/s is attained. Standard views are obtained in different projections using a gamma camera with a low-energy parallel hole collimator. The ventilation defects are indicative of airway obstruction.

Studies of Nonembolic Lung Diseases

^{67}Ga-Citrate

^{67}Ga-citrate is used in the evaluation of the presence and extent of many nonembolic lung diseases such as tumors, asbestosis, etc. After intravenous administration, gallium is bound to transferrin in plasma and hence its plasma clearance is slow. It is nonspecific in biodistribution and at 48 to 72 hr it is seen in the liver ($\sim 5\%$), kidneys ($\sim 2\%$), and bone and bone marrow ($\sim 25\%$). It is secreted by the large intestine, and the appearance of increased bowel activity on the scan often poses a problem. For this reason,

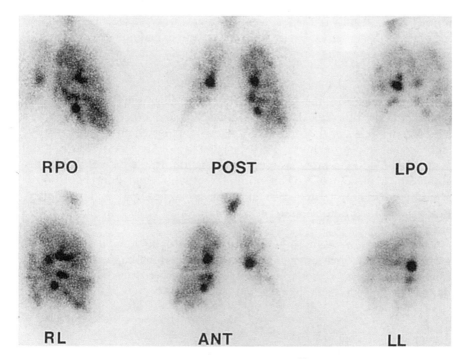

FIGURE 13.12. Lung ventilation images obtained with ^{99m}Tc-DTPA aerosol indicating multiple defects in a patient with chronic obstructive pulmonary disease (see Fig. 13.9 for abbreviations).

patients are often given laxatives before scanning for effective cleansing of the bowel.

The mechanism of localization of ^{67}Ga is supported by a number of hypotheses (Weiner, 1996). A large fraction of ^{67}Ga is found to be bound to lysosomelike organelles in the cytoplasm. The ^{67}Ga uptake in tumor cells is influenced by vascularity, increased permeability of the cells and a decrease in pH in the cytoplasm due to increased glycolytic activity in the cell. In the latter case, the lower pH dissociates ^{67}Ga-citrate, and then gallium ions bind to the intracellular proteins in the tumor cell. Gallium binds to lactoferrin released by polymorphonuclear leukocytes in areas of infections, and so it has been suggested that ^{67}Ga-bound lactoferrin is responsible for gallium localization in inflammatory diseases and abscesses. Another theory supports that the ^{67}Ga uptake is mediated by transferrin-specific receptors present on the cell membrane. The ^{67}Ga uptake is suppressed by chemotherapeutic and radiation treatment.

Approximately 5 to 10 mCi (185–370 MBq) ^{67}Ga-citrate is injected intravenously and the whole body scan is obtained 48 to 72 hr after injection using a large field-of-view scintillation camera equipped with a medium-energy parallel hole collimator. There is only a minimal ^{67}Ga uptake in normal lungs, female breasts, and thymic areas, whereas increased uptake is seen in areas where infection, inflammation, and carcinoma are involved.

Diagnosis

Perfusion imaging of the lungs is effective in diagnosing pulmonary embolism, tumor, tuberculosis, fibrosis, infection, and other related diseases. Ventilation studies of the lungs indicate airway patency, airway obstruction, emphysema, and bronchitis. A combined study of lung perfusion (Q) and ventilation (V) often provides useful information. In the case of pulmonary embolism, a mismatch V/Q of normal ventilation and poor perfusion is typically observed. In the case of emphysema, asthma, and pulmonary fibrosis, both ventilation and perfusion are poor, giving a matched V/Q sean.

^{67}Ga scans are useful in evaluating nonembolic lung disorders such as inflammatory diseases, infections, sarcoidosis, lung cancers, pulmonary fibrosis, asbestosis, silicosis, and tissue damage by drugs such as amiodarone, bleomycin, methotrexate, and vincristine.

Liver

Anatomy and Physiology

The liver is the largest organ in the body, weighing about 1.5 to 1.7 kg in normal adults. It is located under the right side of the rib cage and is attached to the interior surface of the diaphragm (Fig. 13.13). Its size and shape can vary considerably from individual to individual. The liver consists of several lobes, each of which is subdivided into lobules. The lobes are delineated from one another by fissures.

The lobules possess sinusoids whose walls consist of two types of cells: hepatocytes or polygonal cells, and Kupffer or reticuloendothelial cells

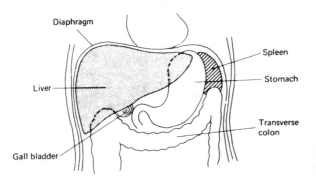

FIGURE 13.13. Position of the liver in the body.

(phagocytes); 70% of the total liver mass consists of hepatocytes and the remaining 30% is made up of phagocytes. Hepatocytes maintain many metabolic processes, whereas phagocytes are responsible for the removal of any foreign particle from the circulation. The liver receives almost 70% of its blood supply from the portal vein and 30% from the hepatic arteries. The hepatic arteries carry oxygenated blood to the liver, whereas the portal vein carries blood rich in products of digestion (e.g., simple sugars and amino acids) from the gastrointestinal tract for further metabolism in the liver.

The major functions of the liver include metabolism, storage, and synthesis of fibrinogen, albumin, heparin, and some globulins; detoxification by conjugation and methylation; formation and excretion of bile into the intestine; and removal of foreign particles by phagocytes. Bile is excreted into the hepatic duct, concentrated in the gallbladder, and finally discharged through the cystic duct into the common bile duct, which delivers it into the duodenum. Bile contains pigments, bile salts, cholesterol, biliverdin, and bilirubin produced from red blood cell destruction in the spleen and the liver. An excess of bilirubin in the plasma and tissue fluids gives a yellow color to the skin, a condition known as jaundice. Excess bilirubin can result from obstruction of the bile duct, damage to the liver, or excessive breakdown of red blood cells.

Radiopharmaceuticals and Imaging Techniques

The radiopharmaceuticals used for liver imaging are divided into two groups based on the physiologic function of the liver they are designed to evaluate. One group is used to evaluate the functional status of the hepatocytes and the patency of the biliary duct, and the other group the phagocytic function of the Kupffer cells. Lipophilic compounds labeled with radionuclides form the first group, and labeled colloids form the second. The characteristics of these radiopharmaceuticals are discussed below and summarized in Table 13.4.

TABLE 13.4. Radiopharmaceuticals for liver imaging.

Characteristics	^{99m}Tc-IDA derivatives	^{99m}Tc-sulfur or albumin colloid
$t_{1/2}$(physical)	6 hr	6 hr
Photon energy (keV)	140	140
Usual dosage (mCi)	5–10	2–15
Usual dosage (MBq)	185–370	74–555
Usual time to start imaging (min)	5	5–10
Uses	Liver function Gallbladder	Liver morphology

^{99m}Tc-Labeled IDA Derivatives

^{99m}Tc-labeled IDA derivatives (^{99m}Tc-DISIDA, ^{99m}Tc-mebrofenin) are commonly used for hepatobiliary imaging. These tracers are extracted by the hepatocytes, excreted into the bile duct and the gallbladder and ultimately into the intestine. Only a small fraction of the injected dosage is eliminated in the urine. Lengthening the alkyl chain on the benzene ring of the IDA molecule results in increased hepatobiliary extraction and decreased renal excretion. Bilirubin competes with IDA derivatives, which leads to poor-quality images when bilirubin level is high (greater than 20–30 mg/100 ml). Of all IDA derivatives, ^{99m}Tc-DISIDA (Hepatolite) and ^{99m}Tc-mebrofenin (Choletec) are the agents of choice for hepatobiliary imaging.

Following intravenous injection of ^{99m}Tc-DISIDA or ^{99m}Tc-mebrofenin, about 8% to 17% of the injected activity remains in the circulation 30 min after injection. Approximately 1% to 9% of the administered activity is excreted in the urine over the first 2 hr after injection. In fasting individuals, the maximum liver uptake occurs by 10 min postinjection and the peak gallbladder activity by 30 to 60 min after injection.

Approximately 3 to 5 mCi (111–185 MBq) ^{99m}Tc-IDA derivative is injected intravenously into patients who have fasted for 4 to 6 hr prior to administration. Serial images are obtained with a scintillation camera fitted with a low-energy parallel hole collimator every 5 min for 30 min followed by 45- and 60-min images. This procedure is called cholescintigraphy. Each view includes the liver, gallbladder, common bile duct, duodenum, and jejunum. The gallbladder is easily visible by 30 min in normal subjects, because the activity is cleared rapidly from the liver. If any part of the above is not seen in 1 to 1.5 hr, then delayed pictures are taken for up to 4 hr.

The mechanism for the clearance of ^{99m}Tc-IDA derivatives involves hepatic extraction, hepatocyte binding and storage, and excretion into biliary canaliculi by an active transport mechanism. There are a number of receptor binding sites on the hepatocytes that are responsible for hepatic uptake. Bilirubin competes for these binding sites more avidly than ^{99m}Tc-IDA derivatives, and therefore at high bilirubin levels the ^{99m}Tc-IDA derivative uptake is compromised. ^{99m}Tc-IDA derivatives are neither conjugated nor metabolized by the liver.

Cholescintigraphy with ^{99m}Tc-IDA derivatives is useful in differentiating between acute and chronic cholecystitis. In acute cholecystitis which is mainly caused by cystic duct obstruction, the gallbladder is not visualized for as long as 4 hr after administration of the tracer as opposed to the normal visualization of the liver, the common bile duct, and the duodenum. Prolonged fasting, acute pancreatitis, and severe liver disease also can lead to nonvisualization of the gallbladder. In chronic cholecystitis, the gallbladder may not be seen in the first hour, but is visualized on delayed images at 4 hr.

Cholecystokinin (CCK) is a polypeptide hormone, endogenously released by the duodenal mucosa or synthetically produced, that causes the gallbladder to contract and the sphincter of Oddi to relax, and increases gastro-intestinal motility and the secretion of bile. Synthetic CCK is available commercially under the name sincalide (Kinevac). At times, investigators have substituted fatty meal for CCK. CCK is administered in conjunction with the ^{99m}Tc-IDA imaging to delineate different status of the gallbladder and biliary tract diseases. In the case of acute cholecystitis, the gallbladder does not clear upon stimulation with CCK because CCK does not have any effect on cystic duct obstruction, whereas in chronic cholecystitis the gall-bladder does clear with CCK stimulation. Some investigators administer CCK prior to imaging particularly to patients fasting more than 24 to 48 hr, in which case the gallbladder is visualized ruling out acute cholecystitis.

Post-CCK cholescintigraphy is useful in determining the gallbladder ejec-tion fraction to differentiate subjects with a partially obstructed, chronically inflamed or functionally impaired gallbladder from those with normal gallb-ladder. Following the ^{99m}Tc-IDA image, CCK is injected at the time when the gallbladder is maximally filled and images are obtained at 5, 10, 15, and 20 min post-CCK. Using appropriate regions of interest on both pre-CCK and post-CCK images and with the proper choice of background at different time intervals, the gallbladder ejection fraction is calculated as the differ-ence between pre-CCK and post-CCK counts divided by the pre-CCK counts (expressed as percentage). A gallbladder ejection fraction of less than 35% indicates abnormalities in the gallbladder function.

Morphine enhances the sphincter of Oddi tone and increases intraluminal common bile duct pressure by 50% to 60%. Based on this, investigators administer morphine intravenously by slow administration, when the gall-bladder is not seen up to 60 min after ^{99m}Tc-IDA derivative administration. The gallbladder is clearly seen on postmorphine images.

A normal cholescintigram and an abnormal cholescintigram without CCK are shown in Fig. 13.14 and 13.15, respectively.

^{99m}Tc-Sulfur Colloid and ^{99m}Tc-Albumin Colloid

The low radiation dose and other favorable characteristics have made ^{99m}Tc-sulfur colloid and ^{99m}Tc-albumin colloid (nanocolloid) the agents of choice for liver imaging. The plasma clearance half-time is approximately 2 to 5 min. Colloids are removed by phagocytes and the maximum hepatic uptake takes place within 20 min. Approximately 80% to 85% of the colloi-dal particles accumulate in the liver, 5% to 10% in the spleen, and the remainder in the bone marrow. Because it is permanently trapped by the phagocytes in the liver, the effective half-life of ^{99m}Tc-colloid is almost equal to the physical half-life of ^{99m}Tc.

The size of the colloid particles is important in imaging the reticuloen-dothelial system. Whereas larger particles (>100 nm) accumulate preferen-tially in the liver and spleen, smaller particles (<20 nm) tend to accumulate in relatively higher concentrations in the bone marrow.

Images of the liver are obtained 5 to 10 min following intravenous injec-

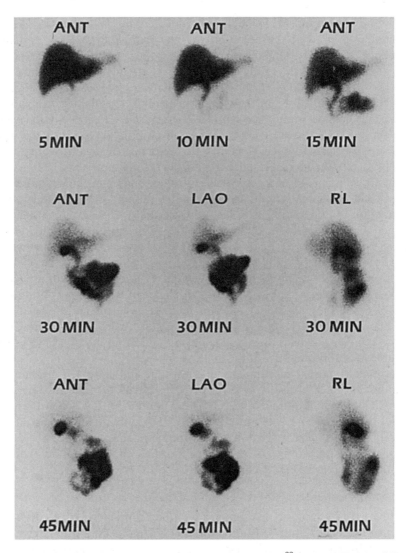

FIGURE 13.14. Normal hepatobiliary images obtained with ^{99m}Tc-DISIDA in different projections. The gallbladder is seen within 15 min after administration of the radio-activity. The radioactivity clears almost completely from the hepatobiliary system into the gut within 45 min (see Fig. 13.9 for abbreviations). (Courtesy of the late Dr. Robert A. Johnson, Albuquerque, NM.)

tion of 2 to 4 mCi (74–148 MBq) ^{99m}Tc-sulfur colloid or ^{99m}Tc-albumin colloid (nanocolloid) into the patient. Anterior, posterior, left lateral and right lateral images are obtained at 15 to 20 min postinjection by the use of a scintillation camera fitted with a low-energy all-purpose parallel hole collimator. Liver flow studies can be performed to assess the vascularity of focal lesions such as tumors or abscesses. In these studies, a bolus injection

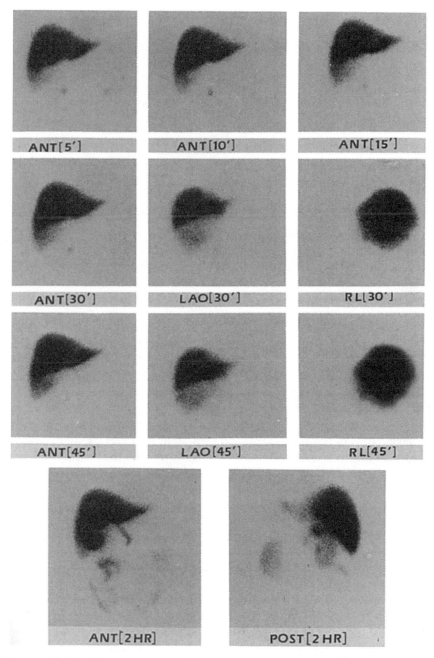

FIGURE 13.15. Abnormal hepatobiliary images obtained with ^{99m}Tc-DISIDA in different projections showing common bile duct obstruction. The gallbladder is not visualized on the 30-min images. The activity is not cleared well into the gut even at 2 hr after administration, even though the gallbladder can be seen (see Fig. 13.9 for abbreviations). (Courtesy of the late Dr. Robert A. Johnson, Albuquerque, NM.)

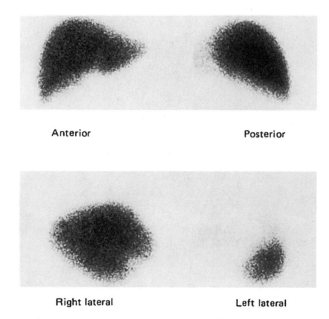

Anterior   Posterior

Right lateral   Left lateral

FIGURE 13.16. Normal liver images obtained with ^{99m}Tc-sulfur colloid in different projections.

of 10 to 15 mCi (370–555 MBq) ^{99m}Tc-sulfur colloid or ^{99m}Tc-albumin colloid (nanocolloid) is given, and rapid sequential images are taken at 2- to 4-s intervals. Normal liver images obtained with ^{99m}Tc-sulfur colloid are shown in Figure 13.16.

Phagocytosis of colloids is governed by a number of factors, that is, blood flow to the organ, reticuloendothelial cell integrity, and the size, charge, and number of particles administered. It has been postulated that after administration, the colloid particle is immediately coated with a serum protein, called the opsonin, and the opsonized colloid is recognized by phagocytes for ingestion. However, it has been found that opsonization is not absolutely necessary for phagocytosis of colloids. There are two receptors on the phagocytic cells—Fc receptor that accepts the Fc (carboxy terminal) end of IgG, and complement 3 (C3) receptor, a foreign surface receptor. Two mechanisms of phagocytosis are postulated based on these two receptors. In one mechanism, the colloid is opsonized and then attached to the Fc receptor, whereupon the cell membrane rises over the particle to engulf it. In the second mechanism, the colloid is attached to the C3 receptor without prior opsonization and is drawn into the cell through invagination of the cell wall.

Other Radiopharmaceuticals

The compound ^{67}Ga-gallium citrate is used in liver imaging, particularly for the detection of abscesses and tumors. Both tumors and abscesses are seen as

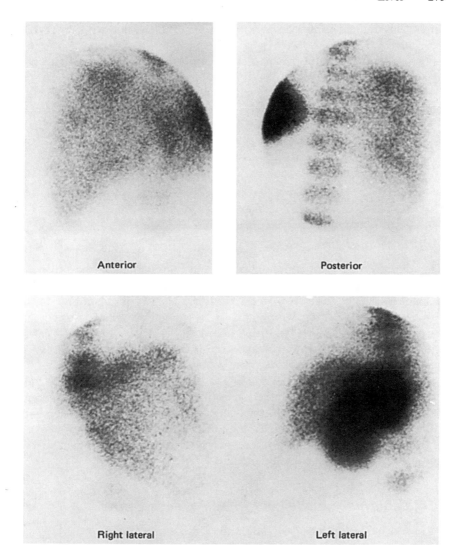

FIGURE 13.17. Liver images showing cirrhosis in a patient. Images were obtained with ^{99m}Tc-sulfur colloid in different projections. Diffuse, patchy, and decreased uptake of the tracer in the liver is indicative of cirrhosis.

hot spots due to increased accumulation of ^{67}Ga. Because the ^{67}Ga accumulation in these lesions is nonspecific and there is also a considerable uptake in normal liver tissue, the value of ^{67}Ga imaging is limited in these cases.

Diagnosis

Various diseases related to liver function, such as jaundice and biliary obstruction, are diagnosed by the use of ^{99m}Tc-labeled IDA derivatives. Chronic and acute cholecystitis can be differentiated with ^{99m}Tc-IDA derivatives.

Diseases involving the morphology of the liver are diagnosed with high accuracy by the use of ^{99m}Tc-sulfur colloid and ^{99m}Tc-albumin colloid. Among these are cirrhosis, abscess, tumor, metastatic lesion, hepatomegaly, hepatitis, and other diffuse and focal lesions. Liver images obtained with ^{99m}Tc-sulfur colloid demonstrating cirrhosis in a patient are shown in Figure 13.17. Tumors and abscesses in the liver are detected with limited success by imaging with ^{67}Ga-gallium citrate.

Spleen

Anatomy and Physiology

The spleen is the largest lymphoid organ and is located under the left side of the rib cage. In adults, its weight varies from 50 to 400 g. It is not normally palpable and is covered by visceral peritoneum. As a result of certain diseases, such as leukemia, lymphoma, typhoid, and so on, the spleen may become very enlarged—a condition called splenomegaly—in which case it can be palpated below the rib cage. The spleen is very fragile and can be ruptured easily by trauma.

Although it is not essential for life, it performs certain important functions. It contains reticuloendothelial or phagocytic cells that remove foreign particles from the circulation, produces lymphocytes and antibodies, and removes damaged and aged red blood cells. It splits hemoglobin from the red blood cells and stores the iron, while it releases bilirubin into the circulation for removal in the bile by the liver.

Radiopharmaceuticals and Imaging Techniques

^{99m}Tc-Sulfur Colloid or ^{99m}Tc-Albumin Colloid

Imaging of the spleen is usually performed with colloids less than 1 μm in size. Approximately 2 to 3 mCi (74–111 MBq) ^{99m}Tc-sulfur colloid or ^{99m}Tc-albumin colloid (nanocolloid) is injected intravenously and imaging is begun about 15 to 30 min after injection. Images are obtained in the anterior, posterior, and left lateral projections with a scintillation camera.

^{99m}Tc-Labeled Red Blood Cells

A dosage of 2 to 3 mCi (74–111 MBq) heat-denatured ^{99m}Tc-labeled red blood cells is injected and imaging can be performed 30 to 60 min after injection to demonstrate the structure of the spleen and any abnormality therein.

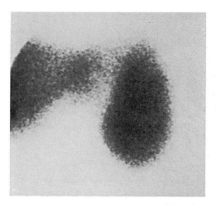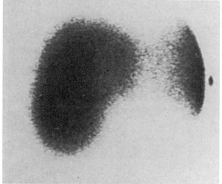

FIGURE 13.18. Images of the spleen obtained with ^{99m}Tc-sulfur colloid demonstrating splenomegaly. Left, anterior; right, posterior.

Diagnosis

Splenomegaly due to tumors, cysts, infarcts, abscesses, and ruptures can be diagnosed by ^{99m}Tc-sulfur colloid or ^{99m}Tc-albumin colloid imaging. Images of the spleen with ^{99m}Tc-sulfur colloid demonstrating splenomegaly are shown in Figure 13.18.

Kidney

Anatomy and Physiology

The urinary system consists of the two kidneys, the ureters, the bladder, and the urethra. Urine is formed by the kidneys, stored in the bladder, and finally discharged through the urethra. The kidneys lie against the posterior wall of the abdominal cavity, one on either side of the vertebral column. Morphologically, each kidney has an outer zone called the cortex, an inner zone called the medulla, and a pelvis (Fig. 13.19). The basic functional unit of the kidney is the nephron, which consists of a glomerulus and a renal tubule (Fig. 13.20). There are about 2 million nephrons in both kidneys. The renal tubule has three segments: the proximal tubule, the loop of Henle, and the distal tubule. The distal tubule empties into the collecting duct, which in turn merges into the renal pelvis.

The nephron performs three functions in the formation of urine: filtration of blood plasma by the glomeruli, selective absorption by the tubules of materials required in the body, and secretion of certain materials by the tubules for addition to the urine.

The blood supply is maintained by the renal artery, and in normal adults the kidneys receive nearly 25% of the cardiac output. The total blood

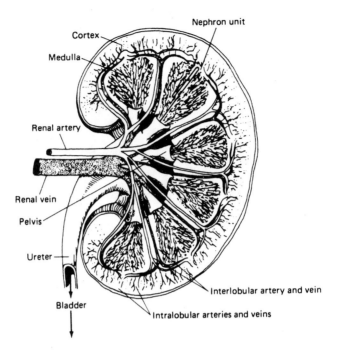

FIGURE 13.19. Internal structure of the kidney, vertical median section.

volume passes through the kidneys in approximately 3 to 5 min. Glomeruli filter about 180 liters of plasma per day, of which 2 liters appear as urine in normal adults. Proteins and organic compounds are not filtered, whereas water and electrolytes are filtered by glomeruli into renal tubules, where almost 95% to 98% of the filtrate is reabsorbed. Certain materials are not filtered by glomeruli but are secreted by renal tubules. The three segments of the renal tubule carry out uniquely coordinated functions of absorption and secretion of materials from and into the filtrate to balance the electrolyte concentration and the pH in the urine.

Radiopharmaceuticals and Imaging Techniques

The characteristics of various radiopharmaceuticals used in renal imaging are summarized in Table 13.5.

^{123}I- or ^{131}I-Orthoiodohippurate (Hippuran)

^{123}I- or ^{131}I-Hippuran is used primarily in renography, in which a time-activity curve is obtained over each kidney after the administration of the tracer. After intravenous administration, the extraction efficiency of ^{131}I-Hippuran is about 88% initially and declines to 60% at 1 hr (McAfee et al.,

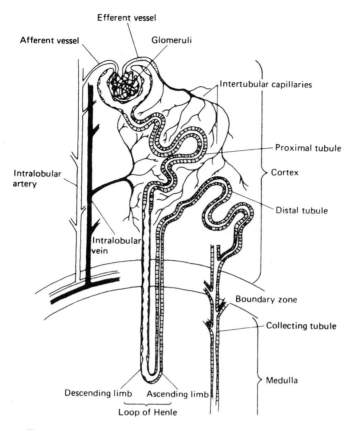

FIGURE 13.20. Structure of a nephron and its blood supply.

1981). It is secreted primarily by the tubules (80%), with the remaining 20% being filtered by the glomeruli. The plasma clearance is rapid with a $t_{1/2}$ of 30 min. Protein binding is ~70%. Radioactivity in the kidneys reaches a peak value in 3 to 5 min and then follows an exponential decrease with a $t_{1/2}$ of 7 to 10 min. No activity is seen in the kidneys 24 hr postinjection. Fecal excretion is negligible.

The functional status of the kidneys is determined by obtaining serial images and a renogram. A renogram is simply an activity versus time curve demonstrating the passage of radiopharmaceutical through the kidneys. Approximately 250 to 300 μCi (9.25–11.1 MBq) ^{131}I-Hippuran or 400 to 500 μCi (14.8–18.5 MBq) ^{123}I-Hippuran is injected intravenously and serial images are obtained immediately and later, using a gamma camera equipped with a medium energy collimator, with both kidneys in the field of view. Images depict the tracer flow through the kidneys. The computer data are then used to construct the renogram, using a selected region of interest on each kidney. The details of the renogram are given later under [99m]Tc-

TABLE 13.5. Radiopharmaceuticals for renal imaging.

Characteristics	^{131}I-orthoiodohippurate	^{99m}Tc-MAG3	^{99m}Tc-DTPA	^{99m}Tc-gluceptate	^{99m}Tc-DMSA
$t_{1/2}$ (physical)	8 day	6 hr	6 hr	6 hr	6 hr
$t_{1/2}$ (effective)	1 hr	—	1 hr	—	—
Photon energy (keV)	364	140	140	140	140
Usual dosage (mCi)	0.25–0.3	5–10	10–15	10–15	2–5
Usual dosage (MBq)	9.25–11.1	185–370	370–555	370–555	74–185
Time to start imaging	Serial imaging	Serial imaging	Serial imaging	3–5 hr	3–5 hr

MAG3. However, ^{131}I-Hippuran is not preferred because of high radiation dose to the patients nor ^{123}I-Hippuran because of the high cost of production of ^{123}I in the cyclotron.

[99M]Tc-Mercaptoacetylglycylglycylglycine(MAG3)

Because millicurie amounts of ^{99m}Tc-MAG3 can be administered providing more photon flux, and because radiation dose is much less than ^{131}I-Hippuran, the former is now the preferable agent for renal function studies. However, there are some differences in the physiologic behavior of the two agents, such as plasma clearance, protein binding, and so forth. ^{123}I-Hippuran also is not preferred because ^{123}I is a cyclotron-produced radionuclide and, therefore, quite expensive.

After intravenous administration, the blood clearance of ^{99m}Tc-MAG3 is rapid and biphasic with a $t_{1/2}$ of 3.18 min for the first component and 16.9 min for the second component (Taylor et al, 1986, 1988). The renal extraction is close to 54%. The protein binding is almost 90%. It is primarily secreted by the tubules to the extent of greater than 90%. The urinary excretion is about 73% in 30 min and about 94.4% in 3 hr after injection. At 3 hr postinjection, only 2% of the activity remains in the blood pool and 2% in the liver, gallbladder, and gut.

^{99m}Tc-MAG3 is used for both flow and function studies of the kidneys. Approximately 5 to 10 mCi (185–370 MBq) of the agent is injected intravenously, and dynamic images are obtained initially, followed by delayed static images using a gamma camera with a low-energy parallel hole collimator. Visual interpretation of the images provides diagnosis of unilateral or bilateral obstructive or functional abnormalities of the kidneys.

The renograms are generated by choosing appropriate regions of interest in each kidney. A schematic normal renogram is shown in Figure 13.21. As can be seen in the figure, the renogram has three segments: segment A represents the arrival of the tracer (vascular phase) and lasts for only approximately 30 s; segment B represents the renal accumulation of the tracer before its excretion; and segment C indicates the excretion of the tracer into the urine. The second and third phases of the renogram are very important in the diagnosis of obstructive diseases of the kidneys. The period between injection and peak renal activity is called the renal transit time, the normal value of which is about 3 to 5 min for adults.

If the transit time is prolonged, the second phase of the renogram is less steep. Renal arterial stenosis, dehydration, or any pooling in the renal pelvis lengthens the transit time. The excretory phase depends on the state of dehydration, capacity of the renal pelvis, or any obstructive tubular abnormality. Various obstructive diseases, such as acute tubular necrosis and ureteral obstruction due to stenosis, may result in delayed excretion of the tracer and thus flatten the third segment of the renogram. Figure 13.22

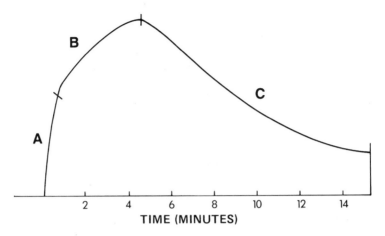

FIGURE 13.21. A schematic normal renogram. **A**: Arrival of tracer. **B**: Renal accumulation of tracer. **C**: Excretion of tracer into urine.

shows serial images and the renogram of a patient with right arterial occlusion and normal left kidney function.

If the obstruction is noted in the excretory phase, often furosemide (Lasix) is administered intravenously a few minutes after peak renal activity is reached in order to differentiate between functional and mechanical obstructions. Furosemide is a diuretic and therefore alleviates functional obstruction, whereby the renogram showing excretory obstruction becomes normal. On the other hand, if the obstruction is mechanical (e.g., calculus), little change in the renogram will occur after furosemide administration.

Effective Renal Plasma Flow (ERPF)

The ERPF or plasma clearance of a radiotracer is the rate of plasma flow through the kidneys, irrespective of whether it is filtered or secreted, and it refers to the volume of plasma that would account for measured quantity of a reagent excreted per minute in the urine. ^{131}I-Hippuran, ^{123}I-Hippuran and, ^{99m}Tc-MAG3 are ocmmonly used for the measurement of ERPF. There are two methods of measuring ERPF: the constant infusion technique and the single injection technique.

In the constant infusion technique, a continuous intravenous infusion of ^{131}I-Hippuran, ^{123}I-Hippuran, or ^{99m}Tc-MAG3 is maintained at a certain flow rate to keep a constant level of plasma radioactivity. An equilibrium is established when the rate of infusion is equal to the rate of excretion of the radiotracer in urine. At equilibrium, the plasma concentration (P) in counts per milliliter, urine concentration (U) in counts per milliliter, and the urine flow rate (V) in milliliters per minute are measured. The ERPF is then

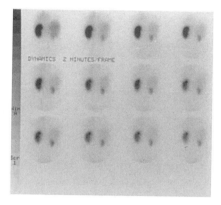

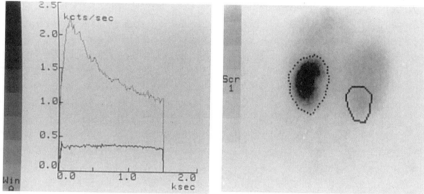

FIGURE 13.22. Renogram with ^{99m}Tc-MAG3. Serial images and renogram of a female patient with right renal arterial occlusion and normal left kidney function. (Courtesy of Andrew Taylor, Jr., M.D., of Emory University School of Medicine, Atlanta, GA.)

calculated from

$$\text{ERPF} = \frac{UV}{P} \qquad (13.2)$$

The value of ERPF is 600 to 700 ml/min for ^{131}I-Hippuran and about 340 ml/min for ^{99m}Tc-MAG3 in normal adults. In obstructive diseases, the value is smaller due to the decreased urine flow.

In the single injection technique, a bolus injection of ^{131}I-Hippuran or ^{99m}Tc-MAG3 is given and the plasma disappearance of the tracer is followed over a period of several hours. The plasma disappearance curve usually has two components. The ERPF is calculated from the administered dosage I, the slopes λ_1, and λ_2, and intercepts A_1 and A_2, of the two components as follows (Sapirstein et al., 1955):

$$\text{ERPF} = \frac{I\lambda_1\lambda_2}{\lambda_1 A_2 + \lambda_2 A_1} \tag{13.3}$$

The reader is referred to other books on nephrology for more details on this subject.

^{99m}Tc-DTPA

^{99m}Tc-DTPA is a useful agent for renal imaging. Following intravenous administration, it is entirely filtered by glomeruli in the kidneys. For this reason, it can be used for the measurement of glomerular filtration rate (GFR) using the techniques employed in measuring ERPF with ^{131}I-Hippuran or ^{99m}Tc-MAG3. Both the constant infusion and single injection techniques can be employed, and Eqs. (13.2) and (13.3) can be used to calculate the renal chearance or GFR of the kidneys. The normal value of renal clearance is about 125 ml/min for a 70-kg man, but it varies with the weight of the body.

The plasma clearance of ^{99m}Tc-DTPA is rapid and its half-time is about 70 min. Its biological half-life is about 1 to 2 hr. Urinary excretion amounts to about 90% in 24 hr and its plasma protein binding is 5% to 10% in 1 hr (Hauser et al., 1970). The renal uptake is about 7% in 1 hr after injection, but it clears rapidly.

Approximately 10 to 15 mCi (370–555 MBq) ^{99m}Tc-DTPA is injected intravenously in a bolus form, and flow pictures (posterior views) are taken with a scintillation camera using a low-energy parallel hole collimator at 1- to 2-s intervals for up to 1 to 2 min. The flow study provides information about blood perfusion in the kidneys. Then the dynamic pictures are acquired every 30 to 120 s for the next 30 min. Renograms can be generated from these dynamic data, which provide information about the renal function. A static image, taken 30 to 60 min later, demonstrates the structure of the kidneys. Serial images obtained with ^{99m}Tc-DTPA are shown in Figure 13.23.

^{99m}Tc-Gluceptate

^{99m}Tc-gluceptate has been employed successfully in renal imaging. Following intravenous administration, ^{99m}Tc-gluceptate is excreted by both glomerular filtration and tubular secretion. Its plasma clearance half-time is only a few minutes. Within 1 to 2 hr after injection, the radioactivity in both kidneys reaches a maximum of about 12% of the administered dosage. Urinary excretion is nearly 50% in 2 hr and 70% in 24 hr following administration, and its protein binding in the plasma is about 50% to 75% (Arnold et al., 1975).

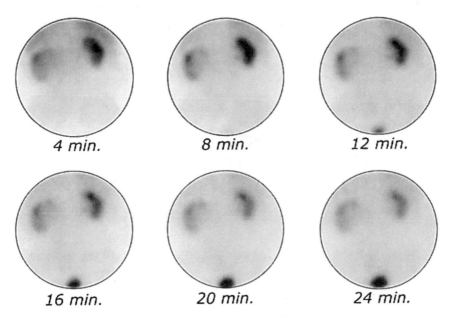

FIGURE 13.23. Posterior images of the kidneys with [99mTc]-DTPA indicating mildly impaired renal uptake in both kidneys, the left kidney being somewhat more impaired than the right kidney.

Approximately 10 to 15 mCi (370–555 MBq) [99mTc]-gluceptate is administered intravenously to the patient. Serial images of both kidneys are obtained at 5-min intervals for up to 30 min after injection using a gamma camera with a low-energy parallel hole collimator. Static images in different projections (posterior, lateral, and lateral oblique) are obtained 3 to 4 hr postinjection. Initial images depict the renal parenchyma well without any radioactivity in the pelvis. The later images, however, reveal the renal structure as a whole, including the pelvis.

[99mTc]-DMSA

[99mTc]-DMSA is another [99mTc]-labeled complex frequently used as a renal imaging agent. Following intravenous injection, it is excreted in the urine via glomerular filtration and tubular secretion. The plasma clearance half-time is about 10 min, which is longer than that of [99mTc]-gluceptate. Plasma protein binding of [99mTc]-DMSA is about 75% in 6 hr and its urinary excretion is about 37% in 24 hr. Renal retention of [99mTc]-DMSA in both kidneys amounts to nearly 24% of the administered dosage 1 hr after injection (Arnold et al., 1975).

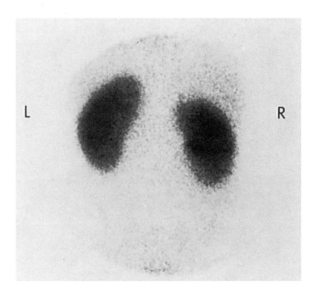

FIGURE 13.24. Normal image of the kidneys (posterior view) obtained with ^{99m}Tc-DMSA at 1 hr after administration.

The usual dosage for intravenous administration is 2 to 5 mCi (74–185 MBq) ^{99m}Tc-DMSA for humans, although an even lower dosage is used to obtain a good image. Images in different projections (posterior, lateral, and oblique) are obtained 3 to 4 hr after injection using a gamma camera with a low-energy parallel hole collimator. A normal image of the kidneys at 1 hr after administration of ^{99m}Tc-DMSA is shown in Figure 13.24.

Captopril Renography

In renal artery stenosis, angiotensin II induces efferent arteriolar vaso-constriction by increasing efferent arteriolar resistance so that the GFR is maintained normal. However, if an angiotensin-converting enzyme (ACE) inhibitor such as captopril is administered, it blocks the formation of angio-tensin II and thus removes the postglomerular efferent resistance, so that the GFR of the affected kidney falls, and tubular tracers accumulate in the tubular lumen without normal excretion. Therefore, a decrease in the uptake of GFR agents such as ^{99m}Tc-DTPA and an accumulation of tubular agents such as ^{99m}Tc-MAG3 are seen after administration of captopril, with pro-longed transit time for both GFR and tubular agents.

Based on these principles, captopril renography is performed to show the presence of renal artery stenosis responsible for renovascular hypertension in patients. Captopril renograms are obtained using ^{99m}Tc-DTPA, or ^{99m}Tc-MAG3. The study is performed using either a 1-day protocol or a 2-day protocol with variations in details from institution to institution.

Initially the patient is asked to withhold any antihypertensive drug at least overnight, diuretics for at least 1 day and any ACE inhibitor for at least 4 days. Some investigators do not suggest hydration, while others hydrate the patient 60 min prior to renography to induce gentle diuresis. In a 1-day protocol, a baseline renogram is obtained using 1 to 3 mCi (37–111 MBq) ^{99m}Tc-DTPA or ^{99m}Tc-MAG3. The patient is asked to void the bladder and is given orally 25 mg captopril in crushed form suspended in water. One hour later, another renogram is obtained with 5 to 10 mCi (185–370 MBq) of the corresponding tracer. In a 2-day protocol, the post-captopril renogram is obtained on a separate day, in which case, higher activities may be used.

In the absence of renovascular hypertension, both pre- and postcaptopril renograms are similar and the renal transit time remains the same. Patients with renal artery stenosis show reduced uptake of ^{99m}Tc-DTPA or increased accumulation of ^{99m}Tc-MAG3 in the postcaptopril renograms and prolonged renal transit time in the affected kidney.

Diagnosis

Renography provides information about the functional status of the kidneys. Abnormal renograms are obtained in cases of ureteral obstruction, acute tubular necrosis, and arterial stenosis. In addition, renal scintigraphy also indicates the presence of any structural defect in the kidneys. Tumors, cysts, abscesses, infarcts, and other space-occupying lesions are seen as cold spots on the image, characterized by decreased uptake of the ^{99m}Tc-labeled compound. The viability and rejection of renal transplants are evaluated by the ^{99m}Tc-DTPA flow study and the functional study using ^{99m}Tc-MAG3. Renal artery stenosis causing renovascular hypertension can be diagnosed by captopril renography.

Skeleton

Anatomy and Physiology

The skeletal system serves as a framework to support the soft tissues of the body. In contrast to popular belief, the bone is a live functional tissue undergoing continuous metabolic changes. The bone serves as a storehouse for calcium and phosphorus, protects soft organs, and works as a lever for muscles.

Bone tissues consist of organic and inorganic constituents, the organic matrix accounting for almost one third of the weight of the bone, and the inorganic matrix forming the rest. The inorganic matrix is called hydroxyapatite crystal and is primarily composed of calcium phosphate and, to a small extent, carbonate and hydroxide. Inorganic calcium salts deposit within the frame of the organic matrix and give strong rigidity to the bone. The blood supply is essential for the growth of new bone; a continuous exchange of minerals takes place between bone and plasma, and the minerals are used in now bone formation. This process of mineral exchange and new bone formation, by which new bone gradually replaces old bone, is called bone accretion. A fracture repairs itself by new bone formation.

Radiopharmaceuticals and Imaging Techniques

^{99m}Tc-Phosphonate and Phosphate Complexes

The ^{99m}Tc complexes such as PYP, MDP, and HDP are the agents used for bone imaging. Several studies have shown superiority of one agent over another, but the general consensus is that ^{99m}Tc-MDP, and ^{99m}Tc-HDP exhibit essentially similar behavior in vivo, whereas ^{99m}Tc-PYP bone scans are somewhat inferior in quality. Currently, ^{99m}Tc-MDP is most commonly used for bone scanning.

The plasma clearance half-time of these compounds is about 3 to 4 min, although it is slightly longer for ^{99m}Tc-PYP. The plasma protein binding of ^{99m}Tc-PYP is more than those of ^{99m}Tc-MDP and ^{99m}Tc-HDP by almost a factor of two; hence, there is a slower plasma clearance of the former. Urinary excretion of ^{99m}Tc-MDP is nearly 75% to 85% in 24 hr, whereas it is about 60% for ^{99m}Tc-PYP (Subramanian et al., 1975). The skeletal retention of ^{99m}Tc-HDP is about 50% of the injected dosage in 24 hr.

Approximately 10 to 20 mCi (370–740 MBq) ^{99m}Tc-MDP or ^{99m}Tc-HDP is injected intravenously and scanning is performed with the patient supine 2 to 3 hr after injection. The 2- to 3-hr waiting period is needed to reduce the background against the bone, and the patient is asked to void before imaging so that the bladder activity does not blur the pelvic region on the image. Whole-body scanning is performed by moving the detector from head to toe of the patient using either a single-head or a dual-head camera equipped with a low-energy, all-purpose parallel hole collimator. Static spot images are obtained with a single-head camera, whereas both anterior and posterior scans are obtained simultaneously using a dual-head whole-body camera.

To distinguish between cellulitis and osteomyelitis in the distal extremities, three-phase bone images (flow, blood pool, and bone uptake) are obtained by giving a bolus injection of 30 mCi (1.11 GBq) ^{99m}Tc-MDP. In the flow phase, images are obtained every 2 s for 60 s, followed by blood pool imaging immediately and bone uptake imaging at 3 to 5 hr after injection. Due to hyperemia in cellulitis, the tracer locallizes in both the flow and blood pool phases, but disappears in the delayed bone uptake phase. On the other hand, in osteomyelitis, wherein some associated hyperemia exists, the tracer uptake is seen in the flow and blood pool phases, with a further increase in localization in the bone uptake phase. In some cases, the background clearance is not optimum because of vascular insufficiency; a fourth phase bone image may be required, which is usually performed the next day to delineate bone uptake better.

Regional bone blood flow rate, bone formation rate, and extraction efficiency are the major factors that influence the bone uptake of phosphonate complexes. In general, the higher the rates of blood flow and bone formation, the greater the bone uptake of radiotracer. There are two hypotheses on the bone uptake mechanism of phosphonate compounds: hydroxyapatite uptake and collagen uptake. In the hydroxyapatite uptake theory, it has been suggested that hydroxyapatite crystal removes the phosphonate component successfully from ^{99m}Tc-phosphate complexes, thus setting the reduced technetium free to bind independently to hydroxyapatite at another binding site. In the collagen uptake theory, it has been suggested that ^{99m}Tc-phosphonate complexes localize in both inorganic and organic matrices of bone, the latter uptake depending on the amount of immature collagen present. It has also been found that ^{99m}Tc-phosphonate complexes localize in soft tissues and tumors to a variable degree.

Diagnosis

Various diseases that are diagnosed by increased uptake of ^{99m}Tc-phosphonate compounds include metastatic lesion, Paget's disease, fracture, osteomyelitis, bone tumor, rheumatoid arthritis, and any other disorder that results in active bone formation. A normal whole-body bone scan obtained with ^{99m}Tc-MDP is shown in Figure 13.25. A typical whole-body bone scan obtained with ^{99m}Tc-MDP indicating metastatic lesions is presented in Figure 13.26.

Heart

Anatomy and Physiology

The cardiovascular system consists of the heart and blood vessels (arteries and veins) and governs the circulation of blood in the body. The heart works as a pump and circulates the blood through blood vessels to the different parts of the body.

The heart is divided into four chambers: the right atrium, left atrium, right ventricle, and left ventricle (Fig. 13.27). Deoxygenated blood from the systemic circulation is received by the right atrium from the superior and inferior vena cavae and then passes into the right ventricle via the tricuspid valve. Blood is then pumped from the right ventricle via the pulmonary artery into the lungs, where it is oxygenated by diffusion of oxygen from the alveoli, and carbon dioxide from the blood is released. Oxygenated blood passes through the pulmonary veins into the left atrium and then to the left ventricle via the mitral valve. The left ventricle pumps the blood into the aorta, which distributes it to the systemic circulation.

The heart goes through a cycle of diastole and systole that maintains appropriate blood pressures in its four chambers as well as in the blood vessels. Diastole is the period of dilatation or expansion of the heart, and

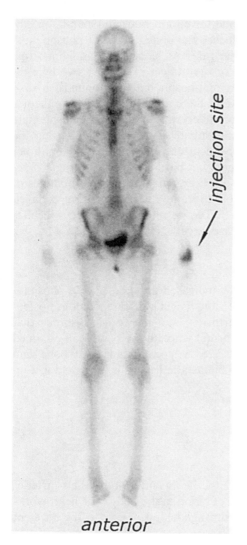

injection site

anterior

FIGURE 13.25. Normal whole-body bone scan obtained with ^{99m}Tc-MDP 2 hr after injection indicating normal distribution of the tracer throughout the bone structure.

systole is the period of contraction of the heart during which blood is forced into the aorta and pulmonary artery. The passage of blood from the right atrium up to the aorta is governed by the above cardiac cycle and by a number of valves present between different atrial and ventricular chambers. The valves are so constructed that only one-way passage of blood is allowed and regurgitation is prevented. The cardiac cycle is a well coordinated function of the heart and any deviation from it leads to a variety of cardiac abnormalities.

The cardiac output is the amount of blood pumped by the heart per unit time. It is 4 to 6 liters/min for a man at rest. The cardiac output depends on

FIGURE 13.26. Typical whole-body bone scan obtained with ^{99m}Tc-MDP 2 hr after injection indicating metastatic lesions at various sites in the body.

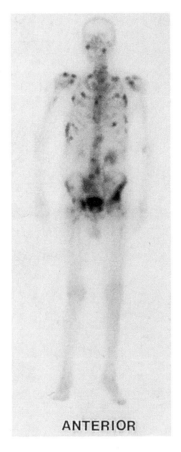

ANTERIOR

the amount of blood the ventricles expel during systole, the heart rate, and the degree of venous filling.

The heart muscle receives its blood supply from the coronary arteries, which arise from the first part of the aorta. The coronary arteries penetrate the mass of cardiac muscle and end in capillaries. The latter connect to venules and finally to the coronary veins. About 5% of the cardiac output (200–300 ml/min) passes through the coronary circulation. However, during severe exercise the coronary blood flow may increase to 1 to 1.5 liters/min.

Radiopharmaceuticals and Imaging Techniques

Various radiopharmaceuticals for myocardial imaging are listed in Table 13.6.

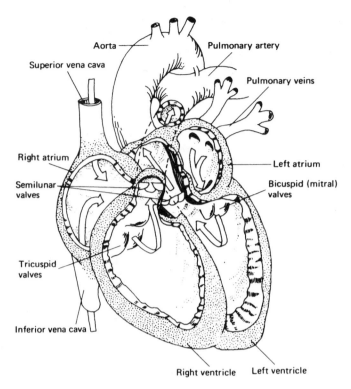

FIGURE 13.27. Anatomic structure of the heart showing interrelationships of the four chambers.

TABLE 13.6. Radiopharmaceuticals for myocardial imaging.

Radiopharmaceuticals	Dosage (mCi)	Dosage (MBq)	Imaging technique	Type of study
^{201}Tl-TlCl	2–3	74–111	Planar or SPECT	Perfusion
^{99m}Tc-sestamibi	10–30	370–1110	SPECT	Perfusion
^{99m}Tc-PYP	10–15	370–555	Planar	Infarct
^{99m}Tc-tetrofosmin	5–25	185–925	SPECT	Perfusion
^{123}I-MIBG	5–10	185–370	Planar or SPECT	cardiac innervation
^{99m}Tc-N-NOET	15–25	555–925	SPECT	Perfusion
^{82}Rb-RbCl	60	2220	PET	Perfusion
^{13}N-NH$_3$	15–20	555–740	PET	Perfusion
^{18}F-FDG	10–15	370–555	PET	Metabolism

TABLE 13.7. Comparative characteristics of different perfusion radiopharmaceuticals

	^{201}Tl	^{99m}Tc-sestamibi	^{99m}Tc-tetrofosmin	^{99m}Tc-N-NOET
Lipophilicity (charge)	hydrophilic cation (1^+)	lipophilic cation (1^+)	lipophilic cation (1^+)	lipophilic neutral ($1°$)
Extraction fraction (%)	73	38	37	48
Capillary permeability—surface area product (ml/g/min)	1.30	0.44	~0.44	1.02
Blood clearance ($t_{1/2}$)	two components (a few minutes)	two components (a few minutes)	two components (a few minutes)	two components (a few minutes)
Myocardial uptake at rest (%)	4	1.0 (1 hr)*	1.0 (2 hr)	2.1 (2 hr)
Myocardial uptake at stress (%)	—	1.4 (1 hr)	1.0 (2 hr)	2.1 (2 hr)
Myocardial washout ($t_{1/2}$)	4 hr	minimal	minimal	minimal
Urinary excretion (%)	~4 (24 hr)	37 (48 hr)	40 (48 hr)	0.8 (24 hr)
Redistribution	yes	unlikely	unlikely	possible
Lung uptake (%) (at rest)	0.9 (24 hr)	2.6 (5 min)	1.7 (5 min)	8 (5 min)
Liver uptake (%) (at rest)	4–7 (24 hr)	19.6 (5 min)	7.5 (5 min)	14 (2 min)

*time in parenthesis is the time postinjection

Perfusion Imaging

Characteristics of different SPECT myocardial perfusion radiopharmaceuticals are given in Table 13.7.

^{201}Tl-Thallous Chloride

^{201}Tl-thallous chloride is used for myocardial perfusion imaging. After intravenous administration, nearly 85% of the administered dosage is extracted by the myocytes during the first pass of the tracer. Blood clearance is rapid, with only 5% remaining in the blood 5 min after injection. It is mostly excreted by the kidneys and the whole-body biological half-life is about 10 days. Maximum myocardial uptake ($\sim$4%) of ^{201}Tl occurs about 5 to 10 min after injection (Atkins et al., 1977). Its myocardial washout has a $t_{1/2}$ of about 4 hr. The myocardial uptake of ^{201}Tl is linearly proportional to the blood flow, arterial concentration of the tracer, and myocardial mass, but can be reduced at high flow rates.

Although thallium belongs to group IIIA, thallous ion behaves like K^+, because they are both monovalent and have similar ionic radii. The extraction of thallium ions by myocytes requires that cations traverse the capillary wall, interstitial space, and myocyte membrane. The barrier at the capillary wall is blood-flow dependent, and Tl^+ is transported through the cell membrane by active transport by the Na^+-K^+–adenosine triphosphatase

(ATPase) enzyme, which is facilitated by depolarization and repolarization of the cell membrane.

Imaging is performed under resting and stress (e.g., exercise) conditions by means of a gamma camera. Normally, the patient is asked to exercise on a treadmill or a bicycle and 2 to 3 mCi (74–111 MBq) ^{201}Tl is injected at the peak of the exercise period. Imaging of the heart is begun 5 to 10 min after injection and completed in about 30 min. After about 3 to 4 hr of resting, the patient's heart is again imaged under identical conditions. The latter images are called the redistribution images. Images can be either planar or SPECT. In the planar technique, images are obtained in different projections (e.g., anterior, left anterior oblique, and right anterior oblique) by means of a single-head gamma camera using a low-energy parallel hole collimator. In the SPECT technique, data are collected by a single-head or a multihead camera in a 64 × 64 or 128 × 128 matrix, at small angle intervals (3° to 6°) over 180° or 360° around the heart. The data are then used to reconstruct the images in transverse, sagittal, or coronal projections.

Gated SPECT can be performed by collecting the data in 15-ms to 75-ms segments during each cardiac cycle (i.e., between two consecutive R-waves). Normally for SPECT, data are acquired in 8 to 16 frames per cardiac cycle and over many cardiac cycles.

Since ^{201}Tl uptake is blood-flow dependent, during the exercise test the normal tissues accumulate more thallium (due to high blood flow) than ischemic tissues (reduced blood flow), thus the latter resulting in a defect on the stress image. In the resting period (redistribution), tissues with high ^{201}Tl uptake (normal) have a faster washout than those with low uptake (ischemic but viable), and tissues that have received less thallium relative to the blood concentration will continue to accumulate ^{201}Tl. Furthermore, a large portion of washout thallium comes from tissues other than the cardiac tissues and is presented to myocardium for extraction. Thus, thallium ions undergo continuous exchange between extracellular and intracellular compartments, leading to what is called the redistribution of thallium. At a certain time later, there is an equilibrium between the intracellular and interstitial compartments of activity and the defect seen in the mildly perfused areas on the stress image will disappear on the 3 to 4 hr redistribution images. However, the initial uptake of thallium in infarcted tissues is so low that at equilibrium, the defect does not disappear on the redistribution image. Thus, a defect on both stress and redistribution images indicates an infarct, whereas a defect on stress images that fills in on redistribution images suggests ischemia. Ischemic defects are mostly reversible and viable, and the patient is likely to benefit from revascularization procedures such as bypass surgery or angioplasty. Myocardial SPECT images (both normal and abnormal) obtained with ^{201}Tl are shown in Figure 13.28.

In patients who cannot perform treadmill exercise, myocardial stress is induced by intravenous administration of a vasodilator such as dipyridamole (Persantine) or adenosine. The latter causes more side effects (e.g., chest pain, flushing, headache, etc.) than the former, but they are more

FIGURE 13.28. ^{201}Tl SPECT images (transverse) of the heart during the stress (S) and redistribution (R) separated by 4 hr. **A**: normal. **B**: posterolateral ischemia. **C**: inferoseptal infarct.

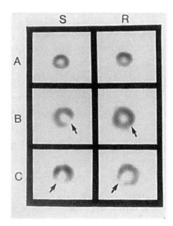

transient. Some of these side effects can be reduced by intravenous administration of aminophylline.

It has been demonstrated that some persistent defects that are seen on the early redistribution images (3–4 hr after injection) are filled in with ^{201}Tl on the delayed distribution images at 8 to 24 hr (Kiat et al., 1988). Time to complete redistribution depends on the severity of stenosis and the blood concentration of ^{201}Tl. To elevate blood concentration of ^{201}Tl, it is suggested that a second injection of 1 mCi (37 **MBq**) ^{201}Tl would facilitate the myocardial uptake in ischemic but viable regions that would otherwise be ·considered as persistent defects (Dilsizian et al., 1990). Three methods are employed: (1) reinjection after the redistribution study and imaging 15 to 20 min later, (2) reinjection immediately before the redistribution study and imaging 15 to 20 min later, (3) reinjection immediately after stress imaging and imaging 3 to 4 hr later. Methods 1 and 2 tend to show increased gut activity, which makes the interpretation of the images somewhat difficult. Method 3 offers the advantage of optimal clearance of the gut activity because of the longer time allowed between the reinjection and redistribution imaging. Using this reinjection technique, almost 40% to 45% of the 3 to 4 hr redistribution defects were identified to be viable, which otherwise would have been considered as persistent defects, and thus these patients benefited from revascularization by coronary artery bypass graft (CABG) and angioplasty.

The radiation characteristics of ^{201}Tl are poor. The low-energy photons (69–80 keV) of ^{201}Tl degrade the spatial resolution of the images due to scattering. The long half-life of 73 hr increases the radiation dose to the patient. It is cyclotron-produced and therefore quite expensive. As substitutes for ^{201}Tl, two ^{99m}Tc-labeled radiopharmaceuticals (^{99m}Tc-sestamibi and ^{99m}Tc-tetrofosmin) are used for SPECT myocardial perfusion imaging. ^{82}Rb-rubidium chloride and ^{13}N-ammonia are used for PET myocardial perfusion imaging.

^{99m}Tc-Sestamibi (Cardiolite)

^{99m}Tc-sestamibi is a lipophilic cationic (1^+) complex that accumulates in the myocardium by passive diffusion, not transported by the Na^+–K^+–ATPase pump. It indicates the myocardial perfusion abnormalities. After intravenous administration, the blood clearance of ^{99m}Tc-sestamibi is rapid with a $t_{1/2}$ of a few minutes both at stress and rest. The first-pass extraction is almost 50% to 60%. Myocardial uptake is proportional to regional myocardial blood flow and amounts to about 1.4% of injected dosage during exercise and about 1.0% at rest. Almost 90% of the activity in the cell is bound to proteins in the mitochondria. The myocardial washout of the activity is slow ($t_{1/2} = 7$ hr). The urinary excretion is 27% at 24 hr and 37% at 48 hr. ^{99m}Tc-sestamibi is not metabolized in vivo (Wackers et al., 1989). There is controversy as to whether, like thallium, ^{99m}Tc-sestamibi redistributes or not. Some investigators reported sestamibi to undergo minimal or no redistribution, while others have demonstrated partial redistribution, which is a factor of 3 lower than that of thallium.

Myocardial imaging is performed by administering intravenously approximately 20 mCi (740 MBq) ^{99m}Tc-sestamibi at both rest and stress conditions. While stress imaging can be performed as early as 15 min after injection, rest imaging should be done at least 45 to 60 min after injection to allow sufficient clearance of the tracer from the liver. SPECT images are obtained in the same manner as in ^{201}Tl imaging. The predominant liver uptake contributes adversely to the images of the heart and therefore administration of fatty meals or milk has been suggested to hasten the clearance of the hepatic activity. However, routine use of fatty meals has not been indicated.

Several imaging protocols have been advocated (Berman et al., 1994): 1-day protocol; 2-day protocol; stress first, rest second, and vice versa; and finally a dual-isotope technique. In all protocols, a gamma camera equipped with a low-energy parallel hole collimator is used for imaging.

In the same-day protocol, 8 to 10 mCi (296–370 MBq) ^{99m}Tc-sestamibi is injected at rest and 22 to 30 mCi (814–1110 MBq) administered at stress 3 to 4 hr later. This method is commonly used by many nuclear physicians. Some investigators have suggested a same-day protocol with the stress study done first, followed by the rest study. In this case, it is useful to subtract the residual background of the first injection from the image of the second.

In the 2-day protocol, stress and rest studies are performed on separate days using 20 to 25 mCi (740–925 MBq) ^{99m}Tc-sestamibi each. Although the detection of hibernating myocardium using this method is suboptimal because of the lack of redistribution of this agent and also because of the short period (1 hr) after injection allowed for imaging, overall this protocol is better than the same-day protocol.

In the dual-isotope technique, a rest thallium study is first performed by injecting 3 to 3.5 mCi (111–130 MBq) ^{201}Tl followed by imaging the heart 15 min later. Soon after the completion of the rest study, the patient is stressed and 25 mCi (925 MBq) ^{99m}Tc-sestamibi is injected at peak stress.

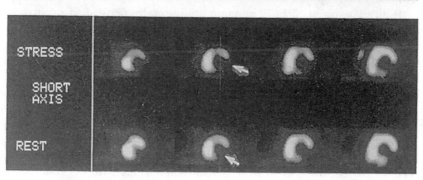

FIGURE 13.29. Transverse SPECT images obtained with ^{99m}Tc-sestamibi during stress and resting separated by 3 hr. **A**: Septal ischemia. **B**: Lateral and posterolateral infarct. Eight mCi (296 MBq) was administered in stress study followed by 24 mCi (888 MBq) administration in resting study 3 hr later. (Courtesy of Steven Port, M.D., Milwaukee, WI.)

Stress imaging is performed 15 to 60 min after injection. This technique, although well appreciated because of the relatively short time needed for the entire protocol, suffers from the differences in physical imaging characteristics of the two tracers.

Typical examples of rest and stress SPECT images of patients with ischemic and infarcted myocardium obtained with ^{99m}Tc-sestamibi are shown in Fig. 13.29.

^{99m}Tc-Tetrofosmin (Myoview)

^{99m}Tc-tetrofosmin is a lipophilic cationic (1^+) perfusion tracer that accumulates in the myocardium in proportion to blood flow. After intravenous administration, it is rapidly cleared from the blood with only less than 5% remaining by 10 min. The urinary excretion is about 9% in the resting study and about 13% in the stress study 2 hr after administration. But by 48 hr postinjection, the urinary excretion is approximately 40% in both conditions (Higley et al., 1993). The myocardial uptake is about 1.2% of the injected dosage at 5 min and 1% at 2 hr after injection, indicating a slow clearance of the tracer from the myocardium. The cumulative fecal excretion is nearly 25% after exercise and 34% at rest. The liver uptake is around 1.2% at stress versus 7.5% at rest by 5 min after injection, compared to 0.5% at stress versus 2.1% at rest by 60 min after administration. The early uptake in the gallbladder and the lungs is high but diminishes with time.The fast clearance of the hepatic, lung and gallbladder activity and the relatively slow clearance of myocardial activity provide good images of the heart. There is minimal, if any, redistribution of the tracer over time.

The myocardial uptake of tetrofosmin has been explained by a membrane potential–driven diffusion mechanism that is independent of cation channel transport but dependent on the metabolic status of the myocytes, and by its relatively high lipophilicity.

Both planar and SPECT imaging are normally performed using a same-day protocol, in which the rest study is followed by the stress study. At rest, 8 to 10 mCi (296–370 MBq) ^{99m}Tc-tetrofosmin is administered and the heart of the patient is imaged 45 to 60 min later with a gamma camera using a low-energy, all-purpose parallel hole collimator. A second injection of 15 to 24 mCi (555–888 MBq) is given to the patient 4 hr later at peak exercise and imaging of the heart is performed 30 to 60 min after injection. Similar to ^{99m}Tc-sestamibi imaging, stress imaging with a smaller dosage followed by rest imaging with a larger dosage or a dual-isotope technique using a combination of a rest ^{201}Tl study and a stress ^{99m}Tc-tetrofosmin study has been reported. Typical SPECT myocardial images with ^{99m}Tc-tetrofosmin are shown in Figure 13.30.

[99m]Tc-N-NOET

[99m]Tc-N-NOET is a lipophilic neutral complex used for the detection of myocardial perfusion abnormalities in patients with coronary artery disease. After intravenous administration, it is cleared rapidly with less than 5% of the injected activity present 5 min postinjection. The 24-hr urinary excretion is about 5.5% of the injected activity at rest and about 3.89% after exercise. The 2-hr lung uptake is 8% at rest and 6.1% after exercise, which falls to 5% at 24 hr after injection (Vanzetto et al, 2000). The 2-hr myocardial uptake is about 2.1% at rest and 2.4% after exercise. The liver activity and renal activity remain constant at 13% to 14% and 3% to 4%, respectively, over a 24-hr period. It has been found that this tracer has a considerable redistribution like thallium, and therefore a second injection may not be warranted.

Approximately 15 to 25 mCi (555–925 MBq) ^{99m}Tc-N-NOET is administered intravenously by slow injection to patients after 12-hr fasting. Both planar and SPECT images are obtained by a gamma camera using a low-energy parallel hole collimator. Initially the exercise imaging is performed and then the rest imaging 2 to 4 hr later. Since there is considerable redistribution of the tracer, like thallium, the rest image may be obtained without a second injection of ^{99m}Tc-N-NOET. Since it is a new tracer and has not yet been approved by the FDA, various protocols of imaging are warranted to obtain the optimal imaging of the coronary artery diseases.

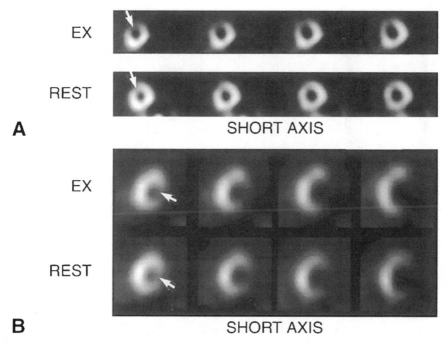

FIGURE 13.30. Transverse SPECT myocardial images obtained with ^{99m}Tc-tetrofosmin at rest and after exercise. A: Reversible ischemia in septum and anterior wall. B: Large infarcts in inferior and lateral walls. (Courtesy of Diwakar Jain, M.D., Drexel University Medical School of Medicine, Philadelphia, PA.)

^{82}Rb-Rubidium Chloride

^{82}Rb is a positron emitter ($t_{1/2} = 75$ s) and a monovalent cationic analog of potassium, and therefore it is used in PET imaging of the heart. This tracer is available from the ^{82}Sr-^{82}Rb generator. Because of the short half-life of ^{82}Rb, it is administered to the patient by means of an infusion system (Saha et al., 1990).

After intravenous administration, the first-pass extraction of ^{82}Rb by the myocardium is about 65% to 75% at normal blood flow. In vivo it behaves like K$^+$ ion. Myocardial uptake occurs by the active transport mechanism via the Na$^+$-K$^+$-ATPase pump. For PET studies, initially attenuation correction data are acquired before ^{82}Rb infusion by using a rotating ^{68}Ge transmission source. For the resting study, 60 mCi (2.22 GBq) ^{82}Rb is then administered by the infusion pump to the subject lying supine with the heart in the field of view, and the data are collected by the PET camera. After completion of the resting study (4–6 min), the subject is administered dipyridamole, adenosine, or dobutamine to induce myocardial stress, followed by infusion of an additional 60 mCi (2.22 GBq). Data are then collected by the PET camera for stress images. All data (both resting and stress) are corrected for attenuation of 511 keV photons using the transmission data,

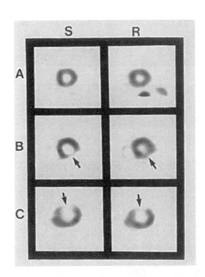

FIGURE 13.31. Transverse ^{82}Rb PET images of the heart during stress (S) and rest (R). A: normal. B: posterolateral ischemia. C: anterior infarct. Myocardial stress was induced by dipyridamole.

which are then used to reconstruct the images in transverse, coronal, and sagittal projections. Patterns of images are similar to those of SPECT studies, with improved contrast resolution, and thus can delineate better between the ischemic and infarcted myocardium. Typical PET images of the heart obtained with ^{82}Rb are shown in Figure 13.31.

Gould et al. (1991) suggested that the cell membrane must be intact for in and out transport of intracellular contents, and thus cell membrane integrity is a good marker of viability of the cell. ^{82}Rb ion apparently washes out of the necrotic cells faster than out of the viable cells and thus ^{82}Rb kinetics in myocardium provides a test for the cell membrane integrity and in turn cellular integrity.

^{13}N-Ammonia

^{13}N ($t_{1/2} = 10$ min) is a positron emitter and is cyclotron produced. ^{13}N-NH$_3$ is used in myocardial perfusion imaging by the PET technique. Administered intravenously, ammonia circulates as NH$_4^+$, which is taken up by the myocytes via initial diffusion across the cell membrane and then through the metabolic fixation by the glutamic acid–glutamine pathway. It is cleared from the blood rapidly with less than 2% of the administered dosage remaining at 5 min after injection. The first-pass extraction is about 100% but decreased at higher flows (Schelbert et al., 1981).

Approximately 15 to 20 mCi (555–740 MBq) ^{13}N-NH$_3$ is injected intravenously and PET images are obtained in the same fashion as in ^{82}Rb PET studies. Ischemia and myocardial infarcts can be detected by this technique. Because of the short half-life, repeat studies can be made in the same sitting of the patient. CMS has approved reimbursement for ^{13}N-NH$_3$-PET for myocardial perfusion imaging.

Other Perfusion Radiopharmaceuticals

^{99m}Tc-teboroxime (Cardiotec) is a neutral lipophilic complex that has been used for myocardial perfusion imaging. After intravenous administration, it clears from the blood rapidly with a $t_{1/2}$ of less than a minute (Narra et al, 1989). The 24-hr urinary excretion is 22% ± 13%. The maximum myocardial uptake is about 2.3% in 2 to 3 min postinjection, the majority of which washes out rapidly in 5 min (Johnson and Seldin, 1990). Because of the rapid washout, this agent has not been successful in myocardial perfusion imaging. However, it has been proposed that the washout kinetics of the tracer is different in normal and abnormal areas of the myocardium. Based on this assumption, investigators have measured the washout rates of ^{99m}Tc-teboroxime to differentiate between normal and abnormal myocardium, but the method has not gained favorable acceptance.

^{15}O-H$_2$O has been used to measure the myocardial blood flow in patients. Because it has a short half-life ($t_{1/2} = 2$ min) and is produced in the cyclotron, its availability is limited.

Metabolic Imaging

^{18}F-Fluorodeoxyglucose (FDG)

Both nonesterified free fatty acid and glucose supply energy to the heart for its expansion and contraction. In the fasting state, free fatty acid is the primary energy substrate, whereas in the fed state glucose becomes the predominant energy source. Based on this concept, ^{18}F-FDG is used for myocardial metabolic imaging.

After intravenous administration, the blood clearance of FDG is triexponential with three components having half-times of 0.2 to 0.3 min, 11.6 ± 1.1 min, and 88 ± 4 min (Phelps et al., 1978). FDG crosses the cell membrane into the cell and is phosphorylated to FDG-6-phosphate mediated inside the myocyte by hexokinase. FDG-6-phosphate is not further metabolized and therefore remains trapped in the myocardium. As mentioned under Brain Imaging, evidence has been reported that ^{18}F-FDG undergoes further metabolism and is incorporated into glycogen (Virkamaki et al., 1997) and also FDG metabolites diffuse into the blood pool (Dienel et al., 1993). The myocardial uptake in normal adults is 1% to 4%. The heart-to-lung, heart-to-blood, heart-to-liver activity ratios are 20:1, 14:1, and 10:1, respectively.

For metabolic imaging, the patient is given 50 g glucose orally 1 hr before administration of ^{18}F-FDG. About 10 to 15 mCi (370–555 MBq) of the tracer is then injected intravenously, and imaging is performed 40 to 45 min postinjection using a PET camera keeping the heart in the field of view and employing the technique similar to that in brain imaging. Attenuation correction is applied using a rotating ^{68}Ge rod source.

Investigators have employed the SPECT technique in FDG imaging using high-energy collimators suitable for 511 keV photons. The results of myocardial viability using FDG SPECT are comparable to those of FDG PET. However, the sensitivity and contrast resolution of PET are much higher than those of SPECT. The SPECT spatial resolution improves with 511 keV collimators but does not approach that of PET.

FDG uptake is governed by five factors: myocardial blood flow, blood concentration of glucose, myocardial demand of glucose, oxygenation of myocytes, and viability of the cells (Saha et al., 1996). After glucose loading or feeding, the energy substrate shifts from fatty acid to glucose and enhances FDG uptake in the myocardium. Myocardial FDG uptake is variable in normal as well as different disease states. In mildly ischemic and hypoxic myocardium, glucose becomes the major energy substrate, and therefore shows increased uptake in these areas relative to the normal areas. In infarcted areas, blood flow and oxygen supply are extremely restricted, and glycolysis is almost totally stopped. These areas do not show any FDG uptake, relative to the normal and mildly ischemic areas. A typical ^{18}F-FDG PET image obtained after glucose loading is illustrated in Figure 13.32. The ^{18}F-FDG-PET study of myocardial viability, which has been nonspecific and nondiagnostic by SPECT, is approved for reimbursement by CMS in the U.S.

Overall, FDG uptake in poorly perfused areas indicates the viability of the myocardium and thus serves as an index for the selection of patients with coronary artery diseases either to treat with medication (infarcted

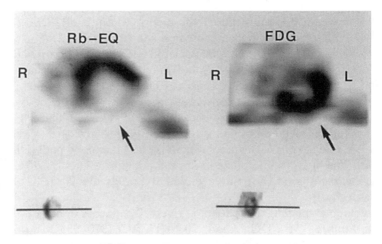

FIGURE 13.32. Transverse ^{18}F-FDG PET image (right) of the heart after glucose loading demonstrating increased FDG uptake in the posterolateral fixed defect identified by ^{82}Rb (equilibrium) PET image (left) to indicate the viability of the tissues. Glucose was administered 1 hr before the administration of ^{18}F-FDG, and PET imaging was performed 40 min after the adminstration of ^{18}F-FDG.

myocardium) or to revascularize by CABG or angioplasty (mildly ischemic but viable myocardium).

Other Metabolic Radiopharmaceuticals

[123]I-labeled fatty acids (iodo-heptadecanoic and para-iodophenyl pentadecanoic acids) have been used for myocardial metabolic imaging. ^{11}C-palmitic acid, ^{13}N-labeled amino acid (glutamic acid), and ^{11}C-acetate have been used for metabolic imaging of the heart by the PET technique. Success was limited with iodinated fatty acids because of beta oxidation and deiodination raising background activity in the blood pool. While ^{11}C-palmitic acid and ^{13}N-glutamic acid offer some success, ^{11}C-acetate is undergoing much research and appears to have a great potential as a metabolic marker. The latter tracer undergoes oxidative metabolism in the heart, is not influenced by the type of substrate present, and can distinguish between viable and necrotic myocardium in coronary artery diseases. ^{11}C-accetate gives a measure of oxygen consumption by the myocardium.

Myocardial Infarct Imaging

[99m]Tc-Pyrophosphate

[99m]Tc-pyrophosphate is used for imaging myocardial infarcts. The physiologic handling of ^{99m}Tc-pyrophosphate has been described in the section on the skeleton in this chapter. Approximately 10 to 15 mCi (370–555 MBq) ^{99m}Tc-pyrophosphate is injected intravenously. Imaging is performed 1 to 2 hr after administration by means of a scintillation camera equipped with a low-energy parallel hole collimator. Anterior, left anterior oblique, and left lateral views of the heart are obtained and myocardial infarcts are seen as areas of increased uptake of the tracer in the infarcted areas. A minimum of 12 to 24 hr after the onset of infarction is needed for infarcts to accumulate an appreciable amount of ^{99m}Tc-pyrophosphate. Maximum uptake is obtained 24 to 72 hr after infarction, and infarct sites remain detectable for 6 to 10 days. Myocardial infarct imaging with ^{99m}Tc-pyrophosphate is shown in Figure 13.33.

The mechanism of uptake of ^{99m}Tc-pyrophosphate by the damaged myocardium is not clearly understood. Increased uptake of the tracer has been attributed to the deposition of granules in enlarged mitochondria of the damaged myocardium. The granules are composed of calcium and phosphate groups similar to the hydroxyapatite crystals in bone. Perhaps ^{99m}Tc-pyrophosphate is absorbed on the calcium phosphate groups of the granules and thus accumulates in the mitochondria. It has also been suggested that the tracer binds to various soluble proteins in the damaged myocardium. It has been found that myocardial uptake of the phosphate is inversely proportional to regional blood flow except at very low values, in which case it decreases with the decrease in blood flow.

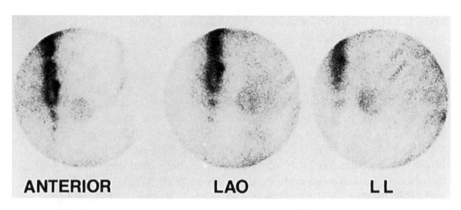

ANTERIOR   **LAO**   **L L**

FIGURE 13.33. Myocardial infarct image obtained with ^{99m}Tc-pyrophosphate in different projections 2 hr after injection, indicating increased uptake in the infarcted area at the anterior apical left ventricular wall. Imaging performed 24 hr after onset of infarction. LAO, left anterior oblique; LL, left lateral.

Cardiac Innervation Imaging

^{123}I-MIBG

MIBG behaves like norepinephrine (NE) as far as the uptake and storage mechanism is concerned. Norepinephrine is synthesized in neuronal cells, stored in large and small vesicles in the heart, and released by the action of acetylcholine. As a neurotransmitter, norepinephrine mediates the function of adrenergic neurons. A rise in adrenergic neuron activity is then associated with increased NE secretion by the sympathetic terminals of the nerves and with accentuated loss of NE from the innervated tissue. In patients with congestive heart failure, the sympathetic nerve terminals in the myocardium are destroyed and the NE stores are depleted. In ischemic heart disease, and particularly in infarcts, a similar situation occurs showing decreased concentration of NE. Depletion of NE stores is also observed in heart transplants, idiopathic dilated cardiomyopathy and hypertrophic cardiomyopathy.

   Because of the similar properties, ^{123}I-MIBG has been used to image patients with diseases related to impairment in NE concentration (Sisson et al., 1987). The patient is given Lugol's solution orally 1 day before and for 4 days after the administration of ^{123}I-MIBG to block the thyroid. Approximately 5 to 10 mCi (185–370 MBq) ^{123}I-MIBG is injected intravenously. Planar or SPECT images are obtained at 3, 24, and 48 hr after injection using a scintillation camera with a low-energy parallel hole collimator. In patients with heart failure, transplants, cardiomyopathy, and infarcts, ^{123}I-MIBG uptake in the heart is poor relative to the normal patients. The uptake is inhibited by drugs such as imipramine and phenylpropanolamine.

Radionuclide Angiography

The application of radionuclide angiography to the determination of ejection fraction and wall motion abnormalities of the heart is well-established. Two important techniques employed in these studies are (1) the first-pass method and (2) the gated equilibrium cardiac blood pool method. These methods are based on the measurement of radioactivity in the left or right ventricular chamber at the end of diastole (ED) and at the end of systole (ES). The ejection fraction (EF) is calculated as

$$EF(\%) = \frac{A_{ED} - A_{ES}}{A_{ED}} \times 100 \tag{13.4}$$

where A_{ED} and A_{ES} are the maximum end-diastolic and minimum end-systolic activities, respectively.

First-Pass Method

In the first-pass technique, the transit of an injected tracer is tracked through the heart chambers that allows detection of abnormalities in transit in diseases such as congenital heart disease, shunts, and valvular insufficiency. In this technique, ^{99m}Tc-pertechnetate, ^{99m}Tc-DTPA, or any ^{99m}Tc-labeled compound can be used as the radiotracer.

The detector of the scintillation camera equipped with a high-sensitivity, parallel hole collimator is placed over the heart in the anterior position before the injection is made. Detectors capable of counting high count rates ($>200,000$ counts/s) are necessary for adequate image quality. Approximately 20 to 30 mCi (740–1110 MBq) of the radiopharmaceutical in a small volume is injected intravenously in a bolus form. After injection, the precordial activity is measured and stored in a computer during the first 40 to 60 s of the first pass of the tracer through the heart. A composite picture of the right or left ventricle is constructed from the stored data, and two regions of interest (ROI) are selected—one corresponding to the ventricle and the other to the background. The time-activity curves are then generated for both regions by the computer, and the background activity is subtracted from the ventricular activity point by point on the corresponding curves. Thus, a corrected (subtracted) curve, representing the net counts within the ventricular activity, is generated. The maximum counts at end-diastole and the minimum counts at end-systole are read from the curve to calculate the ejection fraction of the ventricle by Eq. (13.4). The first-pass technique is the method of choice for the assessment of right ventricular function.

Gated Equilibrium Cardiac Blood Pool Method

The gated equilibrium cardiac blood pool method is also termed the multigated acquisition (MUGA) method or radionuclide ventriculography

(RNV). The aim of this technique is to obtain images of the cardiac chambers and great vessels with high resolution that help evaluate the ventricular function. This technique is commonly used for the left ventricle and the most common radiopharmaceutical is the in vivo labeled ^{99m}Tc-RBC. In in vivo labeling, the contents of a stannous pyrophosphate kit vial (containing about 1–1.5 mg of stannous ion for a 70-kg subject) are injected intravenously after reconstitution with isotonic saline, and then 20 to 30 mCi (740–1110 MBq) ^{99m}TcO$_4^-$ is injected 30 min later. Stannous ions reduce Tc and the reduced Tc binds to hemoglobin in the red blood cells. If necessary, in vitro labeled RBCs also can be used in this method.

In the gated equilibrium study, 5 to 10 min are allowed after administration of ^{99m}TcO$_4^-$ for equilibrium to be achieved. Images are obtained with a scintillation camera equipped with a low-energy parallel hole collimator in the left anterior oblique position. Data are accumulated in synchronization with the R-wave of the QRS complex in the electrocardiogram and stored in a computer in 15 to 75-ms segments during each cardiac cycle (i.e., between two consecutive R-waves) Normally 8 to 16 frames per cardiac cycle are acquired. Data acquisition is continued for many cardiac cycles until counts of statistical accuracy (~100,000–300,000 counts) are accumulated in each frame. Normally, data acquisition requires about 10 to 15 min. Regions of interest corresponding to the left ventricle and the background are selected by the computer. Time-activity curves are then generated for both the ventricle and the background. Background activity is subtracted from ventricle activity point by point from the two curves. Thus, a time-activity curve representing the net activity in the left ventricle is obtained. The maximum activity at end-diastole and the minimum activity at end-systole from the corrected curve are then used to calculate the ejection fraction of the left ventricle by Eq. (13.4). The scintigraphic display of a gated study is presented in Figure 13.34.

Another application of this technique is the detection of any wall motion abnormalities by observing the difference between the end-diastole and end-systole images of the left ventricle. The images are constructed by the computer as usual, and the two images are concentric in a normal heart. An abnormal wall motion, which may result from ischemia, infarction, and other hypokinetic cardiac conditions, is manifested by eccentric differences in the end-diastole and end-systole images.

These studies can also be made by "cineangiography," a movie-type presentation of the cardiac cycle, which can be applied to both right and left ventricles.

Radionuclide Stress Ventriculography

The value of radionuclide ventriculography can be enhanced by inducing stress in patients leading to what is called stress ventriculography. Initially, a first-pass study is performed at rest using 15 mCi (555 MBq) ^{99m}Tc-DTPA. The patient is asked to exercise using a bicycle equipped with an ergometer, and a second first-pass study is obtained using 25 mCi (925 MBq) ^{99m}Tc-

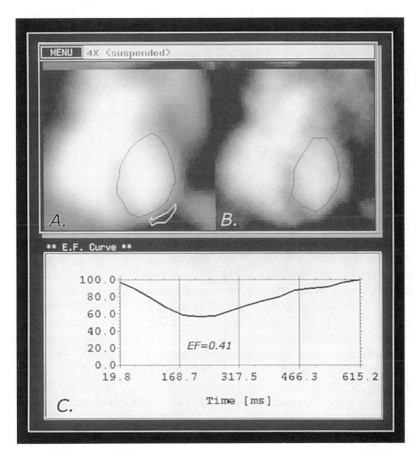

FIGURE 13.34. Gated equilibrium blood pool study of the heart. A: Left anterior oblique image of the heart at end-diastole. B: Left anterior oblique image of the heart at end-systole. C: Composite time-activity curve generated from counts collected over several hundred cardiac cycles from the background subtracted left ventricular region of interest.

DTPA. The difference in wall motion between the two studies would indicate an abnormality in the heart. The absence of activity in the abnormal hypofunctioning areas in the resting myocardium is enhanced by radionuclide stress ventriculography. In exercise, the ejection fraction increases in normal subjects. If it does not increase in a patient, it indicates abnormal ventricular function such as cardiomyopathy and heart failure.

Diagnosis

Perfusion imaging of the heart using ^{201}Tl, ^{99m}Tc-sestamibi, ^{99m}Tc-tetrofosmin, [82]Rb, etc. can delineate the viable ischemic areas from the nonviable infarcted areas in myocardium. ^{18}F-FDG PET imaging is highly accurate in predicting the viability of myocardium. Myocardial infarcts (acute) are detected by ^{99m}Tc-pyrophosphate. Radionuclide angiography during rest or stress provides the ejection fraction of the right or left ventricle, which is 50% to 80% at rest and 55% to 86% at stress in normal adults. In the cases of akinesis, hypokinesis, and dyskinesis of the ventricle due to infarction or ischemia, the ejection fractions are lower than the above limits, whereas they are higher in the case of hyperkinesis.

Miscellaneous Imaging Procedures

Adrenal Gland Imaging

The two adrenal glands are endocrine glands, one situated above each kidney. Each adrenal gland consists of two structures—a central medulla and an outer cortex. The adrenal medulla produces hormones such as adrenaline and noradrenaline, which influence blood pressure. The adrenal cortex secretes various glucocorticoids, of which corticosterone, hydrocortisone, and aldosterone are most essential for life. The production of steroids in the adrenal gland is primarily influenced by adrenocorticotropin hormone (ACTH). Carbohydrate metabolism is greatly influenced by corticosterone and hydrocortisone, whereas renal function and sodium and potassium balance are mainly controlled by aldosterone. It is believed that cholesterol is a precursor of steroid hormones. Addison's disease is manifested by hypofunctioning of the adrenal cortex, and Cushing's disease results from hyperfunctioning of the gland due to ACTH overproduction.

^{131}I-NP-59

^{131}I-NP-59 is an iodinated cholesterol derivative and has been used for imaging of the adrenal cortex. Approximately 1 mCi (37 MBq) ^{131}I-NP-59 is injected intravenously. The thyroid uptake of any free ^{131}I-iodide is blocked by administering Lugol's solution orally 1 day before and for 4 days after ^{131}I-NP-59 administration. The normal adrenal uptake in the cortex is of the order of 0.2% of the administered dosage.

Imaging is performed with a scintillation camera equipped with a medium-energy parallel hole collimator 5 to 7 days after injection of ^{131}I-NP-59. Cushing's syndrome, aldosteronism, and adrenal tumors are diagnosed by increased uptake of the tracer in the adrenal glands. It is not approved by the FDA for clinical use.

^{131}I-MIBG

^{131}I-MIBG is used for imaging the abnormal adrenal medulla. Approximately 0.5 mCi (18.5 MBq) ^{131}I-MIBG is injected intravenously (a higher dosage is given for ^{123}I-MIBG). To block the thyroid uptake of free ^{131}I-iodide, Lugol's solution is given orally 0.8 ml per day 1 day before and for 4 days after the administration of ^{131}I-MIBG. Whole-body images are obtained at 48 hr and 72 hr postinjection using a gamma camera with a medium-energy parallel hole collimator. Normal adrenal glands do not accumulate this tracer. Pheochromocytomas, which are medullary neoplasms, accumulate it significantly and are detected by this technique.

Tumor Imaging

Tumors appear in different parts of the body as a result of the proliferation of abnormal cells. How this abnormal proliferation occurs is not clearly known, although several investigators propose that the high rate of DNA synthesis in the tumor cell is responsible for cell proliferation of some tumors. Various carcinogens (cancer-causing agents) may initiate the increased rate of DNA synthesis. Tumors, either benign or malignant, have some characteristics that are taken advantage of in radionuclide imaging. For example, tumors have increased metabolic activity and blood flow, high vascular permeability, pinocytosis of proteins, and tumor-associated antigen. With a proper choice of radiopharmaceuticals suitable for evaluating any of these characteristics, tumor imaging can be accomplished. In this approach, tumors are seen as hot spots on the image due to increased localization of the tracer. In other cases, tumors are seen as cold spots or areas of decreased activity on the image. This phenomenon results from the fact that tumor cells do not concentrate the particular radiopharmaceutical, whereas normal cells do.

Numerous tumor-imaging radiopharmaceuticals have been developed and used for clinical trials. Many of them are nonspecific; one agent may be somewhat good for one type of tumor, but of no use for other types. Several radiopharmaceuticals used for specific tumor imaging are summarized in Table 13.8.

^{67}Ga-Citrate

Various tumors, benign or malignant, are detected by scintigraphy using ^{67}Ga-citrate. The biodistribution of this tracer has been described in the section on lung imaging.

Gallium behaves like iron and thus binds to transferrin in the blood to form a gallium-transferrin complex in vivo. The tumor uptake of gallium has been explained by the fact that there are transferrin-specific receptors on tumor cells, which have high affinity for gallium. Transferrin receptors are regulated by the cells to meet the need for iron in DNA synthesis. In highly proliferating tumor cells with rapid DNA synthesis, the surface transferrin receptors are upregulated leading to increased gallium uptake. Chemotherapy, radiotherapy, and excess iron reduce the DNA synthesis and hence a decline in ^{67}Ga uptake. Although the transferrin-receptor theory explains the majority of ^{67}Ga uptake, it has been found that a part of ^{67}Ga uptake in tumor is mediated by a means independent of transferrin receptors, i.e., it occurs in the absence of transferrin.

TABLE 13.8. Radiopharmaceuticals for tumor imaging.

Radiopharmaceutical	Dosage (mCi)	Dosage (MBq)	Type of tumor
^{131}I-sodium iodide	0.1	3.7	Thyroid
^{67}Ga-gallium citrate	10	370	Lymphoma, Hodgkin's disease, various neoplastic diseases
^{111}In-Capromab pendetide (ProstaScint)	5	185	Prostate cancer
^{99m}Tc-Arcitumomab (CEA-scan)	20–30	740–1110	Colorectal cancer
^{111}In-Pentetreotide (OctreoScan)	3–6	111–222	Neuroendocrine tumors (carcinoid, gastroma, etc.)
^{111}In-IbritumomabTiuxetan (Zevalin)	5	185	Non-Hodgkin's lymphoma
^{99m}Tc-Sestamibi (Miraluma)	25–30	925–1110	Breast cancer
^{201}Tl-Thallous chloride	5	185	Brain tumor, thyroid cancer
^{131}I-MIBG	0.5	18.5	Pheochromocytoma, neuroblastoma
^{18}F-FDG	10–15	370–555	Brain tumor, breast cancer, lung tumor, head and neck cancer, esophageal cancer, melanoma, colorectal cancer, lymphoma, thyroid follicular cancer
^{99m}Tc^{5+}-DMSA	10	370	Medullary thyroid carcinoma

Another explanation for ^{67}Ga uptake was made on the basis of the formation of a ^{67}Ga-lactoferrin complex. Increased concentration of lactoferrin has been observed in some tumors (e.g., Hodgkin's disease and Burkitt's lymphoma). The affinity of lactoferrin for gallium is higher than that of transferrin, and therefore increased ^{67}Ga uptake is seen in these tumors.

Approximately 10 mCi (370 MBq) ^{67}Ga-citrate is administered intravenously and planar imaging is performed with a gamma camera using a medium- to high-energy collimator. Three separate windows for 93 keV, 184 keV, and 300 keV photons are preferred to one single broad-energy window for imaging, because the latter admits excessive scatter radiations and degrades image quality. Images are obtained 48 to 72 hr after administration. Although many investigators use planar imaging, SPECT imaging has been used in delineating small and deep-seated tumors.

^{67}Ga is secreted by the large intestine and the appearance of increased activity in the bowel often causes difficulty in identifying the abdominal tumors. For this reason, patients are given laxatives before scanning for effective cleansing of the bowel.

A variety of tumors are detected by ^{67}Ga imaging, among which lymphoma, lung tumor, melanoma, hepatoma, and head and neck tumors are most common. Tumor masses greater than 1 cm are usually well seen by ^{67}Ga scintigraphy. While the sensitivity and specificity of detecting lym-

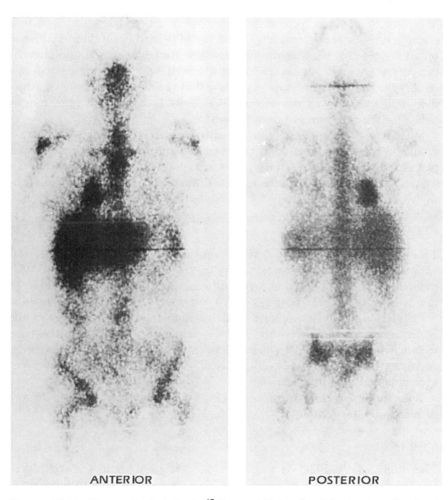

ANTERIOR   POSTERIOR

FIGURE 13.35. Abnormal whole-body ^{67}Ga scan 48 hr after injection showing focal increased uptake in the right lower lobe of the lung due to squamous cell carcinoma.

phoma, melanoma, and hepatoma are good, those of lung tumors are poor except for mediastinal metastatic diseases. A ^{67}Ga scan showing increased uptake in the lower lobe of the right lung due to squamous cell carcinoma is shown in Figure 13.35.

^{99m}Tc-Sestamibi (Miraluma)

^{99m}Tc-sestamibi accumulates nonspecifically in various tumors, among which breast tumors, lung cancer, bone tumors, medullary thyroid cancer (MTC) and brain tumors have been documented. Approximately 15 to 20 mCi (555–740 MBq) ^{99m}Tc-sestamibi is administered intravenously and imaging is performed of the respective organ at different time intervals (5–60 min postinjection for breast, and 20–30 min for MTC and brain tumors). Planar breast images are obtained in prone positions for better spatial resolution of the defects. Special cut-out tables with a lead bridge separating the two breasts are available for imaging the breast in the prone position. The sensitivity and specificity of this test are 84% to 94% and 72% to 94%, respectively, for the detection of breast tumors.

SPECT imaging of brain tumors with ^{99m}Tc-sestamibi shows increased uptake in the tumor relative to the normal tissue. Some uptake in choroid plexus is also seen. Both primary and metastatic lung cancers are detected by this agent, particularly when SPECT imaging is performed. The sensitivity of detecting MTC using ^{99m}Tc-sestamibi is low at about 50%.

^{201}Tl-Thallous Chloride

This tracer has been used to detect brain tumors, bone tumors, MTC, and various other tumors. Approximately 2 to 5 mCi (74–185 MBq) ^{201}Tl-thallous chloride is injected intravenously and imaging is performed 20 to 30 min later using a gamma camera with a low-energy parallel hole collimator.

^{201}Tl scintigraphy is accurate in delineating the different stages of the brain tumor, particularly when SPECT imaging is performed. Also, this technique successfully differentiates between viable tumors versus radiation necrosis, because thallium localizes avidly in viable tumors, but does not accumulate in radiation necrosis.

Bone tumors, breast cancer, and MTC are detected with variable degrees of success by this technique.

^{18}F-FDG

The utility of ^{18}F-FDG in the detection of various tumors is well documented. FDG uptake in tumors is based on enhanced glucose metabolism in malignant tumors compared to normal tissues. Types of tumors and their metastases that have been detected by FDG PET include lungs, head and neck, breast, bladder, thyroid, colon, liver, lymphoma, musculoskeletal, brain tumors and many others.

The physiological handling of ^{18}F-FDG after intravenous administration has been described (see Central Nervous System above). For imaging, approximately 10 to 15 mCi (370–555 MBq) ^{18}F-FDG is administered intravenously, and PET images are obtained 40 to 60 min later. Attenuation corrections are applied by using the rotating ^{68}Ge source.

Since the brain derives its energy solely from glucose metabolism, normal tissues exhibit FDG uptake, with gray matter accumulating more than white matter. In the case of brain tumors, the malignant areas take up more FDG than normal tissues because of the increased glycolysis in tumors. The FDG-PET can differentiate between low grade and high grade tumors due to the difference in the degree of glucose metabolism related to malignancy.

FIGURE 13.36. An FDG-PET image (transverse) of the brain in a patient obtained with 10 mCi (370 MBq) ^{18}F-FDG indicating increased uptake in the glioblastoma tumor (arrow) in the right hemisphere.

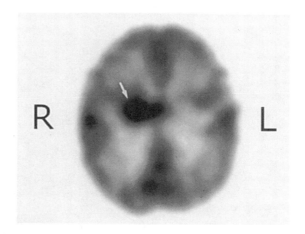

The high-grade tumors show higher FDG uptake than the low-grade tumors. A typical FDG-PET image of a brain tumor is shown in Figure 13.36.

FDG-PET is accurate in the differentiation of recurrent tumors from necrosis after radiotherapy or chemotherapy, since radiation necrosis is detected as hypometabolic areas as opposed to increased uptake of the tracer in tumors. The effects of various therapies of brain tumors can be monitored by FDG-PET so that the progress and prognosis of treatment can be evaluated.

At present, the Centers for Medicare and Medicaid Services (CMS) has approved reimbursement for the ^{18}F-FDG-PET studies of a variety of cancers: lungs, breast, colorectal, head and neck, melanoma, lymphoma, esophageal and recently thyoid follicular cancer. The whole-body images of the patients are obtained using either a PET camera or a coincidence camera 40 to 45 min after injection of 10 to 15 mCi (370–555 MBq) ^{18}F-FDG into the patient. The whole-body images are useful for the detection of metastasis and staging of various cancers. Such studies are also useful for monitoring the response of the treatment of the cancer. A typical example of a whole body image with ^{18}F-FDG-PET is shown in Fig. 13.37.

^{111}In-Pentetreotide

Pentetreotide is a DTPA conjugate of octreotide, a long-acting synthetic analog of natural somatostatin that is present in many tissues of the body. ^{111}In-pentetreotide binds to the somatostatin receptors in various tissues, thus showing an increased uptake.

The plasma clearance of ^{111}In-pentetreotide is initially rapid with 33% of the injected dosage remaining at 10 min postinjection and then slowly declining to 1% at 24 hr postinjection. The biological half-life of ^{111}In-

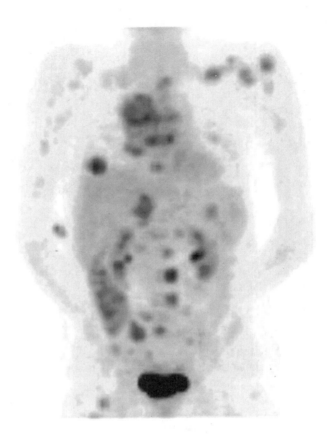

FIGURE 13.37. Whole-body ^{18}F-FDG PET image of a patient showing metastasis in liver, right adrenal, and multiple areas of bone due to primary non–small cell lung carcinoma in right lower lobe and right hilum.

pentetreotide is 6 hr and it is not metabolized in vivo for several hours after administration. It is mostly cleared by the kidneys with 50% excretion in 6 hr and 85% in 24 hr postinjection.

The patient is hydrated and 3 mCi (111 MBq) for planar imaging, or 6 mCi (222 MBq) for SPECT imaging, of ^{111}In-pentetreotide is injected intravenously into the patient. It should not be administered through the total parenteral nutrition (TPN) line, because a complex glycosyl octreotide conjugate may form. Imaging is performed using a gamma camera with a medium-energy parallel hole collimator at 4 and 24 hr after injection.

[111]In-pentetreotide localizes in various primary and metastatic neuro-endocrine tumors bearing somatostatin receptors. Gastrinomas and carcin-

oids are successfully diagnosed by this agent, whereas insulinomas, neuronblastomas, pituitary adenomas, and MTC are detected with limited success. Other tumors that have been successfully detected by this technique include breast cancer, lymphomas, granulomas, and sarcoidosis.

^{99m}Tc-Depreotide (NeoTect)

^{99m}Tc-depreotide is a synthetic peptide that binds with high affinity to somatostatin receptors (SSTRs) in both normal and abnormal tissues. The SSTRs are expressed in various malignancies, but it is approved for the detection of pulmonary masses in patients proven or suspected to have pulmonary lesion by CT and/or chest x-ray. Approximately 15 to 20 mCi (555–740 MBq) is injected intravenously into a patient who has had 8 oz of water. It should not be injected through the TPN line. The plasma disappearance has three components with half-lives: 4.3 min, 43.6 min, and 22.4 hr. The urinary excretion is about 12% in normal subjects.

SPECT imaging is performed by using a gamma camera with a low-energy parallel hole collimator at 2 hr postinjection. Increased uptake of the tracer is seen in areas of high concentration of SSTRs. It is useful for detecting pulmonary lesions complementary to the CT or chest x-ray findings. The sensitivity and specificity are about 70% and 80%, respectively.

Radiolabeled Antibody

Because monoclonal antibody binds to antigen, the former has been used in the radiolabeled form to detect the latter in tumors. Approximately 2 to 5 mCi (74–185 MBq) ^{111}In-labeled Mab, 0.5 to 1 mCi (18.5–37 MBq) ^{131}I-labeled Mab, or 5 to 10 mCi (185–370 MBq) ^{99m}Tc-labeled Mab is administered intravenously to patients suspected of having tumors against which the antibody is produced. The blood clearance is usually slow and the liver uptake is prominent. Tumor uptake of the antibody is normally low with an average value of 0.005% per gram. Planar or SPECT imaging of the whole body is performed at 24, 48, 72, and sometimes 120 to 144 hr after injection in the case of ^{111}In- or ^{131}I-labeled antibodies. Increased uptake of the tumor is seen at the tumor sites and depends on the specificity and concentration of the Mab.

Tumor uptake of antibody is limited by a number of factors: blood flow, vascular volume, diffusion of the antibody through the capillaries, the size of the antibody, and loss of immunoreactivity. If the tumor is more vascular and less necrotic, there will be more blood flow, and hence more antibody uptake. On the other hand, antibodies are large molecules, and hence the diffusion through the capillaries is limited. Smaller fragments Fab' and F(ab')$_2$ have been used to increase the tumor uptake, but their absolute uptake is still low due to rapid blood clearance of these fragments, although the tumor-to-background ratios improve considerably. Loss of immunoreactivity during labeling may compromise the tumor uptake of the antibodies.

A difficulty with the use of murine antibodies is human antimurine antibody (HAMA) response after their administration to humans. The severity of the HAMA response depends on the quantity of murine antibodies administered in one or more injections and the immune condition of the subject. Chimeric antibodies produced by the recombinant methods are less immunogenic and more useful than the murine types.

In vivo deiodination of radioiodinated Mab raises the blood pool background and thus makes at times the image interpretation difficult. Newer techniques of iodination using organometallic agents that give more in vivo stable iodinated compounds have been introduced. ^{111}In-labeled Mab accumulates largely in the liver, and tumor detection by imaging in the vicinity of the liver becomes difficult. Some investigators explained, but others disproved, that ^{111}In-labeled Mab breaks down in vivo and ^{111}In then localizes as colloid in the liver. Using GYK-DTPA, SCN-Bz-DTPA, or DOTA as the bifunctional chelator, the stability of ^{111}In-labeled Mab and hence success in tumor imaging with it have considerably improved. The use of ^{99m}Tc-labeled Mab significantly reduces the radiation dose to the patient, compared to ^{131}I- or ^{111}In-labeled antibody. Also, the Fab$'$ fragments of the antibody are used to reduce the radiation dose to the patient and to improve the target-to-background ratio in scintigraphic imaging.

Numerous antibodies have been developed against various tumors, labeled with radionuclides, and finally used for the detection of tumors. Several Mabs have been approved by the FDA for clinical use and they are described briefly below.

^{111}In-Capromab Pendetide (ProstaScint)

This tracer is used for the detection of prostate cancer. Approximately 5 mCi (185 MBq) is injected intravenously and planar or SPECT images are obtained using a gamma camera equipped with a medium-energy parallel hole collimator at 72 to 120 hr after injection. A cleansing enema is recommended 1 hr before imaging to clear the abdominal background. The plasma clearance half-time is 67 hr and the urinary excretion is about 10% in 72 hr. It primarily localizes in the liver, spleen, and bone marrow.

Prostate cancer and metastasis are detected by this agent with reasonable accuracy. A scintigraphic image obtained with ProstaScint is shown in Fig. 13.38.

^{99m}Tc-Arcitumomab (CEA-Scan)

This agent is the ^{99m}Tc-labeled Fab$'$ fragment of a Mab against carcinoembryonic antigen (CEA), which is expressed in various tumors, particularly colorectal cancer. After intravenous administration, it is cleared from the blood biexponentially with half-times of 1 hr and 13 hr. Approximately 28% of the dosage is excreted in the urine over 24 hr after administration.

FIGURE 13.38. A planar image obtained with ^{111}In-capromab pendetide (ProstaScint) indicating metastatic sites (arrows) due to prostate cancer in a patient.

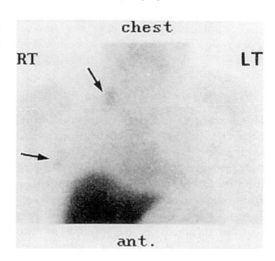

Approximately 20 to 30 mCi (740–1110 MBq) is administered intravenously to the patient and planar or SPECT images of the abdomen and pelvis are obtained using a gamma camera with a low-energy parallel hole collimator at 2 to 5 hr postinjection. The agent is good for detecting colorectal cancer and its metastatic sites.

[111]In-Ibritumomab Tiuxetan (Zevalin)

The majority of non-Hodgkin's lymphomas (NHLs) are of B-cell origin due to their abnormal growth. Ibritumomab tiuxetan and its chimeric analog rituximab are antibodies against CD20 antigen, expressed on normal B cells and most malignant B-cell lymphomas, and therefore bind to the CD20 antigen and lyse the lymphoid B-cells. ^{111}In-ibritumomab tiuxetan is used as an imaging agent prior to therapy of NHL patients with ^{90}Y-ibritumomab tiuxetan in order to predict the biodistribution of the therapeutic dosage.

Approximately 5 mCi (185 MBq) ^{111}In-ibritumomab tiuxetan is administered intravenously over a 10-min period immediately following the infusion of 250 mg/m^2 rituximab. The effective blood half-life of ^{111}In-ibritumomab tiuxetun is 27 hr and urinary excretion is 7.3% and 3.2% over 7 days. The whole-body images are obtained at 2 to 24 hr and 48 to 72 hr, and, if needed, at 90 to 120 hr postinjection. The normal biodistribution of the tracer is demonstrated by blood pool activity on the 24-hr image with high uptake in the normal liver and spleen; low uptake in the kidneys, bladder, and bowel throughout the imaging period; and increased uptake in tumor tissues. Altered biodistribution is indicated by increased lung uptake relative to the blood pool and liver, and greater renal and bowel uptake than the liver uptake. If ^{111}In imaging shows altered rather than normal pattern of distribution, the patient does not receive the ^{90}Y-ibritumomab tiuxetan therapy.

Thrombus Detection

Hundreds of thousands of people die annually from complications of thrombosis and embolism such as heart attack, stroke, and pulmonary embolism. Whereas heart attacks and strokes are caused by arterial thrombus, pulmonary embolisms are caused by venous clots, particularly those originating from the lower extremity veins. Many other complications related to peripheral vascular diseases result from atherosclerosis and thrombosis.

A thrombus is formed in two stages. First, prothrombin reacts with Ca^{2+} to form thrombin in the presence of thromboplastin. Second, fibrinogen reacts with thrombin to form a fibrin monomer, which in turn polymerizes to form a fibrin clot. Thromboplastin is produced from platelets or damaged tissue by the action of a number of factors in the blood.

Pulmonary embolism results mainly from the release of thrombi originating in the deep veins of lower extremities, such as the iliac and femoral veins. Such thrombus formation is highly probable in postoperative patients. Therefore, early detection of actively forming deep-vein thrombi is very important in these patients.

In earlier periods, ^{125}I-labeled fibrinogen was used to detect deep vein thrombus (DVT) in lower extremities, but it is no longer used because it is not commercially available. Since platelets are involved in thrombus formation, ^{111}In-labeled platelets have been used successfully to detect actively forming thrombi. The labeling technique has been described in Chapter 7. Approximately 2 to 4 mCi (74–148 MBq) is injected intravenously into the patient and imaging is performed at 24, 48, and 72 hr after injection using a gamma camera. Increased uptake is seen at the sites of actively forming thrombi.

Other agents such as ^{111}In-, ^{99m}Tc-, or ^{131}I-labeled antifibrin antibody, streptokinase, and urokinase have been employed for detecting clots, but success in imaging is limited for various technical reasons. Recently, ^{99m}Tc-labeled peptides such as P280 and P748, which bind to GPIIb/IIIa receptors in the actively forming thrombi, have been used for the detection of these thrombi, and ^{99m}Tc-apcitide is one of them.

^{99m}Tc-Apcitide (AcuTect)

^{99m}Tc-apcitide is a radiolabeled synthetic peptide that binds to the GP IIb/IIIa adhesion-molecule receptors found on activated platelets. It is therefore used to detect various actively forming thrombi in patients.

Following intravenous administration, the radioactivity of ^{99m}Tc-apcitide clears from the blood in normal subjects biexponentially with a mean $t_{1/2}$ of about 2.5 hr. The mean protein binding in patients is about 75.8% at 30 min postinjection. The urinary excretion is about 60% at 1 hr after injection.

Approximately 20 mCi (740 MBq) ^{99m}Tc-apcitide is administered to patients suspected of lower extremity deep vein thrombosis, intravenously in an upper extremity. Imaging is performed 10 to 60 min after injection using a gamma camera with a low-energy parallel hole collimator. At times, delayed images may be needed at 4 to 6 hr post injection for better contrast. Positive uptake in the thrombi is indicated by the asymmetric localization of the tracer on contrast-enhanced images and in both anterior and posterior projections.

Lymphoscintigraphy

The lymphatic vessels are thin-walled channels lined by endothelium and containing numerous valves preventing backflow of lymph. Lymph is similar to plasma in composition and unlike blood, it flows slowly. The lymphatic system produces lymphocytes and monocytes, destroys aged red blood cells, and transfers a large portion of the fat absorbed in the intestine to the bloodstream. The lymphatic capillaries unite to form lymphatic ducts, which convey the lymph to lymph nodes. Other lymphatic ducts convey lymph from the nodes to the main lymphatic vessels and the thoracic duct, which then discharge it into the subclavian vein. The flow of lymph is caused by contraction of skeletal muscles, respiratory movement, heart beats, and intestinal movement.

Lymph nodes are usually small structures about 1 cm in diameter. They are usually situated at the proximal ends of the limbs and in the neck, groin, abdomen, and thorax. Lymph nodes provide protection against bacterial infection by phagocytic digestion of bacteria in the lymphatic vessels. A severely infected lymph node becomes swollen and tender.

The lymphatic system provides the paths for the spread (metastasis) of cancer from one part of the body to another. Hodgkin's disease, lymphocytic leukemia, various metastatic diseases, and many lymph node disorders can be assessed by lymphoscintigraphy. Lymph node pathology is demonstrated by diminished or absent flow of lymph.

The most common radiopharmaceuticals used for lymphoscintigraphy are ^{99m}Tc-SC, ^{99m}Tc-antimony sulfide colloid, and ^{99m}Tc-albumin colloid (nanocolloid). The latter two are preferable because of their smaller particle size, but they are not available commercially in U.S. However, filtered ^{99m}Tc-SC, as described in Chapter 7, provides optimal particle size for reasonable lymphoscintigraphy. The usual dosage for administration is about 450 μCi (16.7 MBq) filtered ^{99m}Tc-SC divided into one to four injections in small volume. Some investigators use a higher dosage of 1 to 2 mCi (37–74 MBq). Injections are given subcutaneously around the tumor site followed by gentle massage around the area. The colloid drains out rapidly from the injection site, however, depending on the particle size, injection site, and pathophysiologic conditions. Small particles are drained to the extent of about 40% to 60%, whereas the larger particles are retained at the injection site. The lymph node activity reaches a plateau in 2 hr after injection. Approximately 3% of the injected activity is retained in all visualized nodes.

Imaging is performed with a gamma camera using a low-energy parallel hole collimator, and time for imaging is site-specific. Images are obtained immediately after injection for melanoma and at 30 to 40 min later in case of breast lymphoscintigraphy. Some investigators wait for 4 to 24 hr before breast imaging.

Normal lymphoscintigraphy demonstrates the normal nodes in inguinal, iliac, and periaortic regions, several lymph nodes in the parasternal regions, and other lymph nodes depending on the site of injection. Sentinel nodes are easily seen by this technique. At times, the liver is also seen due to lymphatic blockage or poor injection. Discontinuity in the drainage may result from metastasis; increased activity in an area may be due to lymphoma, or blockage of the lymphatics. In case of melanoma, delineation of specific sites of lymphatic drainage by lymphoscintigraphy leads to decision on the surgical removal of the involved regional lymph nodes. In breast lympho-scintigraphy, poor uptake in lymph nodes and absent distant lymphatic filling may indicate intranodal tumor in the breasts.

Gastric Emptying Imaging

Abnormal rates of gastric emptying are associated with many disease states, and their determination offers useful information in assessing these diseases. Radionuclidic techniques have been successfully employed in determining the gastric emptying half-time.

Various kinds of ^{99m}Tc-labeled meals in solid or liquid form have been used to measure the gastric emptying time. In one solid meal, approximately 1 mCi (37 MBq) ^{99m}Tc-SC is mixed with a bowl of oatmeal. In another type of solid meal, the same amount is cooked with scrambled eggs and given as a sandwich with bread to the patient. In a liquid type of meal, 1 mCi (37 MBq) ^{99m}Tc-DTPA or 0.5 mCi (18.5 MBq) ^{111}In-DTPA in 300 ml water solution is commonly used for drinking.

The patient is allowed after 6 hr of fasting to take any of the above meals. In the case of solid meals, the patient is asked to drink additional 8 ounces of milk or orange juice. For dual isotope liquid-solid gastric emptying studies, liquid meal with ^{111}In-DTPA and solid meal with ^{99m}Tc-SC are given to the patient simultaneously. The patient's stomach is imaged at 5 and 10 min after administration using a gamma camera with an appropriate collimator and using appropriate windows for respective photon energies, and then every 5 to 15 min until the stomach activity reaches half its original activity. In each image, about 50,000 counts are obtained. Assuming the initial image activity in the stomach is 100%, the activity in each subsequent image can be expressed as a percentage of the original stomach activity. From a plot of percent activity versus time, the gastric emptying half-time can be determined. The normal values are 50 to 80 min for solid meals and 10 to 15 min for liquid meals. Delayed emptying time is found in gastric ulcers, pyloric stenosis, vagotomy, and malignancies.

Meckel's Diverticulum Imaging

Approximately 2% of the population has Meckel's diverticulum, and symptomatic Meckel's diverticulum (i.e., rectal bleeding) is found in one fourth of this population, who are primarily young. Ectopic gastric mucosa lines the symptomatic diverticuli, and the latter are usually imaged with ^{99m}Tc-pertechnetate, which is concentrated by the gastric mucosa.

Approximately 10 to 15 mCi (370–555 MBq) ^{99m}Tc-pertechnetate is injected intravenously into a patient who has received 300 mg of cimetidine orally every 6 hr for 1 day, or 6 μg/kg pentagastrin 15 min before the injection. Cimetidine inhibits acid secretion and thus prevents ^{99m}Tc activity from the gastric mucosa into gastric contents. This decreases the background activity. Pentagastrin stimulates pertechnetate accumulation in gastric mucosa. Imaging is performed with a scintillation camera fitted with a low-energy parallel hole collimator immediately and every 10 min for 1 hr after administration. Sometimes, lateral and delayed views are obtained in equivocal situations. A persistent focal activity on the images indicates Meckel's diverticulum.

Gastrointestinal Bleeding Detection

Gastrointestinal (GI) bleeding is a common clinical problem. Upper GI bleeding mostly results from esophageal varices, peptic ulcers, hemorrhagic gastric ulcers, neoplasms, and drug-induced gastric erosions. Lower GI bleeding may be caused by diverticular diseases, inflammatory bowel diseases, or neoplasms.

The success rate of detection of GI bleeding by endoscopic and other clinical methods is limited. The scintigraphic technique has gained considerable success in the detection and localization of GI bleeding. The most commonly used radiopharmaceuticals are ^{99m}Tc-SC and ^{99m}Tc-RBCs. After injection, a fraction of the activity from the circulation extravasates at the bleeding site.

Ten mCi (370 MBq) ^{99m}Tc-SC is injected intravenously and the patient's upper and lower GI tracts are imaged with a gamma camera fitted with a low-energy parallel hole collimator at 2-min intervals for 20 min. If a bleeding site is seen, more images are taken to localize definitely the site of bleeding. Sometimes delayed images are necessary to obtain an accurate diagnosis. At times, the liver and spleen activity may blur the bleeding sites in the surrounding areas. Because of the rapid clearance of ^{99m}Tc-SC from the circulation, the background is minimal and the sites with bleeding rates as low as 0.05 to 0.1 ml/min can be detected by ^{99m}Tc-SC.

Most GI hemorrhages are intermittent and may be missed with ^{99m}Tc-SC because of the rapid clearance of the colloid. Several investigators argue that it is preferable to use a tracer that remains in the intravascular space for a longer period for the localization of the bleeding site. The ^{99m}Tc-RBCs labeled by the in vitro technique or by the modified in vivo technique (Chapter 7) are considered to be the agents of choice for GI bleeding imaging.

Approximately 20 mCi (740 MBq) ^{99m}Tc-RBC is administered intravenously and the abdomen is imaged by a scintillation camera using a low-energy parallel hole collimator. Images are taken, one immediately and then every 15 min for about 1 hr. Images are repeated at intervals of several hours up to 24 hr if the bleeding site is not detected by the first hour. Images are considered positive when a focus of activity is noticed. Detection of bleeding sites with ^{99m}Tc-RBC is possible when the bleeding rate exceeds 6 to 12 ml/min.

Inflammatory Diseases and Infection Imaging

Inflammatory diseases and infections such as sepsis and abdominal abscesses form a group of diseases that need early detection for patient management. Most inflammatory diseases result from a response to infections, although conditions such as arthritis and synovitis also involve inflammatory processes without the presence of infections. Most of these conditions are detected by the use of ^{67}Ga-citrate, ^{99m}Tc-leukocytes, or ^{111}In-leukocytes. The techniques of labeling of leukocytes with ^{99m}Tc and ^{111}In have been described in Chapter 7.

^{67}Ga-citrate

Gallium uptake by inflammatory diseases is explained by the formation of complexes between ^{67}Ga and lactoferrin which is released by leukocytes, and between ^{67}Ga and siderophores. Leukocytes are attracted to infected areas in large concentrations and release lactoferrin in response to stimulation by infection. Also present in infections is a group of compounds called siderophores produced by bacteria in infections that avidly bind to gallium.

Approximately 5 to 10 mCi (185–370 MBq) ^{67}Ga-citrate is injected intravenously and imaging is performed initially 24 hr postinjection and, if necessary, later using a gamma camera with a medium-energy collimator. Gallium scan is useful in the detection of abscess, cellulitis, and peritonitis. This test is highly sensitive in the detection of osteomyelitis. Other indications for ^{67}Ga scanning include various lung diseases associated with inflammatory process such as asbestosis, toxicity due to chemotherapy, bacterial nephritis, and *Pneumocystis carinii pneumonia* in AIDS patients.

^{111}In- or ^{99m}Tc-Leukocytes

Leukocytes are a mixed population of polymorphonuclear granulocytes (neutrophils), lymphocytes, and monocytes, and they defend the body against infection. Neutrophils are attracted to the infected area by chemotaxis and kill microorganisms by phagocytosis. Lymphocytes and monocytes are primarily responsible for defense against infection by immune reactions. Based on these functional attributes of leukocytes, ^{111}In- or ^{99m}Tc-leukocytes are found useful in the detection of infections in patients.

Approximately 0.5 mCi (18.5 MBq) ^{111}In-leukocytes containing about 10^8 leukocytes is injected intravenously, and imaging of the whole body or the region of interest is performed 18 to 24 hr after injection using a scintillation camera with a medium-energy collimator. At times, delayed images at 48 hr are obtained for better resolution of images. The plasma disappearance half-time of the tracer is of the order of 6 to 7 hr. Approximately 50% of the cells accumulate in the liver, $\sim$11% in the spleen, and $\sim$8% in the lungs.

In the case of ^{99m}Tc-leukocytes, 8 to 10 mCi (296–370 MBq) is injected intravenously and images are obtained 1 to 4 hr later using a gamma camera with a low-energy parallel hole collimator. The biodistribution of this tracer is similar to that of ^{111}In-leukocytes.

^{99m}Tc-sulesomab, the Fab' fragment of anti–NCA-90 antibody which is an anti-granulocyte antibody, is used as an in vivo granulocyte labeling agent for imaging inflammation and infection. It is approved for clinical use in European countries but not in the U.S. Approximately 10 to 15 mCi (370–555 MBq) is injected intravenously, and images are obtained at 1 to 4 hr later using a gamma camera with a low-energy parallel hole collimator. The blood clearance $t_{1/2}$ of ^{99m}Tc-sulesomab is about 23 min. Infection or inflammation is seen on the images as increased uptake of the tracer. It is interesting to note that localization in inflammation or infection does not occur by binding to circulating granulocytes. It diffuses into the affected area nonspecifically via increased vascular permeability and then binds to only activated granulocytes in inflammation or infection (Skehan et al, 2003).

Various infectious diseases are well detected by labeled leukocyte imaging. It is particularly useful in fever of unknown origin where the infected area is clinically unidentified. Osteomyelitis is correctly identified by this technique. ^{111}In-leukocyte imaging is preferred to ^{99m}Tc-leukocyte imaging in abdominal abscess areas. This is primarily because of the partial breakdown of the ^{99m}Tc-leukocytes that leads to increased ^{99m}Tc background in the abdominal areas. However, early imaging with ^{99m}Tc-leukocytes helps to detect inflammatory bowel disease better than ^{111}In-leukocytes, because of the avid accumulation of the tracer in the diseased area and less background. On the other hand, leukocyte accumulation in intraabdominal sepsis is low, and in this situation ^{111}In-leukocyte imaging is preferable. Bacterial endocarditis, rejection of vascular grafts, and various lung infections have been successfully documented by this technique. A typical ^{111}In-

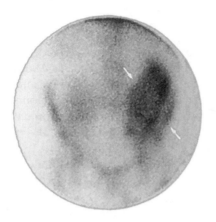

FIGURE 13.39. A 24-hr anterior ^{111}In-leukocyte image of an abscess in the left abdomen (arrows). Pelvic uptake is normal.

leukocyte image of an abscess in the pelvic area of a patient is shown in Figure 13.39.

Parathyroid Imaging

There are normally four parathyroid glands (two upper and two lower) situated on the posterolateral sides of the two thyroid glands. These glands secrete parathyroid hormone (PTH), which regulates and maintains normal serum calcium level (9–11 mg/dl) by its action on bone, the small intestine, and the kidneys. Overfunctioning of the parathyroid glands leads to hyperparathyroidism manifested by higher serum calcium level (hypercalcemia), whereas underfunctioning of the glands results in hypoparathyroidism indicated by low serum calcium level. Various disease entities such as hyperplasia, adenoma, parathyroid carcinoma, and multiple gland diseases can cause hyperparathyroidism in patients.

Several imaging protocols are in use for the diagnosis of abnormal parathyroid. In most cases, a dual-isotope technique is employed based on the principle of delineating the parathyroid from the thyroid using the two different tracers for the two types of glands. Combinations such as $^{99m}TcO_4^-/^{201}Tl$, $^{123}I/^{201}Tl$ and $^{123}I/^{99m}Tc$-sestamibi are used as the dual isotopes. Inherent in these techniques is the fact that $^{123}I^-$ or $^{99m}TcO_4^-$ localizes in the thyroid, whereas ^{201}Tl or ^{99m}Tc-sestamibi localizes in both the thyroid and parathyroid glands. Thus by subtracting the image of ^{123}I or $^{99m}TcO_4^-$ from the image of ^{201}Tl or ^{99m}Tc-sestamibi after normalization with respect to maximum ^{123}I or $^{99m}TcO_4^-$ counts, one obtains a true image of the parathyroid glands.

In practice, 300 μCi (11.1 MBq) ^{123}I-NaI orally or 2 mCi (74 MBq) $^{99m}TcO_4^-$ intravenously is administered to the patient followed by planar imaging of the glands 4-hr postinjection with a gamma camera equipped with a pinhole collimator. The patient is then injected with 2 mCi (74 MBq)

^{201}Tl and imaged again 15-min postinjection. This procedure can be reversed with ^{201}Tl first and ^{123}I or ^{99m}TcO$_4^-$ next. SPECT imaging may be performed with a scintillation camera using a low-energy all-purpose parallel hole collimator. In the alternative protocol, 25 to 30 mCi (925–1110 MBq) ^{99m}Tc-sestamibi is substituted for ^{201}Tl. Some investigators use simultaneous imaging by setting two separate windows for the two isotopes. After image processing, either separately or simultaneously, the data on the ^{201}Tl or ^{99m}Tc-sestamibi image are normalized with respect to maximum counts on the ^{123}I or ^{99m}TcO$_4^-$ image, and the latter image is subtracted from the former. The net image gives the details of the parathyroid uptake of the tracer, which in turn indicates the presence or absence of abnormal parathyroid.

In another technique, a single dosage of 10 to 20 mCi (370–740 MBq) ^{99m}Tc-sestamibi is injected and the patient's parathyroid is first imaged 10 to 15 min postinjection and then 2 to 3 hr later. The early image shows anatomy in and around the thyroid and the delayed image shows increased uptake in pathologically enlarged parathyroid glands with minimal uptake in the thyroid. Because of the easy methodology, this technique has gained wide acceptance.

Questions

1. What are the radiopharmaceuticals commonly used in brain imaging? What is the mechanism of localization of these tracers? Do you expect an increased or decreased uptake of radioactivity in the normal and abnormal brain?
2. What are the primary uses of ^{18}F-FDG in brain imaging?
3. In bone and brain imaging, 10 to 15 mCi (370–555 MBq) ^{99m}Tc-labeled compounds are injected, whereas in liver imaging, only 2 to 4 mCi (74–148 MBq) are injected. Why?
4. Elucidate the mechanism of synthesis of thyroid hormones (T3 and T4) in the thyroid.
5. In a 24-hr iodine uptake test, the thyroid count is 34,500 cpm and the thigh count is 3020 cpm. The thyroid phantom count is 90,500 cpm and the room background count is 200 cpm. Calculate the 24-hr uptake value. Is it euthyroid, hypothyroid, or hyperthyroid?
6. Name various drugs that affect the thyroid uptake of ^{131}I.
7. What is the mechanism of localization of ^{99m}Tc-MAA in lung imaging? How many particles are usually administered per dosage to the patient and what fraction of the pulmonary capillaries is occluded by these particles?
8. A physician requests a lung scan for a patient suspected of pulmonary embolism. As a nuclear pharmacist, which radiopharmaceutical would you prepare and how much would you dispense? When is a ^{133}Xe ventilation study indicated?

9. When is the use of ^{99m}Tc-mebrofenin and ^{99m}Tc-sulfur colloid indicated in liver imaging? What are the plasma disappearance half-times of these two tracers? How much would you inject of each tracer?

10. What are the radiopharmaceuticals that are used for hepatobiliary imaging? How does bilirubin level affect the hepatic uptake of ^{99m}Tc-IDA derivatives?

11. Describe the method of cholescintigraphy. When is the gallbladder seen in a normal patient?

12. What is the effect of CCK or morphine on cholescintigraphy?

13. Make a table of all radiopharmaceuticals used in renal studies, including information such as the quantity of the tracer, the plasma clearance half-time, urinary excretion, optimum time to begin imaging after injection, and clinical information obtained.

14. Discuss the three phases of a renogram in the normal and abnormal states of the kidneys.

15. In glomerular filtration rate measurement by the constant infusion method, the plasma concentration and urinary concentration of ^{111}In-DTPA are 1200 cpm/ml and 15,600 cpm/ml, respectively. The urine flow rate is 9 ml/min. Calculate the glomerular filtration rate.

16. What are the different ^{99m}Tc-phosphonate compounds used in bone scintigraphy? Explain the mechanism of bone uptake of ^{99m}Tc-phosphonate compounds. Why do you have to wait 2 to 3 hr after injection before imaging? Explain the differences in plasma clearance and urinary excretion of different ^{99m}Tc-phosphonate compounds.

17. In myocardial infarct imaging with ^{99m}Tc-pyrophosphate, how soon after the onset of infarction is the infarct site seen on the image? When does the maximum uptake in the myocardial infarct occur? How soon after injection can this imaging begin?

18. In myocardial imaging, how is the infarct seen on the image with ^{99m}Tc-pyrophosphate and ^{201}Tl-thallous chloride—as increased or decreased activity in the infarct? Explain the observations.

19. Compare the biological properties of ^{201}Tl, ^{99m}Tc-sestamibi, and ^{99m}Tc-tetrofosmin.

20. What are the salient features of difference between ^{201}Tl SPECT and ^{82}Rb PET imaging?

21. How does glucose loading help ^{18}F-FDG uptake in the myocardium? Spell out the mechanism of myocardial uptake of ^{18}F-FDG.

22. What are the agents used for the gated equilibrium blood pool study of the heart? Describe the measurement of the ejection fraction of the left ventricle by this method. What is the normal value of the ejection fraction? What is the role of stress ventriculography?

23. What are the different agents of choice for tumor imaging? What is the mechanism of localization of gallium in tumor?

24. What is the common radiopharmaceutical for lymphoscintigraphy? What are the common diseases that can be diagnosed by lymphoscintigraphy?

25. What are the different radiopharmaceuticals used for (a) gastric emptying, (b) Meckel's diverticulum, (c) gastrointestinal bleeding, and (d) inflammatory diseases?
26. When is captopril renography indicated and how is it performed?
27. What is the rationale for the use of ^{123}I-MIBG in myocardial imaging?
28. Describe the different radiopharmaceuticals employed for adrenal imaging.
29. Describe the role of radiolabeled antibodies in tumor imaging. Elucidate the different FDA approved antibodies for various tumor imaging.
30. Discuss the relative importance of ^{99m}Tc-sestamibi, ^{201}Tl, and ^{18}F-FDG in tumor imaging. Which one is the best tracer in delineating tumors from radiation necrosis?
31. What are the types of tumors that are imaged with ^{111}In-pentetreotide?
32. Describe the methods of imaging parathyroids with different radiopharmaceuticals.
33. Why is ^{99m}Tc-RBC preferred to ^{99m}Tc-SC in GI bleeding scintigraphy?

References and Suggested Reading

Anthony CP, Thibodeau GA. *Textbook of Anatomy and Physiology*. St. Louis: Mosby; 1979.

Arnold RW, Subramanian G, McAfee JG, et al. Comparison of ^{99m}Tc complexes for renal imaging. *J Nucl Med*. 1975; 16:357.

Atkins HL, Budinger TF, Lebowitz E, et al. Thallium-201 for medical use. Part 3: Human distribution and physical imaging properties. *J Nucl Med*. 1977; 18:133.

Barrio JR, Huang SC, Melega WP, et al. 6-[^{18}F]fluoro-L-dopa probes dopamine turnover rates in central dopaminergic structures. *J Neurosci Res*. 1990; 27:487.

Berman DS, Kiat HS, Van Train KF, et al. Myocardial perfusion imaging with technetium-99m-sestamibi: comparative analysis of imaging protocols. *J Nucl Med*. 1994; 35:681.

Delbeke D, Martin WH, Patton JA, et al., eds. *Practical FDG Imaging. A Teaching File*. New York: Springer Verlag; 2002.

Dienel GA, Cruz NF, Sokoloff F. Metabolites of 2-deoxy-[^{14}C]-glucose in plasma and brain: influence on rate of glucose utilization determined with deoxyglucose method in rat brain. *J Cereb Blood Flow Metab*. 1993; 13:315.

Dilsizian V, Rocco TP, Freedman NMT, et al. Enhanced detection of ischemic but viable myocardium by the reinjection of thallium and stress-redistribution imaging. *N Engl J Med*. 1990; 323:141.

Early PJ, Sodee DB, eds. *Principles and Practice of Nuclear Medicine*. 2nd ed. St. Louis: Mosby; 1995.

Freeman LM, ed. *Freeman and Johnson's Clinical Radionuclide Imaging*. 3rd ed. New York: Grune & Stratton; 1984.

Gould KL, Yoshida K, Hess MJ, et al. Myocardial metabolism of fluorodeoxyglucose compared to cell membrane integrity for the potassium analogue rubidium-82 for assessing infarct size in man by PET. *J Nucl Med*. 1991; 32:1.

Harbert J, Eckelman WC, Neumann RD, eds. *Nuclear Medicine: Diagnosis and Therapy*. New York: Thieme Medical; 1996.

Hauser W, Atkins HL, Nelson KG, et al. Technetium-99m-DTPA: a new radio-pharmaceutical for brain and kidney imaging. *Radiology*. 1970; 94:679.

Henkin RE, Boles MA, Dillehay GL, et al., eds. *Nuclear Medicine*. St Louis: Mosby; 1996.

Higley B, Smith FW, Smith T, et al. Technetium-99m-1,2-bis[bis(2-ethoxyethyl)-phosphino]ethane: human biodistribution, dosimetry and safety of a new myocardial perfusion imaging agent. *J Nucl Med*. 1993; 34:30.

Johnson LL, Seldin DW. Clinical experience with technetium-99m teboroxime, a neutral, lipophilic myocardial perfusion imaging agent. *Am J Cardiol*. 1990; 66: 63E.

Kiat H, Berman DS, Maddahi J, et al. Late reversibility of tomographic myocardial Tl-201 defects: an accurate marker of myocardial viability. *J Am Coll Cardiol*. 1988; 12(6):1456.

Kuhl DE, Barrio JR, Huang SC, et al. Quantifying local cerebral blood flow by N-isopropyl-p-^{123}I-iodoamphetamine (IMP) tomography. *J Nucl Med*. 1982; 236:196.

Leveille J, Demonceau G, DeRoo M, et al. Characterization of technetium-99m-L,L-ECD for brain perfusion imaging, Part 2: Biodistribution and brain imaging in humans. *J Nucl Med*. 1989; 30:1902.

Maisey MN, Britton KE, Collier BD. *Clinical Nuclear Medicine*. 3rd ed. London: Chapman & Hall; 1998.

McAfee JG, Grossman ZD, Gagne G, et al. Comparison of renal extraction efficiencies for radioactive agents in the normal dog. *J Nucl Med*. 1981; 22:333.

Mejia AA, Nakamura T, Masatoshi I, et al. Estimation of absorbed dose in humans due to intravenous administration of fluorine-18-fluorodeoxyglucose in PET studies. *J Nucl Med*. 1991; 32:699.

Mettler FA Jr, Guiberteau MJ. *Essentials of Nuclear Medicine Imaging*. 4th ed. Philadelphia: Saunders; 1998.

Murray IPC, Ell PJ. *Nuclear Medicine in Clinical Diagnosis and Treatment*. 2nd ed. Edinburgh: Churchill Livingstone; 1998.

Narra RK, Nunn AD, Kuczynski, et al. A neutral technetium-99m complex for myocardial imaging. *J Nucl Med*. 1989; 30:1830.

Phelps ME, Hoffman EJ, Selin C, et al. Investigation of F-18-fluoro-2-deoxyglucose for the measure of myocardial glucose metabolism. *J Nucl Med*. 1978; 19:1311.

Ruhlmann J, Oehr P, Biersack HJ, eds. *PET in Oncology. Basics and Clinical Applications*. Heidelberg: Springer Verlag; 1999.

Saha GB, Go RT, MacIntyre WJ, et al. Use of ^{82}Sr/^{82}Rb generator in clinical PET studies. *Nucl Med Biol*. 1990; 17:763.

Saha GB, MacIntyre WJ, Brunken RC, et al. Present assessment of myocardial viability by nuclear imaging. *Semin Nucl Med*. 1996; 26:315.

Sandler MP, Coleman RE, Walkers FJT, et al., eds. *Diagnostic Nuclear Medicine*. 3rd ed. Baltimore: Williams and Wilkins; 1996.

Sapirstein LA, Vigt DG, Mandel MJ, et al. Volumes of distribution and clearances of intravenously injected creatinine in the dog. *Am J Physiol*. 1955; 181:330.

Schelbert HR, Phelps ME, Huang SC, et al. N-13 ammonia as an indicator of myocardial blood flow. *Circulation*. 1981; 63:1259.

Sharp PF, Smith FW, Gemmell HG, et al. Technetium-99m HMPAO stereoisomers as potential agents for imaging regional cerebral blood flow: human volunteer studies. *J Nucl Med*. 1986; 27:171.

Sisson JC, Shapiro B, Meyers L, et al. Metaiodobenzylguanidine to map scintigraphically the adrenergic nervous system in man. *J Nucl Med*. 1987; 28:1625.

Skehan SJ, White JF, Evans JW, et al. Mechanism of accumulation of ^{99m}Tc-sulesomab in inflammation. *J Nucl Med.* 2003; 44:11.

Subramanian G, McAfee JG, Blair RJ, et al. Technetium 99m methylene diphosphonate—a superior agent for skeletal imaging; comparison with other technetium complexes. *J Nucl Med.* 1975; 16:744.

Taylor A Jr, Eshima D, Christian PE, et al. Technetium-99m kit formulation; preliminary results in normal volunteers and patients with renal failure. *J Nucl Med.* 1988; 29:616.

Taylor A Jr, Eshima D, Fritzberg AR, et al. Comparison of iodine-131 OIH and technetium-99m MAG3 renal imaging in volunteers. *J Nucl Med.* 1986; 27:795.

Vallabhajosula S, Zimmerman RE, Pickard M, et al. Technetium-99m ECD: a new brain imaging agent. In vivo kinetics and biodistribution studies in normal human studies. *J Nucl Med.* 1989; 30:599.

Vanzetto G, Fagret D, Pasqualini R, et al. Biodistribution, dosimetry, and safety of myocardial perfusion imaging agent ^{99m}Tc-N-NOET in healthy volunteers. *J Nucl Med.* 2000; 41:141.

Virkamaki A, Rissanen E, Hamalainen S. Incorporation of [3-sup^{3}H]glucose and 2-[1-sup^{14}C]deoxyglucose into glycogen in heart and skeletal muscle in vivo: Implications for the quantitation of tissue glucose uptake. *Diabetes.* 1997; 46:1106.

Wackers FJT, Berman DS, Maddahi J, et al. Technetium-99m hexakis 2-methoxy-isobutyl isonitrile: human biodistribution, dosimetry, safety and preliminary comparison to thallium-201 for myocardial perfusion imaging. *J Nucl Med.* 1989; 30:301.

Wagner HN, Jr, Szabo Z, Buchanan JW. *Principles of Nuclear Medicine.* 2nd ed. Philadelphia: Saunders; 1995.

Weiner RE. The mechanism of ^{67}Ga localization in malignant disease. *Nucl Med Biol.* 1996; 23:745.

14
Molecular Imaging

Basics of Molecular Imaging

Molecular imaging is an emerging discipline that provides techniques to image specific molecular pathways in various diseases in living species. Such imaging can reveal the causes of diseases and provide clues to their prevention and cure. Although certain imaging modalities can be considered as "molecular" (such as monoclonal antibody, receptors imaging, etc.), only recently has the true design of molecular imaging drawn considerable interest. The current strategy in molecular imaging is to identify a target molecule in a specific organ or its disease state in a living organism, develop a high-affinity probe for the molecule, and ultimately use the probe to detect the distribution and pharmacodynamics of the molecule. Genes composed of deoxyribonucleic acid (DNA) molecules are responsible for many diseases and therefore have been the primary target of investigation in molecular imaging. A brief description of the subject is presented here.

Deoxyribonucleic acid molecules encode genetic information required to sustain life in living organisms. DNA is composed of four nucleotide bases: adenine (A), thymine (T), cytosine (C), and guanine (G). The structure of the DNA molecule is a double helix formed by two complementary strands of base-pair nucleotides (Fig. 14.1A). The base pairs are formed in a very specific manner: adenine pairs with only thymine, and cytosine pairs only with guanine. The base pairs form complexes with deoxyribose sugar bearing 3' hydroxyl groups and 5' phosphate groups in each strand of the DNA helix. The two strands are connected by hydrogen bonds between the bases of each strand.

Somatic cells divide by a process called mitosis in which two exact daughter cells are produced. The daughter cells must have an exact number of chromosomes with the same genes, i.e., identical sequence of bases on the DNA molecules as the parent cell. During a period, called the synthetic (S) phase, prior to mitosis, the DNA molecule must be duplicated. As seen in Fig. 14.1, in the replication process, the double-strand DNA molecule

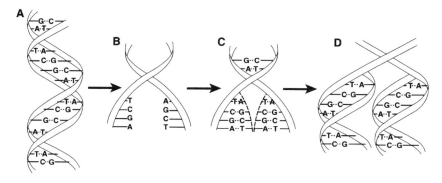

FIGURE 14.1. Replication of a DNA molecule. **A:** DNA molecule before replication. Note the base pairing between A and T, and C and G. **B:** Unwinding and separation of a portion of the DNA molecule resulting in unpaired bases on two strands. **C:** Free available bases in the cell join appropriately with the unpaired bases on each open strand. **D:** New backbones are constructed, producing two complete DNA molecules that are identical to the parent molecule. The replication continues along the DNA chain until the whole molecule is replicated. A, adenine; T, thymine; C, cytosine; G, guanine.

unfolds into two separate strands that act as templates, upon which new complementary strands of DNA are synthesized. Within the cell, there is a "storehouse" of new bases that pair correctly with the bases on the two unfolded strands of the original DNA molecule. Thus, two DNA molecules are produced, which are exact replicas of the parent DNA molecule.

Genes are composed of segments of DNA molecules, and many genes form a thread-like structure called the chromosome. Genes are the basic units of heredity in the cells of all living organisms. A single gene typically consists of several thousand base-pair nucleotides and occupies a fixed position (locus) on the chromosome. There are estimated 20,000 to 30,000 genes consisting of nearly 6 billion nucleotides (or 3 billion base pairs) in the human genome, all packaged into 23 pairs of chromosomes, half of which are derived from each parent. The information encoded within the DNA structure of a gene directs the manufacture of proteins that are essential for life-supporting activities within a cell. Structurally, a gene is arranged into segments of DNA coding sequences called exons, which are separated by noncoding sequences called introns. While the exons carry all genetic codes for making proteins, introns do not have any known genetic information.

When a gene is turned on, a protein is produced with its genetic sequences. The main mechanism of activating a gene is the binding of an inducer protein to a promoter site in the front part of the gene. Normally the gene remains in an activated state, guiding the synthesis of proteins as needed, unless some factor turns it off. Negative feedback is a mechanism to switch off the gene. In this case, the presence of excess protein from a specific gene

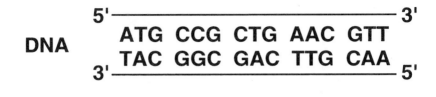

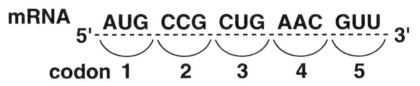

FIGURE 14.2. A genetic message starts with a double-strand DNA molecule that is read in three-letter words called "codons." When a gene is activated, the DNA molecule unfolds and all codons in one of the strands are copied to produce mRNA, which directs the order of amino acid in protein.

can inactivate the gene, while a lesser amount would turn it on, thus maintaining a balanced supply of the desired protein. Another mechanism of gene regulation is external signaling, in which case an extraneous molecule binds to a gene specific protein (e.g., receptors), necessitating its replacement and thus turning on the specific gene.

The genetic message is not read as single letters, but as three-letter words, which are called "codons." When a gene is activated, the two DNA strands unfold and all codons containing the genetic message encoded in one of the strands are first copied to produce ribonucleic acid (RNA) by the enzyme, RNA polymerases, in a process called transcription (Fig. 14.2). The RNA transcript is stabilized by adding a cap of 5-methyl guanine to 5′ end, and a cap of a series of adenines to the 3′ end. This single-strand RNA is complementary to the DNA strand and differs from the DNA molecule by having uracil instead of thymine in its structure. This is called the primary transcript or the pre–messenger RNA (mRNA). The pre-mRNA molecule is released, while the two original strands of DNA recombine to form the original DNA molecule. Since introns are not needed for protein production, they are spliced out of the pre-mRNA molecule to create the so-called messenger RNA (mRNA). The mRNA molecules are typically several hundred to many thousand base-pair long. After the transcription in the nucleus, the mRNA molecule crosses the nuclear membrane and moves into the cytoplasm (Fig. 14.3). The mRNA molecule binds to polyribosome present on endoplasmic reticulum in the cytoplasm and then the translation process takes place to produce proteins. In the translation process, each codon of

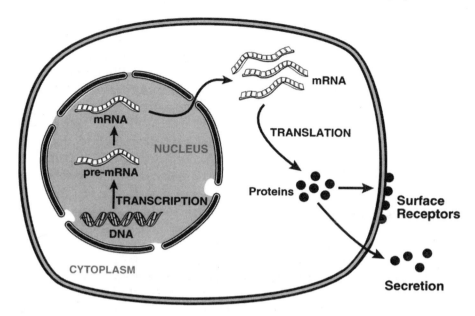

FIGURE 14.3. A schematic pathway of DNA replication to protein formation. A DNA molecule unfolds and one of the two strands is copied to form a pre-mRNA molecule. The nonessential introns are spliced out of pre-mRNA to produce an mRNA molecule, which then directs the synthesis of a protein via a process called translation. The proteins are enzymes, receptors, etc., that either bind to the cell surface or are released in the vascular compartment.

mRNA attracts a specific carrier molecule, called transfer RNA (tRNA), which carries a specific amino acid. On approach to the vicinity of the mRNA molecule, the tRNAs attach the amino acids like beads on a string, one at a time, thus forming a peptide. The translation process is stopped by a stop codon at the end of the RNA molecule. Both mRNA and peptide fall off the polyribosome, followed by rapid degradation of mRNA, and aggregation of many peptides into proteins (Fig. 14.3). There are estimated 115,000 proteins that carry out all essential functions of life inside and outside cells. A typical cell weighs about a nanogram and contains 1 to 5 picogram (pg) of DNA and 10 to 50 pg of total RNA that has 10,000 to 50,000 mRNAs; 2% to 4% of total RNA is mRNA. The RNA/DNA ratio in a cell is about 10.

Alterations in the DNA molecule that predispose to diseases may exist from birth (genetic defects) or may be acquired during the course of life (mutation). The DNA molecule replicates countless times during protein synthesis, and occasional mistakes in DNA replication can cause damages to DNA. Also, extraneous factors, such as radiations, chemicals, viruses etc., can damage the DNA molecules. These changes lead to mutations of the genes, which, at times, cannot be corrected by the cells. Consequently, gene expression is altered in the cell, resulting in specific diseases related to the mutated genes. Molecular biologists are pursuing challenging research to identify genes responsible for various diseases. Once identified, the genes can be manipulated directly by transferring new or missing genes (gene therapy). Specific therapies targeted at specific proteins (e.g., protease inhibitors, receptor agonists) manufactured by specific genes can be developed. Screening can be used for assessment of disease risk in groups of people with specific genetic disorder. Radiolabeled probes can be designed to detect various diseases caused by specific genes.

Methodology of Molecular Imaging

Application of gene-related information in the detection of human diseases forms the basis of molecular imaging. The impact of knowledge of gene sequences in the human genome is widespread both in experimental research and clinical applications. Identification of new targets for early disease detections, development of specific molecular markers for therapy assessment, and imaging gene expressions are only a few of the many important applications in molecular imaging.

It is understood from Fig. 14.3 that imaging at the molecular level can be accomplished by targeting DNA in the nucleus, mRNA or protein molecules in the cytoplasm, or protein molecules (receptors) on the cell surface. Targeting DNA is difficult because of limited accessibility to the nucleus and also only a limited number of DNAs are available in the cell. Targeting mRNA in the cytoplasm and extra- or intracellular proteins can be accomplished experimentally and is discussed below.

Conventional Imaging of Proteins

Radiolabeled substrates that interact with proteins manufactured from specific genes are used to image the receptors on the cell surface or enzymes in the cytoplasm. ^{11}C-labeled methylspiperone is used to image the distribution of dopamine-2-receptors in the brain. In ^{111}In-labeling of leukocytes, ^{111}In binds to cytoplasmic proteins by intracellular ligand exchange reaction with ^{111}In-oxine. Although this type of imaging is very common in nuclear medicine, it is limited by a lack of suitable substrates for many proteins. Antibodies have been developed against many antigens (proteins) of specific genes, which are radiolabeled and used to detect the antigens in different normal and abnormal tissues in humans. However, these agents are primarily applicable to proteins on the cell surface and in the vascular compartment because antibodies barely cross the cell membrane. Success has been achieved with radiolabeled antibodies and their fragments in detecting such cell surface proteins in many clinical situations.

Oligodeoxynucleotide Antisense Probes to Image mRNA

As already mentioned, only one of the two DNA strands is transcribed into a single-strand mRNA. Because the sequence of base pairs in the mRNA determines the series of amino acids that will string together to make proteins, the mRNA sequence is said to contain genetic message in correct "sense" orientation. A group of molecules called the "antisense" oligonucleotides (ASON) that are a complementary or genetic mirror to a portion of the much longer mRNA molecules have been developed. The ASONs are typically 15 to 30 base-pair-long DNA segments and bind to their complementary portions of the mRNA molecule, producing a short double-strand sequence along the otherwise long single-strand mRNA molecule. This ASON-mRNA complex prevents the translation process and in turn the production of protein on polyribosome (Fig. 14.4). Moreover, the cell considers the double-strand portion of the complex as abnormal and so an enzyme, called ribonuclease H, degrades them, and consequently the gene expression stops.

Investigators have explored the use of ASONs as both therapeutic and diagnostic agents against mRNAs from various genes including those of human immunodeficiency virus (HIV). In vivo, the ASONs containing phosphodiester linkages are rapidly degraded by enzymes in serum. To prevent this degradation, various changes have been manipulated on their structures. In vivo hybridization of ASONs with mRNA occurs at the picogram (10^{-12} g) concentration, and small tumors (0.5 cm in size) can be imaged in 1 to 2 hr postinjection. In vivo uptake of ASONs by the cells involves endocytosis (either receptor mutation or adsorption) and pinocytosis, but no passive diffusion through the cell membrane. These ASONs have high affinity for mRNA, but they bind to only a fraction of all base pairs (several hundred to thousand) of mRNA due to its secondary and tertiary structure. The biodistribution study of an ASON, phosphorothioate, in animals

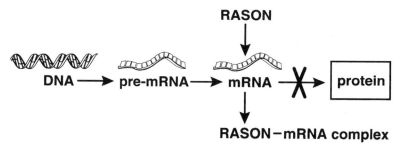

FIGURE 14.4. A schematic representation of how radiolabeled antisense oligonucleotides (RASONs) stop the synthesis of protein by forming a complex with an mRNA molecule.

showed that the plasma disappearance was extremely rapid and had two components. The highest accumulation occurred in the kidneys and liver, and a minimal localization in the brain. Since gene expression can be arrested by ASONs at the transcription level before protein synthesis in a cell, many diseases (cancer, cardiovascular diseases, etc.) can be treated using an appropriate ASON for specific mRNA responsible for a disease. ASONs targeting mRNAs in HIV, c-*myc*, c-*erbB2*, c-*fos*, and Ha-*ras* oncogenes have been developed and employed to monitor and prevent the progression of malignancy related to these genes by noninvasive imaging.

While the treatment of a variety of diseases related to gene expression using ASONs has great importance in clinical practice, the use of ASONs for diagnostic purposes has equal importance in detecting these diseases prior to their full expression. Changes in the smooth muscle hyperplasia after coronary artery angioplasty and cardiac bypass surgery have been detected by using ASONs. Many investigators have developed radiolabeled antisense oligonucleotides (RASONs) to image diseases at the mRNA level using nuclear imaging techniques.

Dewanjee et al. (1994) successfully used the first RASON probe for nuclear imaging of amplified c-*myc* oncogenes. The RASONs were phosphodiester and monothioester labeled with ^{111}In using bifunctional chelating agent, diethylenetriaminepentaacetic acid (DTPA). Similar labeling has been reported with ^{99m}Tc , ^{125}I, and ^{18}F, and most of these studies involved animals with only a few human experiments.

Reporter Genes for Imaging

Measurement of gene expression is accomplished by several methods such as Southern, Northern, and Western blot methods and the hybridization technique. A new technique has been introduced to monitor gene expression using the so-called reporter genes. A reporter gene is a defined encoded nucleotide sequence that upon introduction into a biologic system forms proteins following its expression. Reporter genes are introduced into target cells of interest by the transfection technique. The end product (protein) of the reporter gene, after transcription and translation processes, can be detected by a number of analytical assays. Some examples of the reporter genes are glucuronidase, green fluorescent proteins (GFPs), luciferase, β-galactosidase, alkaline phosphatase, cytosine deaminase (CD), and herpes simplex virus Type 1 thymidine kinase (HSV1-tk). For example, when alkaline phosphatase is introduced into a cell, the final protein produced from this gene is secreted in the blood. Similarly, if the cells are infected with a HSV1-tk reporter gene, the viral thymidine kinase is expressed, which phosphorylates pyrimidine and purine nucleoside derivatives, causing them to be trapped intracellularly.

Monitoring of the reporter gene expression can be accomplished by assaying their phenotype substrates (enzymes, receptors, etc.) using a variety of

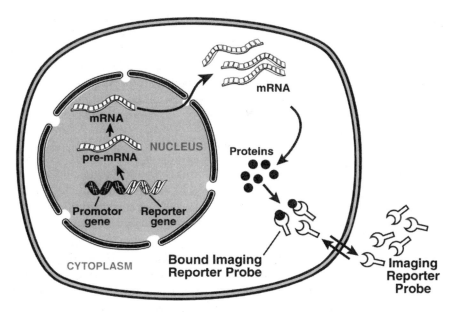

FIGURE 14.5. A schematic presentation of the use of a radiolabeled reporter gene probe to detect a specific gene expression.

methods, namely, fluorescence, chemiluminescence, absorbance, magnetic resonance imaging, and radiolabeled probes. The use of radiolabeled reporter probes to monitor and quantitate gene expression has brought considerable interest among research scientists (Fig. 14.5).

Synthetic purine nucleosides such as acyclovir and ganciclovir are used to treat herpes simplex virus infection. These analogs are phosphorylated to triphosphate analogs by various cellular enzymes, which are then incorporated into DNA to form templates that bind to and inactivate viral DNA polymerases, thus preventing the replication of the viruses. Based on this concept, ^{18}F-labeled fluoroacyclovir (9-[2-hydroxyethoxymethyl] guanine) (FACV), fluoroganciclovir (9-[[2-hydroxy-1-(hydroxymethyl)ethoxy] methyl] guanine) (FGCV), and fluoropenciclovir (9-[4-hydroxy-3-hydroxy-methylbutyl] guanine) (FPCV) have been used as reporter gene probes to image and monitor the HSV1-tk viral expression. Two other nucleosides, 9-[(3-fluoro-1-hydroxy-2-propoxyl) methyl] guanine (FHPG) and 9-(4-fluoro-3-hydroxymethylbutyl) guanine (FHBG), both labeled with ^{18}F, have been used as reporter probes for positron emission tomography (PET) imaging of HSV1-tk expression. Uracil nucleoside derivatives such as 5-iodo-2′-fluoro-2′-deoxy-1-β-D-arabinofuranosyluracil (FIAU) and 2′-fluoro-5-methyl-β-D-arabinofuranosyluracil (FMAU) labeled with ^{124}I, ^{123}I, and ^{131}I have been utilized as probes to study the HSV1-tk expression. In typical studies, a virus containing HSV1-tk was introduced in vivo into animals, and 24 to 48 hr later the radiolabeled reporter probe was injected intravenously. The animals were then imaged 24 to 48 hr later by single photon emission computed tomography (SPECT) or PET, and good correlation between the level of gene expression and the uptake of the probe was obtained. The possibility of assessment of endogenous gene expression is also under investigation, provided an appropriate probe is available.

Another well-recognized reporter gene is dopamine-2-receptor (D2R) reporter gene, which is expressed mainly in the brain. Several D2R ligands labeled with ^{18}F [e.g., 3-(2'-^{18}F-fluoroethyl)spiperone (^{18}F-FESP)] and with ^{123}I (e.g., ^{123}I-iodobenzamide) have been used as reporter probes to image D2R expression.

Gene Therapy

Gene therapy is one of the most rapidly evolving areas in medicine. The strategy of gene therapy is based on the understanding of different diseases caused by defects in genetic constructs. In genetic deficiency, therapy is aimed at restoring the function that is caused by genetic mutation. In oncology, appropriate genes causing the cancer can be used to modify the tumor cells to prevent their growth, or to prime host cells to generate antitumor activity. Gene therapy also can be employed to delay or inhibit the progression of chronic diseases caused by specific genes.

Gene Delivery

Gene therapy calls for delivery of the respective gene by ex vivo or in vivo routes. Each of these methods is unique in its approach, embracing both advantages and disadvantages. In the ex vivo technique, the target cells are removed from the host, transfected with the respective gene, and then redelivered to the host. In the in vivo technique, some carriers are used to carry the gene in vivo to the appropriate target cells. These carriers are called "vectors," in which a gene of interest is packaged for delivery to the target cells. Viruses are ideal vectors. Vectors can be either viral or nonviral, and their delivery can be made via inhalation and intramuscular or intravenous injection. Several approaches of gene delivery are briefly discussed below.

Adenoviral Vectors

Adenoviruses are viruses with a double-strand DNA that rarely integrates into the host DNA but elicits strong immune response that worsens with repeated administrations. Although various cells can be transfected by these vectors, the respiratory tract cells are most vulnerable. Genes required for replication are deleted from these viruses and genes of interest for transfection are inserted into them, after which the infected viruses are delivered to the cells that are vulnerable to infection by adenoviruses. High titers of these viruses can be produced in in vitro culture media, allowing the possibility of efficient gene transfer.

Retroviral Vectors

Retroviruses contain a single-strand RNA genome. It is converted into DNA, which, unlike adenoviruses, is incorporated into the host DNA. These viruses are replication-deficient and are the widely used viruses both experimentally and clinically. Retroviral genes, namely, *gag, pol,* and *env,* are substituted with genes of specific interest to be delivered by the virus to the host cell. These viruses are available in high titers for efficient transfection, but are limited by their small size (so large genes cannot be inserted) and by the fact that they infect only dividing cells.

A group of retroviral vectors, called lentiviruses, also are used for transfecting the cells. The human immunodeficiency virus (HIV) is a lentivirus that can be used for the delivery of an intended gene. These vectors can infect both dividing and nondividing cells without any appreciable immune response.

Nonviral Vectors

One of the nonviral vector techniques is to inject DNA directly into the bloodstream. But hydrolysis of naked DNA and its degradation by serum nucleases are the major drawbacks in this approach. Plasmid vectors (an autonomously replicating molecule) have been investigated for the gene delivery but limited by the poor efficiency in transfection of the host cells. Liposomes carrying the desired gene have been prepared and used for the gene delivery, but are markedly less efficient than virus-mediated transfer.

Specific Diseases

Cystic fibrosis is developed by mutations in the cystic fibrosis transmembrane regulator (CFTR) gene causing abnormal transmembrane conductance. The disease is characterized by increased pulmonary infections and obstructions to bowel transit due to abnormal secretions in pulmonary and gastrointestinal epithelium. Gene therapy is aimed at restoring CFTR gene expression by using liposomal and adenoviral vectors to deliver the CFTR gene to bronchial epithelium.

Severe combined immunodeficiency disorder is encountered when adenosine deaminase gene is deficient, resulting in the accumulation of a toxic level of deoxyadenosine to cause T-cell death. This disorder has been treated by injecting the adenosine deaminase gene in vivo into the peripheral blood lymphocytes.

Several malignant tumors have been treated by gene therapy by either arresting the cell proliferation or enhancing the cell apoptosis. Oncogenes are genes that promote cellular growth and proliferation. These oncogenes can be inhibited by antisense RNA, antibodies, and catalytic RNA that digest oncogene RNA. Antioncogenes, also called tumor suppressor genes, normally suppress tumor malignancy and so their absence would result in proliferation of the malignant cells. The suppressor genes can also regulate tumor cell apoptosis. The deficiency of a suppressor gene, *p53*, causes primary non–small cell lung carcinoma. Injection of retroviral *p53* gene complexes showed tumor regression in patients having this malignancy.

Apoptosis is a normal cellular process by which cells undergo programmed death, eliminating aged or damaged cells from the system. This process keeps a balance between cell growth and cell death. It has been shown that the absence or aberration of apoptosis is responsible for the development of malignancy in several instances. The *fas* gene is involved in triggering apoptosis, and so inserting this gene can shift the balance from cell proliferation in malignancy to apoptosis. ^{99m}Tc-labeled annexin V has been used to image apoptosis in acute transplant rejection.

Another paradigm of gene therapy is the use of cytokines to increase antitumor immunity. These cytokines include interleukin-2 (IL-2), IL-4, IL-12, granulocyte-monocyte colony-stimulating factors (GM-CSFs), tumor necrosis factors (TNFs), and interferons. When appropriate genes are inserted into the peripheral blood, lymphocytes or tumor-infiltrating lymphocytes are activated, and antitumor activity is induced, inhibiting the cell growth.

Suicide genes induce production of a chemical by the tumor cell itself that turns out to be lethal to the cell. A specific example of a suicide gene is HSV1-tk that easily infects the tumor cells. If a prodrug (e.g., acyclovir or ganciclovir) is injected systematically, it is converted by cellular kinases into toxic triphosphate derivatives. The latter are incorporated into DNA that leads to DNA chain termination, causing cell death. Colon carcinoma has been treated with a suicide gene, cytosine deaminase gene, that upon expression produces 5-fluorouracil, which has antitumor activity.

Peripheral limb ischemia and atherosclerosis are caused by endothelial cell dysfunction due to lack of angiogenic factors such as vascular endothelial growth factor (VEGF). In an approach to improve blood flow by promoting angiogenesis in ischemic vessels, VEGF encoding DNA has been applied onto angioplasty catheters and a reduction in restenosis rates obtained due to early endothelialization. Similar VEGF gene therapy has also been applied to the cases of bypass grafts, where inserted genes alter the thrombogenicity of the prosthetic grafts by stimulating neoendothelialization.

The above is a brief synopsis of the tremendous potential that molecular genetics and gene therapy can offer. Many new techniques, probes for imaging, discovery of genes responsible for various diseases, and various vectors for gene delivery are only a few of the numerous issues that will unfold in the future, and provide clues to solving many diagnostic and therapeutic problems related to a variety of diseases.

Questions

1. Describe how a protein is synthesized by the activation of a gene.
2. What are the estimated number of genes in a human genome, and how many proteins carry out the functions of life?
3. Describe different methodologies used in molecular imaging and discuss their merits and disadvantages.
4. Discuss different techniques of gene delivery.
5. Elucidate some specific diseases that can be diagnosed or treated by gene technology.

Suggested Reading

Blasberg R. PET imaging of gene expression. *Eur J Cancer*. 2002; 38:2137.

Dewanjee MK, Ghafouripour AK, Kapadvanjwala M, et al. Noninvasive imaging of c-*myc* oncogene messenger RNA with indium-111-antisense probes in a mammary tumor-bearing mouse model. *J Nucl Med*. 1994; 35:1054.

Gambhir SS. Imaging gene expression. In: Schiepers C, ed. *Diagnostic Nuclear Medicine*. New York: Springer-Verlag; 1998:253.

Gambhir SS. Molecular imaging of cancer with positron emission tomography. *Nature Reviews*. 2002; 2:683.

Luker GD, Piwnica-Worms D. Beyond the genome: Molecular imaging in vivo with PET and SPECT. *Acad Radiol*. 2001; 8:4.

Ross DW. *Introduction to Molecular Medicine*. New York: Springer-Verlag; 1992.

Sharma V, Luker GD, Piwnica-Worms D. Molecular imaging of gene expression and protein function in vivo with PET and SPECT. *J Magn Reson Imaging*. 2002; 16:336.

Urbain JLC. Reporter genes and Imagene. *J Nucl Med*. 2001; 42:106.

Voss SD, Kruskal JB. Gene therapy: a primer for radiologists. *Radiographics*. 1998; 18:1343.

Weissleder R, Mahmood U. Molecular imaging. *Radiology*. 2001; 219:316.

15
Therapeutic Uses of Radiopharmaceuticals in Nuclear Medicine

Treatment of Hyperthyroidism

Hyperthyroidism is a disease manifested by excessive thyroid hormone activity and can arise from a number of pathogenic processes. Several strategies are employed in the treatment of hyperthyroidism, e.g., use of antithyroid drugs such as propylthiouracil or methimazole, thyroidectomy, and use of ^{131}I. Each of these methods has its own merits and disadvantages, but drug therapy and ^{131}I treatment are the most common choices.

The rationale for radioiodine therapy is that it accumulates in the thyroid and irradiates the glands with its β^- and γ radiations, about 90% of the total radiation dose being delivered by β^- particles. Several methods of choosing the treatment dosage of ^{131}I are currently used. The simplest method is to administer the same amount of ^{131}I-NaI, nominally 3 to 7 mCi (111–259 MBq), to all patients having the similar clinical condition of hyperthyroidism. Almost 60% of the patients benefit from a remission of hyperthyroidism within 3 to 4 months, and a second treatment cures another 25% to 30%. This fixed activity method has limitations, because the activity administered is arbitrary and has no correlation with either the severity of the disease or the weight of the gland.

The most common method of ^{131}I treatment is to administer a specified amount of ^{131}I in microcuries per gram of the thyroid, based on the estimate of the 24-hr thyroid uptake and the mass of the glands. An assumption is made that an average biologic half-life of ^{131}I is essentially constant for all patients. The empirical formula for this method is given by

$$\text{Administered } \mu\text{Ci} = \frac{\mu\text{Ci/g} \times \text{mass of thyroid (g)} \times 100}{24\text{-hr uptake (\%)}} \tag{15.1}$$

Many clinicians use a dosage of 55 to 80 μCi (2–3 MBq) per gram for Graves' disease. If one assumes 1 μCi (37 kBq) deposited in the thyroid gives 1 rad (0.01 Gy) of radiation dose, then a dosage of 80 μCi (2.96 MBq) per gram, for example, would give 6400 rad (64 Gy) to 60-g thyroid glands with 75% uptake. The mass of the thyroid is estimated by palpation or by thyroid imaging. For very enlarged glands and severely hyperthyroid patients, larger dosages of 160 to 200 μCi (5.9–7.4 MBq) per gram are given to achieve rapid response.

[131]I treatment is contraindicated in pregnant women because ^{131}I crosses the placental barrier and can cause radiation damage to the fetal thyroid. The fetal thyroid starts to accumulate iodine around the 10th week of gestation, and therefore ^{131}I treatment at or after this time should be avoided. Also, in the period before the 10th week of gestation, such treatment may give radiation exposure to the fetus and therefore should not be given. It is recommended that a pregnancy test be obtained prior to ^{131}I treatment for all women of child-bearing age. Patients treated with ^{131}I are advised to delay conception for at least 6 months after treatment.

In Graves' disease, complete remission of hyperthyroidism is achieved in 60% of the patients after treatment. Patients with severe hyperthyroidism, particularly older patients, are treated with antithyroid drugs before ^{131}I treatment to obtain better results following treatment.

Recurrence of hyperthyroidism after the first treatment is found in about 6% to 14% of the patients and requires repeat treatments with [131]I. Hypothyroidism is observed in 25% to 40% of the patients treated, mostly in those patients treated with high dosages of [131]I. To reduce the prevalence of hypothyroidism, smaller or divided dosages of ^{131}I are given over a longer period of time. After ^{131}I treatment, drugs such as thiomides, stable iodine, and β-adrenergic blocking agents (propranolol, metoprolol, etc.) are given to patients to control hyperthyroidism.

Toxic multinodular goiters (Plummer's disease) are highly resistant to ^{131}I treatment and so are treated with higher and multiple dosages of [131]I. The incidence of hypothyroidism is low in this group of patients, because of the resistance to treatment. These patients should be prepared for ^{131}I therapy with prior antithyroid medication.

In a small number of patients, exacerbation of hyperthyroidism resulting in conditions such as heart failure and thyroid crisis is noted within 3 to 5 days after ^{131}I treatment. This results from excessive release of T3 and T4 from the treated thyroid gland. However, nowadays the incidence of worsening of hyperthyroidism is lessened by the use of propranolol prior to treatment.

Treatment of Thyroid Cancer

Well-differentiated thyroid cancers that include papillary and follicular cancers are treatable with ^{131}I, because they are capable of concentrating ^{131}I, although very little. Anaplastic and medullary thyroid cancers do not concentrate ^{131}I, and therefore ^{131}I therapy is of no value in the treatment of these cancers. The papillary and follicular cancers metastasize in various parts of the body and the extent of metastasis often needs to be assessed prior to ^{131}I treatment.

Prior to ^{131}I treatment, most patients undergo total or near-total thyroidectomy surgically in which the cancerous tissues plus some normal tissues are removed. The removal of normal tissues causes hypothyroidism that results in an increase in endogenous TSH, which stimulates residual cancer to localize ^{131}I. All oral medication of thyroid hormone (T4) is stopped for 6 weeks prior to treatment to raise the level of TSH. Since stable iodine in the blood interferes with ^{131}I accumulation, a low-iodine diet is also recommended to augment the ^{131}I uptake by the thyroid. No radiographic contrast examination should be done 6 to 8 weeks prior to treatment. Sometimes lithium carbonate is administered before ^{131}I treatment because lithium inhibits the release of ^{131}I from thyroid cancers.

Whole-Body Imaging

The purpose of whole-body imaging is to detect functioning metastatic thyroid cancer and/or residual normal thyroid tissue, and is accomplished by administering ^{131}I-NaI orally. The dosage for administration is debatable, varying from 2 to 10 mCi (74–370 MBq). However, in our institution, a 5-mCi (185-MBq) dosage is administered and whole-body images are obtained 24 to 72 hr later using a gamma camera with a medium-energy parallel hole collimator. At times, spot images need to be taken and also imaging may be extended for as long as 7 days for equivocal metastatic sites.

Interpretation of whole-body images requires experience and knowledge in the biodistribution of ^{131}I in the body. Normally, iodide accumulates in the nose, salivary glands, mouth, esophagus, stomach, bladder, colon, and liver, and therefore hot spots in these areas should be interpreted carefully. Hair and clothes contaminated with urine may cause artifacts on the images. Residual thyroid neoplasms occasionally concentrate ^{131}I and should be correlated with x-ray findings as well as the surgeon's report. Metastatic foci are recognized by the increased uptake of ^{131}I.

Treatment with ^{131}I

Patients for ^{131}I treatment fall into two broad groups: those with normal residual thyroid tissue with or without occult metastases, and those with functioning primary or metastatic carcinoma. The treatment of the first group is called ablation, and most physicians use 25 to 30 mCi (925–1110 MBq) ^{131}I-NaI, although dosages as high as 150 mCi (5.55 GBq) have been used. For the second group of patients, most clinicians use a standard amount of activity, which varies between 100 mCi (3.7 GBq) and 200 mCi

(7.4 GBq) depending on the extent of metastatic sites. Smaller dosages are given for cancer remnants in the thyroid bed or cervical lymph node metastasis, whereas larger dosages are given for lung and bone metastases.

Accurate estimation of the radiation dose to the tumor sites is impossible because of the difficulty in determining the volume of distant metastases. The size of tumors and lymph node metastases and their ^{131}I uptake can be estimated from scintigraphic images, from which the radiation dose to the area may be calculated. Radiation dose from the common dosages of ^{131}I ranges from 5,000 to 30,000 rad (50–300 Gy).

Although radiation therapy with ^{131}I is safe, there are complications that may be encountered after treatment with [131]I. In the case of ablation of a large amount of thyroid tissues with 30 mCi (1110 MBq) [131]I, acute pain and tenderness of thyroiditis are common. Occasionally, anorexia, nausea, and vomiting are seen as radiation syndromes. Apparently there has been found no increase in the incidence of infertility after treatment with [131]I. Radiation pneumonitis occurs in some patients who have been treated with a high dosage of ^{131}I for lung metastasis of thyroid cancer.

Bone marrow depression is encountered in patients treated with very high dosages of [131]I. These effects are noticeable in 5 to 6 weeks after the administration of the dosage. The incidence of leukemia, although low in frequency, has been reported occurring between 2 and 10 years after the treatment, and repeat treatments with ^{131}I in short intervals increase this frequency.

The parotid and salivary glands concentrate ^{131}I and receive significantly high radiation dose during treatment. Acute inflammation of the salivary glands (sialadenitis) develops in 10% of the patients treated with ^{131}I for thyroid cancer. This incidence is more evident with higher dosages of [131]I.

The effectiveness of ^{131}I therapy for thyroid cancer depends on the location of the metastases. Improvement was found by scanning in 68% of the patients with lymph node metastasis, in 46% of the patients with lung metastasis and only in 7% of the patients with bone metastasis. Response to treatment is related to the mass of cancer present in a given location. While the treatment of functioning thyroid cancers is of value in the overall management of the patient, the value of ablation therapy is questionable.

Recurrence of thyroid carcinoma takes place in many patients with papillary and follicular carcinoma. For recurrent thyroid carcinoma or remnant metastasis with poor response to previous treatment, repeat treatment with ^{131}I is given at 3-month to 1-year intervals depending on the extent, aggressiveness, and location of the metastatic sites. Whole-body imaging should be done annually after treatment until there is no detectable tumor or metastatic uptake for two consecutive years. Other clinical indicators such as TSH, serum thyroglobulin, and radiographic imaging also are obtained to monitor the progress of the treatment. It should be noted that, according to many investigators, ^{131}I therapy is of no use for the treatment of medullary thyroid carcinoma.

Treatment of Bone Pain

A common complication in cancer patients is the spread of cancer to the bone (bone metastasis) resulting in severe pain. Osseous metastasis is found in 85% of terminally ill patients with breast, prostate, and lung cancer and to a lesser extent with other malignancies. Palliation of bone pain in these patients is the common goal to improve the quality of life. To this end, several strategies are adopted, e.g., use of analgesics, external radiation beam therapy, and internal radionuclide therapy. The latter is discussed below.

Radionuclide therapy in bone pain palliation is based on the avidity of various radiopharmaceuticals preferentially localizing in bone. ^{32}P-orthophosphate has been in use for a long time for bone pain therapy. Two current radiopharmaceuticals, ^{89}Sr-SrCl$_2$ and ^{153}Sm-EDTMP, have been found to be useful in palliative therapy of bone pain, because they preferentially localize in osteoblastic sites and destroy the malignant cells with radiations.

^{32}P-Sodium Orthophosphate

Phosphorus-32 decays by β^- emission with a half-life of 14.3 days. Its maximum β^- energy is 1.70 MeV. Following intravenous administration, 85% of the injected dosage is accumulated in the hydroxyapatite crystals and the remainder localizes in the nonosseous tissues. Since it is incorporated in the structure of DNA and RNA, these structures are damaged by β^- radiations. Bone marrow is the most seriously damaged tissues by ^{32}P radiations.

Approximately 6 to 12 mCi (222–444 MBq) ^{32}P-sodium orthophosphate is administered intravenously and often multiple administrations are made based on the response to the initial treatment. Frequently androgen is given for a week prior to administration of ^{32}P to enhance the bone uptake of the tracer.

The response rate of ^{32}P therapy is about 80% and the mean period of response is about 5.1 ± 2.6 months. The common side effect is hematologic toxicity due to bone marrow suppression. Occasionally, an increase in bone pain (bone flare) is seen, which is primarily due to androgen given prior to ^{32}P administration. However, ^{32}P-therapy has not been accepted widely for palliation of bone pain because of myelotoxicity.

^{89}Sr-Strontium Chloride (Metastron)

Strontium-89 has a half-life of 50.6 days decaying with the emission of a β^- particle, having a maximum energy of 1.43 MeV. After intravenous administration, it localizes in reactive bone and is excreted in the urine (80%) and feces (20%) with a biological half-life of 4 to 5 days. Approximately 30% to

35% of the injected dosage remains in normal bone for 10 to 14 days post-injection. However, the retention in osteoblastic areas is as high as 85% to 90% at 3 months postinjection.

Approximately 4 mCi (148 MBq) ^{89}Sr-SrCl$_2$ is injected into patients for the relief of bone pain due to metastasis from various cancers. Injection is made slowly over a period of 1 to 2 min. Patients should have a platelet count of at least 60,000 and a leukocyte count of 2400 at the time of administration. Myelosuppression may occur particularly with higher dosages, thus reducing the platelet and leukocyte counts by almost 25% to 30%.

Initial relief of pain is usually noticed within 3 days of administration, but it may be as late as 25 days. The mean duration of pain relief is of the order of 3 to 6 months and, therefore, retreatments with ^{89}Sr may be considered every 3 to 6 months. Complete remission of pain is found in 5% to 20% of the patients after ^{89}Sr treatment, and almost 80% of the patients experience some relief of pain from osteoblastic metastasis (Robinson et al., 1995). In 10% of the patients, there is an initial increase in bone pain within ~3 days of therapy that subsides in about a week.

^{153}Sm-EDTMP (Quadramet)

Samarium-153 is a β^- emitter with a maximum energy of 0.81 MeV and decays with a half-life of 1.9 days. It emits a γ-ray photon of 103 keV (28%) that is suitable for scintigraphic imaging. ^{153}Sm-EDTMP is rapidly cleared from the blood and avidly localizes in bone. Almost 35% of the injected tracer is excreted in the urine by 6 hr postinjection. A dosage of 1 mCi/kg (37 MBq/kg) ^{153}Sm-EDTMP is administered intravenously to patients targeted for bone pain palliation. It appears to be deposited as an insoluble complex on the hydroxyapatite crystals. Relief of pain is found in about 65% of the patients within 1 to 11 months and may last for a year (Farhanghi et al., 1992). Further relief of pain is achieved with repeat treatments. Myelotoxicity is observed in these patients, but is related to the dosage administered.

Treatment of Non-Hodgkin's Lymphoma

^{90}Y-Ibritumomab Tiuxetan (Zevalin)

Yttrium-90 decays by β^- emission (100%) with a half-life of 64 hr. It has high-energy β^- rays with an effective path length of 5.3 mm, meaning that 90% of β^- energy is absorbed in a sphere of 5.3-mm radius. ^{90}Y-ibritumomab tiuxetan (Zevalin) is a stable agent used for the treatment of non-Hodgkin's lymphoma (NHL).

In the United States, approximately 35,000 people are diagnosed with

NHL each year, and 65% of them are of the low-grade or follicular type of NHL. Patients with this type of NHL may remain in remission for years, but eventually have bouts of relapses that tend to be resistant to repeat treatments over time. ^{90}Y-ibritumomab tiuxetan is an optional but promising treatment for these patients.

Treatment of NHL patients with ^{90}Y-ibritumomab tiuxetan is performed only after confirmation of no altered biodistribution by ^{111}In-ibritumomab imaging as discussed in Chapter 13 (see Tumor Imaging). Also, the therapy must be preceded by two dosages of 250 mg/m^2 of rituximab—the first before imaging with ^{111}In, and the second before the administration of ^{90}Y-ibritumomab. The administered dosage is based on body weight and baseline platelet counts, and a typical patient dosage range is 20 to 30 mCi (740–1110 MBq) with a maximum limit of 32 mCi (1184 MBq). Both rituximab and ^{90}Y-ibritumomab tiuxetan target the white blood cells (B cells) including malignant B cells involved in the disease, resulting in significant tumor shrinkage. The overall response rate was found to be 74% to 80% in about 2 months after therapy in patients who failed to respond to chemotherapy. The most common side effects are the flu-like symptoms and a marked reduction in blood cell counts.

Polycythemia Vera and Leukemia

Polycythemia vera is a disease characterized by an increased red blood cell mass, frequently associated with bone marrow hyperactivity. ^{32}P-sodium orthophosphate is used for the treatment of polycythemia vera. Therapy results from radiation injury to the cell precursors and the bone marrow due to bone accumulation of ^{32}P.

Usually 3 to 4 mCi (111–148 MBq) ^{32}P in the form of ^{32}P-sodium orthophosphate is administered intravenously, and 12 weeks later the patient's response is evaluated. In the case of marked elevation of red blood cells, phlebotomy is also instituted simultaneously. If the red cell mass is not reduced sufficiently after the first treatment, a second treatment with 3 mCi (111 MBq) ^{32}P may be made.

Cases of leukemia have been reported in patients treated with ^{32}P-sodium orthophosphate. It has been suggested that ^{32}P should not be used for treatment if the platelet count is less than 15,000. Life expectancy after ^{32}P treatment has been reported to be 10 to 12 years.

Leukemia is characterized by a marked increase in leukocytes and their precursors in the blood. Approximately 1 to 2 mCi (37–74 MBq) ^{32}P-sodium orthophosphate is given weekly until the white blood cell count is sufficiently decreased. Life expectancy does not increase to a large extent by this treatment.

Malignant Effusion in Pleural and Peritoneal Cavities

Malignant effusion in the pleural and peritoneal cavities is often treated with ^{32}P-chromic phosphate colloid. Treatment is usually given after drainage of the fluid from the cavity. Ten mCi (370 MBq) ^{32}P-chromic phosphate colloid is instilled in cases of pleural effusion, and double the quantity in cases of peritoneal effusion. Macrophages remove these colloidal particles, which are ultimately fixed on the walls of the fluid cavity and kill the malignant cells by β^- radiations.

Pretargeted Radioimmunotherapy of Cancer

The use of radiolabeled monoclonal antibody (Mab) for the treatment of cancer has the difficulty of higher background activity in the vascular compartment that results in unnecessary radiation dose to normal tissues, particularly bone marrow. To circumvent this situation, investigators have adopted the strategy of pretargeting of tumor cells with an unlabeled Mab, followed later by the administration of a radiolabeled hapten that binds to the antibody in the tumor. The unlabeled antibody in the circulation is removed by complexation with an agent that is injected prior to the administration of the radiolabeled hapten. The complex is rapidly cleared by breakdown in the liver. A review article on this topic has been presented by Boerman et al (2003).

In one common approach, pretargeting is based on the interaction between streptavidin (SA) or avidin and biotin. Avidin, a constituent of the egg white of reptiles, amphibians, and birds, is a protein that can bind up to 4 molecules of vitamin H, D-biotin with an affinity a million times higher than that between antigen and Mab. Streptavidin (SA) is a bacterial analog of avidin with similar characteristics. In practice, a biotinylated Mab is injected first, whereby the tumor is pretargeted with the Mab. Unlabeled avidin or streptavidin (called the "chase") is given to reduce the blood level of the biotinylated Mab. Radiolabeled avidin is then administered, which avidly binds to biotin in the tumor demonstrating increased tumor uptake with a reduced background. Similarly, tumors can be pretargeted with avidin first, followed by the administration of radiolabeled biotin in the last step.

In another approach, Mabs developed against chelating agents such as ethylenediaminetetraacetic acid (EDTA) or dodecanetetraacetic acid (DOTA) are used to pretarget the tumor. The circulating Mab is removed by injection of transferrin substituted with multiple haptens. Radiolabeled EDTA or DOTA (e.g., ^{111}In-DOTA) is then injected and it binds avidly to the tumor and thus results in increased uptake. This method is further improved by using Mabs with dual specificity (called bifunctional or bispecific Mabs). Such bifunctional Mabs or fragments of Mabs have been produced by chemical cross-linking, hybridoma technology, and a genetic engineering technique, by which complexes like Mab-Mab or (Fab′)-(Fab′) are formed. In these conjugated Mabs, one Mab may be against the tumor and the other against a chelating agent.

Tumors are pretargeted with the injection of tumor Mab (or Fab′)-chelate Mab (or Fab′) bifunctional Mab (or fragments). Radiolabeled chelate such as ^{111}In-chelate or ^{90}Y-chelate is injected later, which binds to the bifunctional Mab in the tumor demonstrating increased uptake.

All of the above methods have both merits and disadvantages, and ongoing research is focused on improving each method to increase the tumor-to-background activity ratio for better delineation of tumor localization.

Questions

1. What are the different methods of treatment with ^{131}I of patients with hyperthyroidism? Discuss the merits and disadvantages of each method.
2. Why is ^{131}I contraindicated in pregnant women? How long is it advised for the patients treated with ^{131}I to delay conception?
3. What are the frequency of recurrence of hyperthyroidism and the incidences of hypothyroidism and leukemia in patients after ^{131}I treatment?
4. Describe the rationale for ^{131}I therapy for patients with thyroid cancer. What are the different strategies for ^{131}I therapy of thyroid cancer?
5. What are the complications observed from the ^{131}I therapy of thyroid cancer?
6. Describe the various treatment methods for palliation of pain from bone metastasis of different cancers. What is the important physiological parameter that is to be considered before and during the treatment?
7. Describe the principles of pretargeted radioimmunotherapy in cancers.

References and Suggested Reading

Becker D, Hurley JR. Radioiodine treatment of hyperthyroidism. In: Sandler MP, Coleman RE, Walkers FJT, et al., eds. *Diagnostic Nuclear Medicine*. 3rd ed. Baltimore: Williams and Wilkins; 1996:943.

Boerman OC, van Schaijk FD, Oyen WJG et al. Pretargeted radioimmunotherapy of cancer: Progress step by step. *J Nucl Med.* 2003; 44:400.

Farhanghi M, Holmes RA, Volkert WA, et al. Samarium-153-EDTMP: pharmacokinetics, toxicity and pain response using an escalating dose schedule in treatment of metastatic bone pain. *J Nucl Med.* 1992; 33:1451.

Hurley JR, Becker DV. Treatment of thyroid cancer with radioiodine (^{131}I). In: Sandler MP, Coleman RE, Walkers FJT, et al., eds. *Diagnostic Nuclear Medicine*. 3rd ed. Baltimore: Williams and Wilkins; 1996:959.

Maxon HR III, Smith HD. Radioiodine-131 in the diagnosis and treatment of metastatic well-differentiated thyroid cancer. *Endocrinol Metab Clin North Am.* 1990; 19:685.

Robinson RG, Preston DF, Schiéfelbein M, et al. Strontium-89 therapy for the palliation of pain due to osseous metastases. *JAMA*. 1995; 274:420.

16
Adverse Reactions to and Altered Biodistribution of Radiopharmaceuticals

Adverse Reactions

An adverse reaction due to a radiopharmaceutical is an unusual experience associated with administration of the radiopharmaceutical. Adverse reactions include sensitivity reactions and many systemic and physiologic symptoms. The most common adverse reactions are nausea, dyspnea, bronchospasm, decreased blood pressure, itching, flushing, hives, chills, coughing, bradycardia, muscle cramps, and dizziness. Some adverse reactions appear later in time than others.

The Society of Nuclear Medicine in the United States collects from its members voluntary reports of adverse reactions due to radiopharmaceutical administration to humans. The Joint Committee on Radiopharmaceuticals of the European Nuclear Medicine Society collects reports on adverse reactions with radiopharmaceuticals in Europe. The overall incidence of adverse reactions in the United States is about 2.3 reactions per 100,000 radiopharmaceutical administrations (Silberstein, 1996). However, no death has been reported and the incidence of severe reactions has declined in recent years due to better formulation and manufacturing of radiopharmaceuticals.

Of the different radiopharmaceuticals in use in the United States, ^{99m}Tc-labeled albumin microsphere (although currently not commercially available) had the highest incidence of adverse reactions, with ^{99m}Tc-sulfur colloid next. There are also several reports of adverse reactions with ^{99m}Tc-MAA, ^{99m}Tc-MDP, and ^{99m}Tc-DISIDA. The number of adverse reactions is probably not accurate, because many nuclear medicine institutions do not consistently report them. With a good mechanism of reporting, perhaps a reliable assessment of the safety of a radiopharmaceutical could be made.

Most adverse reactions are mild in nature and require no or minimal treatment. Antihistamines are the mainstay for the treatment of severe anaphylaxis. Epinephrine is the agent of choice and is given subcutaneously or intramuscularly, whereas in severe conditions it is given intravenously. In the case of poor response to antihistamine, aminophylline may be given.

TABLE 16.1. Iatrogenic alteration in the biodistribution of common radiopharmaceuticals.

Imaging	Drug	Effect on localization
Bone imaging with ^{99m}Tc-phosphonate compounds	Chemotherapeutic agents	Increased renal activity
	Melphalan	Increased bone uptake
	Corticosteroids	Decreased bone uptake
	Cytotoxic therapy	Increased uptake in calvarium
	Meperidine	Soft tissue uptake
	Iron dextran	Increased uptake at injection site
	Aluminum ion	Increased liver activity
	Dextrose	Increased renal activity
	Iron	Increased renal activity
	Phospho-soda	Decreased bone uptake
RES imaging with ^{99m}Tc-SC	Al^{3+}, Mg^{2+}	Increased lung activity
	Anesthetics	Increased splenic uptake
	Estrogens	Focal areas of decreased uptake in liver
	BCNU	Decreased splenic uptake
Myocardial perfusion imaging with ^{201}Tl chloride	Dipyridamole	Increased myocardial uptake
	Propranolol	Decreased myocardial uptake
	Digitalis glycosides	Decreased myocardial uptake
	Furosemide	Increased myocardial uptake
	Isoproterenol	Increased myocardial uptake
Hepatobiliary imaging with ^{99m}Tc-IDA derivatives	Cholecystokinin	Increased gallbladder contraction
	Narcotic analgesics	Prolonged liver-to-duodenum transit time
	Atropine	Prolonged gallbladder activity
	Nicotinic acid	Decreased hepatic uptake
Thyroid uptake and imaging with ^{131}I-NaI	TcO_4^-, Br^-, ClO_4^-, SCN^-	Decreased uptake
	Iodide-containing preparations (Lugol's solution, SSKI, cough medicine, kelp, etc.)	Decreased uptake
	Contrast media	Decreased uptake
	Antithyroid drugs (Tapazole, propylthiouracil)	Decreased uptake
	Natural or synthetic thyroid preparation (Cytomel, Synthroid)	Decreased uptake
Tumor and inflammatory process imaging with ^{67}Ga-citrate	Iron dextran (before ^{67}Ga injection)	Decreased uptake
	Iron dextran (after ^{67}Ga injection)	Increased uptake
	Desferoxamine (before ^{67}Ga injection)	Decreased uptake
	Desferoxamine (after ^{67}Ga injection)	Increased uptake
	Chemotherapeutic agents	Diffuse lung uptake
	Antibiotics	Uptake in colon and kidneys
	Estrogens	Uptake in mammary tissue
In-vivo ^{99m}Tc-labeling of RBCs	Heparin	Poor labeling
	Dextran	Poor labeling
	Doxorubicin	Poor labeling
	Penicillin	Poor labeling
	Hydralazine	Poor labeling
	Iodinated contrast media	Poor labeling

Two comprehensive reviews on the adverse reactions to radiopharmaceuticals have been published by Silberstein (1996) and Hesselwood et al. (1997).

Iatrogenic Alterations in the Biodistribution of Radiopharmaceuticals

The effects of various drugs on the biodistribution of radiopharmaceuticals have long been recognized as an important factor in the interpretation of scintigraphic images. Altered biodistribution due to extraneous drugs may be undesirable or intentional. In most cases, however, patients receive several medications that tend to interfere with the distribution of the radiopharmaceutical used in a subsequent nuclear medicine procedure. Some drugs enhance the localization of the radiopharmaceutical in the target organ, whereas others depress uptake. In some cases, biodistribution is shifted to other organs. Knowledge of altered biodistribution due to other drugs helps the physician avoid misinterpretation of the scintigraphic images and thus an incorrect diagnosis. An excellent review article on this issue has been published by Hladik et al. (1987). Different imaging procedures and various drugs that alter the biodistribution of radiopharmaceuticals used in these procedures are listed in Table 16.1.

Questions

1. Which radiopharmaceutical has the highest incidence of adverse reactions? What is the most common drug that is used to alleviate the effects of adverse reactions?
2. Enumerate the drugs that affect adversely the labeling of RBCs.
3. What are the common drugs or agents that affect the thyroid uptake of ^{131}I?

References and Suggested Reading

Hesselwood S, Leung E. Drug interactions with radiopharmaceuticals. *Eur J Nucl Med.* 1994; 21:348.

Hesselwood S, Keeling DH, and the Radiopharmacy Committee of the European Association of Nuclear Medicine. Frequency of adverse reactions to radiopharmaceuticals in Europe. *Eur J Nucl Med.* 1997; 24:1179.

Hladik WB III, Ponto JA, Lentle BC, et al. Iatrongenic alterations in the biodistribution of radiotracers as a result of drug therapy: reported instances. In: Hladik WB III, Saha GB, Study KT, eds. *Essentials of Nuclear Medicine Science.* Baltimore: Williams and Wilkins; 1987:189.

Silberstein EB. Adverse reactions to radiopharmaceutical agents. In: Henkin RE, Boles MA, Dillehay GL, et al., eds. *Nuclear Medicine.* St. Louis: Mosby; 1996:485.

Silberstein EB, Ryan J, and Pharmacopeia Committee of Nuclear Medicine. Prevalence of adverse reactions in nuclear medicine. *J Nucl Med.* 1996; 37:185; erratum, page 1064.

Appendix A
Abbreviations Used in the Text

Ab	antibody
AEC	Atomic Energy Commission
Ag	antigen
ALARA	as low as reasonably achievable
ALI	annual limit on intake
ASON	antisense oligonucleotides
BBB	blood–brain barrier
BET	bacterial endotoxin test
BFC	bifunctional chelating agent
CABG	coronary artery bypass graft
CMS	Centers for Medicare and Medicaid Services
CNS	central nervous system
CSF	cerebrospinal fluid
DAC	derived air concentration
DISIDA	diisopropyliminodiacetic acid
DIT	diiodotyrosine
DMSA	dimercaptosuccinic acid
DNA	deoxyribonucleic acid
DOT	Department of Transportation
DTPA	diethylenetriaminepentaacetic acid
EC	electron capture
ECD	ethyl cysteinate dimer
EDTA	ethylenediaminetetraacetic acid
FDA	Food and Drug Administration
FDG	fluorodeoxyglucose
HAMA	human antimurine antibody
HDP	hydroxymethylene diphosphonate
HEDP	1-hydroxyethylidene diphosphonate
HIDA	N-[N'-(2,6-dimethylphenyl) carbamoylmethyl] iminodiacetic acid
HIV	human immunodeficiency virus
HMPAO	hexamethylpropylene amine oxime

HSV	herpes simplex virus
HVL	half-value layer
HYNIC	hydrazinonicotinamide
ICRP	International Committee on Radiation Protection
IMP	isopropyl-p-iodoamphetamine
IND	Notice of Claimed Investigational Exemption for a New Drug
IRB	Institutional Review Board
IT	isomeric transition
ITLC	instant thin-layer chromatography
kV	kilovolt
LAL	Limulus amebocyte lysate
MAA	macroaggregated albumin
Mab	monoclonal antibody
MAG3	mercaptoacetylglycylglycylglycine
MDP	methylene diphosphonate
MEK	methyl ethyl ketone
MIRD	medical internal radiation dose
MIT	monoiodotyrosine
mRNA	messenger ribonucleic acid
MTC	medullary thyroid carcinoma
MUGA	multigated acquisition
NCA	no carrier added
NCRP	National Council on Radiation Protection and Measurement
NDA	New Drug Application
NP-59	6β-iodomethyl-19-norcholesterol
NRC	Nuclear Regulatory Commission
PET	positron emission tomography
PM	photomultiplier (tube)
PTU	propylthiouracil
QF	quality factor
RASON	radiolabeled antisense oligonucleotide
R_f	ratio in chromatography
RBE	relative biologic effectiveness
RIA	radioimmunoassay
RISA	radioiodinated serum albumin
RSO	radiation safety officer
SPECT	single photon emission computed tomography
T_3	triiodothyronine
T_4	thyroxine
TBG	thyroxine-binding globulin
TEDE	total effective dose equivalent
TIBC	total iron-binding capacity
TLD	thermoluminescent dosimeter
TNF	tumor necrosis factor

TSH	thyroid-stimulating hormone
USAN	United States Adopted Names
USP	*U.S. Pharmacopeia*
V	volt
VEGF	vascular endothelial growth factor

Appendix B
Terms Used in the Text

Absorption. A process by which the energy of radiation is removed by a medium through which it passes.

Absorption coefficient (μ). The fraction of radiation energy absorbed per unit thickness (linear absorption coefficient) or per unit mass (mass absorption coefficient) of absorber.

Accelerator. A machine to accelerate charged particles linearly or in circular paths by means of an electromagnetic field. The accelerated particles such as α particles, protons, deuterons, and heavy ions possess high energies and can cause nuclear reactions in target atoms by irradiation.

Accuracy. A term used to indicate how close a measurement of a quantity is to its true value.

Aerobic. A term used to indicate the growth of microorganisms in the presence of oxygen.

Aliquot. A definite fraction of a measured sample, particularly volume.

Anaerobic. A term used to indicate the growth of microorganisms in the absence of oxygen.

Annihilation radiation. Gamma radiations of 511 keV energy emitted at 180° after a β^+ particle is annihilated by combining with an electron in matter.

Antibody (Ab). A substance that is produced in response to an antigen and forms a specific complex with it.

Antigen (Ag). A substance that can induce the production of an antibody and bind with it specifically.

Atomic mass unit (amu). By definition, one twelfth of the mass of $^{12}_{6}C$, equal to 1.66×10^{-24} g or 931 MeV.

Atomic number (Z). The number of protons in the nucleus of an atom.

Attenuation. A process by which the intensity of radiation is reduced by absorption and/or scattering during its passage through matter.

Auger electron. An electron ejected from the outer electron shell by an x ray by transferring all its energy.

Average life (τ). *See* Mean life.

357

Avogadro's number. The number of molecules in 1 g·mole of any substance or the number of atoms in 1 g·atom of any element. It is equal to 6.02×10^{23}.

Becquerel (Bq). A unit of radioactivity. One becquerel is equal to 1 disintegration per second.

Binding energy. The energy to bind two entities together. In a nucleus, it is the energy needed to separate a nucleon from other nucleons in the nucleus. In a chemical bond, it is the energy necessary to separate two binding partners an infinite distance.

Biological half-life (T_b). The time by which one half of an administered dosage of a substance is eliminated by biological processes such as urinary and fecal excretion.

Bremsstrahlung. Gamma-ray photons produced by deceleration of charged particles near the nucleus of an atom.

Carrier. A stable element that is added in detectable quantities to a radionuclide of the same element, usually to facilitate chemical processing of the radionuclide.

Carrier-free. A term used to indicate the absence of any stable isotopic atoms in a radionuclide sample.

Chelating agent. A compound that binds to a metal ion by more than one coordinate covalent bond.

Collimator. A device to confine a beam of radiation within a specific field of view. Collimators may be converging, pinhole, diverging, and parallel-hole types.

Colloid. A dispersion of a substance in a liquid. The size of the dispersed particles (colloid) ranges from 10 nm to 1 μm.

Committed dose equivalent $(H_{T,50})$. The dose equivalent to organs or tissues of reference (T) that will be received from an intake of radioactive material by an individual during the 50-year period following intake.

Conversion electron (e^-). *See* Internal conversion.

Critical organ. See Organ, critical.

Cross section (σ). The probability of occurrence of a nuclear reaction or the formation of a radionuclide in a nuclear reaction. It is expressed in a unit termed barn; 1 barn $= 10^{-24}$ cm^2.

Curie (Ci). A unit of activity. A curie is defined as 3.7×10^{10} disintegrations per second.

Decay constant (λ). The fraction of atoms of a radioactive element decaying per unit time. It is expressed as $\lambda = 0.693/t_{1/2}$ where $t_{1/2}$ is the half-life of the radionuclide.

Deep-dose equivalent. (H_d). Dose equivalent at a tissue depth of 1 cm (1000 mg/cm^2) due to external whole-body exposure.

Dosage. A general term for the amount of a radiopharmaceutical administered in microcuries or millicuries, or becquerels.

DNA. Deoxyribonucleic acid is a double-strand helical molecule made of base pairs between adenine and thymine and guanine and cytosine. The base pairs in the two strands are connected by hydrogen bonds. DNA molecules imprint the characteristics of living subjects.

Dose. The energy of radiation absorbed by any matter.

Dosimeter. An instrument to measure the cumulative dose of radiation received during a period of radiation exposure.

Dosimetry. The calculation or measurement of radiation absorbed doses.

Effective half-life (T_e). Time required for an initial administered dosage to be reduced to one half due to both physical decay and biological elimination of a radionuclide. It is given by $T_e = (T_p \times T_b)/(T_p + T_b)$, where T_e is the effective half-life, and T_p and T_b are the physical and biological half-lives, respectively.

Electron (e^-). A negatively charged particle circulating around the atomic nucleus. It has a charge of 4.8×10^{-10} electrostatic units and a mass of 9.1×10^{-28} g, equivalent to 0.511 MeV, or equal to 1/1836 of the mass of a proton.

Electron capture (EC). A mode of decay of a proton-rich radionuclide in which an orbital electron is captured by the nucleus, accompanied by emission of a neutrino and characteristic x rays.

Electron volt (eV). The kinetic energy gained by an electron when accelerated through a potential difference of 1 V.

Elution. A method of "washing off" an adsorbed substance from a solid-adsorbing matter (such as ion-exchange resin) with a liquid.

Embolus. A relatively large blood clot released from a blood vessel and lodged in a smaller vessel so as to obstruct blood circulation.

Erg. The unit of energy or work done by a force of 1 dyne through a distance of 1 cm.

Erythropoiesis. The process of formation of red blood cells.

Fission (f). A nuclear process by which a heavy nucleus divides into two nearly equal smaller nuclei, along with the emission of two to three neutrons.

Free radical. A highly reactive chemical species that has one or more unpaired electrons.

Genes. Genes are composed of segments of DNA molecules and are the basic units of heredity in all living systems.

Generator, radionuclide. A device in which a short-lived daughter is separated chemically and periodically from a long-lived parent adsorbed on adsorbent material. For example, ^{99m}Tc is separated from ^{99}Mo from the Moly generator by eluting with saline.

Gray (Gy). The unit of radiation dose in SI units. One gray is equal to 100 rad.

Half-life ($t_{1/2}$). A unique characteristic of a radionuclide, defined by the time during which an initial activity of a radionuclide is reduced to one half. It is related to the decay constant λ by $t_{1/2} = 0.693/\lambda$.

Half-value layer (HVL). The thickness of any absorbing material required to reduce the intensity or exposure of a radiation beam to one half of the initial value when placed in the path of the beam.

Hematocrit. The fractional volume in percentage of red blood cells in the total blood.

Hydrolysis. A process in which a compound splits into two components by reacting with water when water is used as the solvent.

Infarct. An area of dead tissue due to a complete lack of blood circulation.

Internal conversion. An alternative mode to γ ray decay in which nuclear excitation energy is transferred to an orbital electron which is then ejected from the orbit.

Ion. An atom or group of atoms with a positive charge (cation) or a negative charge (anion).

Ionization chamber. A gas-filled instrument used to measure radioactivity or exposure in terms of ion pairs produced in gas by radiations.

Ischemia. A condition in which a region of tissue has a deficiency in blood supply.

Isobars. Nuclides having the same mass number, that is, the same total number of neutrons and protons. Examples are $^{57}_{26}$Fe and $^{57}_{27}$Co.

Isomeric transition (IT). Decay of an excited state of a nuclide to another lower excited state or the ground state.

Isomers. Nuclides having the same atomic and mass numbers but differing in energy and spin of the nuclei. For example, ^{99}Tc and ^{99m}Tc are isomers.

Isotones. Nuclides have the same number of neutrons in the nucleus. For example, $^{131}_{53}$I and $^{132}_{54}$Xe are isotones.

Isotopes. Nuclides having the same atomic number, that is, the same number of protons in the nucleus. Examples are $^{14}_{6}$C and $^{12}_{6}$C.

K capture. A mode of radioactive decay in which an electron from the K shell is captured by the nucleus.

Labeled compound. A compound whose molecule is tagged with a radionuclide.

$LD_{50/60}$. A dosage of a substance that, when administered to a group of any living species, kills 50% of the group in 60 days.

Linear energy transfer (LET). Energy deposited by radiation per unit length of the matter through which the radiation passes. Its usual unit is keV/μm.

Lyophilization. A process by which a liquid substance is rapidly frozen and then dried or dehydrated under high vacuum.

Mass defect. The difference between the mass of the nucleus and the combined masses of individual nucleons of a nuclide.

Mass number (A). The total number of protons and neutrons in the nucleus of a nuclide.

Mean life (τ). The period of time a radionuclide exists on the average before disintegration. It is related to the half-life and decay constant by $\tau = 1/\lambda = 1.44\, t_{1/2}$.

Metastable state (m). An excited state of a nuclide that decays to another excited state or the ground state with a measurable half-life.

Molarity (*M*). Number of g·moles of a solute in 1000 ml of a solution.

mRNA. Messenger ribonucleic acid carries out the production of proteins, when a gene is activated to do so through transcription and translation.

Neutrino (*v*). A particle of no charge and mass emitted with variable energy during β^-, β^+, and electron capture decays of radionuclides.

No carrier added (NCA). A term used to characterize the state of a radioactive material to which no stable isotope of the compound has been added purposely.

Normality (*N*). A unit of concentration of a solution. A $1N$ solution contains 1 g equivalent weight of a substance in 1000 ml of solution. One equivalent weight of a substance is defined by the weight of the substance that releases or reacts with 1 molecule of hydrogen or hydroxyl ion.

Nucleon. A common term for neutrons or protons in the nucleus of a nuclide.

Organ, critical. The organ that is functionally essential for the body and receives the highest radiation dose after administration of radioactivity.

Organ, target. The organ intended to be imaged and expected to receive a high concentration of administered radioactivity.

Oxidation. A chemical process by which an atom or a group of atoms loses electrons to become more positively charged.

Parenteral. A term indicating the route of drug administration other than oral. Examples are intrathecal, intravenous, interstitial, and intramuscular.

pH. The unit of hydrogen ion concentration. It is given by the negative common logarithm of the hydrogen ion concentration in a solution: $pH = -\log_{10} [H^+]$.

Phagocytosis. A process by which phagocytes remove foreign particulate matter from blood circulation. Colloidal particles are removed by phagocytes in the liver.

Phantom. A volume of material artificially made to simulate the property of an organ or part of the body when exposed to radiation.

Physical half-life (T_p). *See* Half-life.

Pinocytosis. Absorption of liquid by cells.

Precision. A term used to indicate the reproducibility of the measurement of a quantity when determined repeatedly.

Quality factor (QF). A factor dependent on linear energy transfer that is multiplied by absorbed doses to calculate the dose equivalents in rem. It is used in radiation protection to take into account the relative radiation damage caused by different radiations. It is 1 for x, γ, and β rays, and 10 for neutrons and protons.

Rad. The unit of radiation absorbed dose. One rad is equal to 100 ergs of radiation energy deposited per gram of any matter, or 10^{-2} J/kg of any medium.

Radiation weighting factor (W_r): see Quality factor.

Radiochemical purity. The fraction of the total radioactivity in the desired chemical form. If ^{99m}Tc-MAA is 90% pure, then 90% of the radioactivity is in the ^{99m}Tc-MAA form.

Radiolysis. A process by which radiolabeled compounds are broken up by radiations from the radionuclide in labeled molecules.

Radionuclidic purity. The fraction of the total radioactivity in the form of the stated radionuclide. Any extraneous radioactivity such as ^{99}Mo in ^{99m}Tc-radiopharmaceuticals is an impurity.

Radiopharmaceutical. A radioactive drug that can be administered safely to humans for diagnostic and therapeutic purposes.

Reduction. A chemical process by which an atom or a group of atoms gains electrons to become more negatively charged.

Relative biological effectiveness (RBE). A factor used to calculate the dose equivalent in rem from rad. It is defined as the ratio of the amount of a standard radiation that causes certain biological damage to the amount of radiation in question that causes the same biological damage.

Roentgen. The quantity of x or γ radiations that produces one electrostatic unit of positive or negative charge in 1 cm^3 of air at 0°C and 760 mm Hg pressure (STP). It is equal to 2.58×10^{-4} C/kg air.

Roentgen equivalent man (rem). A dose equivalent defined by the absorbed dose (rad) times the relative biological effectiveness or quality factor or radiation weighting factor of the radiation in question.

Scintillation scanning or imaging. Recording of the distribution of radioactivity in the body or a section of the body with the use of a detector.

Sequestration. A process of separation of cells, such as removal of aged red blood cells by the spleen.

Shallow-dose equivalent (H_s). Dose equivalent at a tissue depth of 0.007 cm (7 mg/cm^2) averaged over an area of 1 cm^2 due to external exposure to the skin.

Sievert (Sv). The unit of dose equivalent and equal to 100 rem.

Specific activity. The amount of radioactivity per unit mass of a radionuclide or labeled compound.

Thermal neutron. Neutrons of thermal energy 0.025 eV.

Thrombus. A blood clot that remains attached at the point of its formation on a blood vessel.

Tissue weighting factor (W_T): A factor related to the radiosensitivity of different tissues in living systems.

Tracer. A radionuclide or a compound labeled with a radionuclide that may be used to follow its distribution or course through a chemical, physical, or metabolic process.

Vectors. Vectors are carriers of genes for in vivo delivery into living systems. Viruses are examples of vectors to deliver genes.

Appendix C
Units and Constants

Energy

1 electron volt (eV)	$= 1.602 \times 10^{-12}$ erg
1 kiloelectron volt (keV)	$= 1.602 \times 10^{-9}$ erg
1 million electron volts (MeV)	$= 1.602 \times 10^{-6}$ erg
1 joule (J)	$= 10^7$ ergs
1 watt (W)	$= 10^7$ ergs/s
	$= 1$ J/s
1 rad	$= 1 \times 10^{-2}$ J/kg
	$= 100$ ergs/g
1 gray (Gy)	$= 100$ rad
	$= 1$ J/kg
1 sievert (Sv)	$= 100$ rem
	$= 1$ J/kg
1 horsepower (HP)	$= 746$ W
1 calorie (cal)	$= 4.184$ J

Charge

1 electronic charge	$= 4.8 \times 10^{-10}$ electrostatic unit
	$= 1.6 \times 10^{-19}$ C
1 coulomb (C)	$= 6.28 \times 10^{18}$ charges
1 ampere (A)	$= 1$ C/s

Mass and energy

1 atomic mass unit (amu)	$= 1.66 \times 10^{-24}$ g
	$= 1/12$ the atomic weight of ^{12}C
	$= 931$ MeV
1 electron rest mass	$= 0.511$ MeV
1 proton rest mass	$= 938.78$ MeV
1 neutron rest mass	$= 939.07$ MeV
1 pound	$= 453.6$ g

Length

1 micrometer or micron (μm)	$= 10^{-6}$ meter
	$= 10^{4}$ Å
1 nanometer (nm)	$= 10^{-9}$ meter
1 angstorm (Å)	$= 10^{-8}$ cm
1 fermi (F)	$= 10^{-13}$ cm
1 inch	$= 2.54$ cm

Activity

1 curie (Ci)	$= 3.7 \times 10^{10}$ disintegrations per second (dps)
	$= 2.22 \times 10^{12}$ disintegrations per minute (dpm)
1 millicurie (mCi)	$= 3.7 \times 10^{7}$ dps
	$= 2.22 \times 10^{9}$ dpm
1 microcurie (μCi)	$= 3.7 \times 10^{4}$ dps
	$= 2.22 \times 10^{6}$ dpm
1 becquerel (Bq)	$= 1$ dps
	$= 2.703 \times 10^{-11}$ Ci
1 kilobecquerel (kBq)	$= 10^{3}$ dps
	$= 2.703 \times 10^{-8}$ Ci
1 megabecquerel (MBq)	$= 10^{6}$ dps
	$= 2.703 \times 10^{-5}$ Ci
1 gigabecquerel (GBq)	$= 10^{9}$ dps
	$= 2.703 \times 10^{-2}$ Ci
1 terabecquerel (TBq)	$= 10^{12}$ dps
	$= 27.03$ Ci

Constants

Avogadro's number	$= 6.02 \times 10^{23}$ atoms/g·atom
	$= 6.02 \times 10^{23}$ molecules/g·mole
Planck's constant (h)	$= 6.625 \times 10^{-27}$ erg·s/cycle
Velocity of light	$= 3 \times 10^{10}$ cm/sec
π	$= 3.1416$
e	$= 2.7183$

Appendix D
Radioactive Decay of ^{99m}Tc

The decay fator is $e^{-\lambda t}$. The decay constant is calculated as $(0.693/6)$ hr^{-1}. The percentage remaining is calculated as $100 \times e^{-\lambda t}$.

Time	Percentage remaining	Time	Percentage remaining
10 min	98.1	4 hr	63.0
20	96.2	10	61.8
30	94.4	20	60.6
40	92.6	30	59.4
50	90.8	40	58.3
1 hr	89.1	50	57.2
10	87.4	5 hr	56.1
20	85.7	10	55.0
30	84.1	20	54.0
40	82.5	30	53.0
50	80.9	40	51.9
2 hr	79.4	50	50.9
10	77.8	6 hr	50.0
20	76.4	20	48.1
30	74.9	40	46.3
40	73.5	7 hr	44.6
50	72.1	8 hr	39.7
3 hr	70.7		
10	69.3		
20	68.0		
30	66.7		
40	65.5		
50	64.2		

Appendix E
Radioactive Decay of ^{131}I

The decay factor is $e^{-\lambda t}$. The decay constant is calculated as $(0.693/8)$ day^{-1}. The percentage remaining is calculated as $100 \times e^{-\lambda t}$.

Time (days)	Percentage remaining
1	91.8
2	84.1
3	77.1
4	70.7
5	64.8
6	59.5
7	54.5
8	50.0
9	45.8
10	42.1
11	38.6
12	35.4
13	32.4
14	29.7
15	27.3
16	25.0
17	22.9
18	21.0
19	19.3
20	17.7

Appendix F
Answers to Questions

Chapter 1
11. (a) 513.9 MeV
    (b) 7.7 MeV

Chapter 2
5. 170 keV
6. 76.3%
7. (a) 9.3×10^{11} dpm
   (b) 0.42 Ci (15.5 GBq)
8. (a) 1.73×10^{13} atoms
   (b) 2.84 ng
9. (a) 135 mCi (5.0 GBq)
   (b) 60 mCi (2.22 GBq)
11. 71.8 mCi (2.66 GBq)
12. 13.7 days
13. 4.61 days
14. 130 mCi (4.81 GBq)
15. 888 days
16. 88.2 min
18. 63%
19. 12 hr
20. (a) 1033 ± 9.3 cpm
    (b) 983 ± 10.5 cpm
21. 10,000
22. 2 standard deviations
23. 1111 counts

Chapter 4
6. (a) 4.30 mCi (159 MBq)
   (b) 1.09×10^{13} atoms
   (c) 3.14 mCi (116 MBq)
7. 1.25×10^5 mCi/mg ^{131}I or

4.63×10^3 GBq/mg ^{131}I
5.27×10^6 mCi/mg ^{99m}Tc or
1.95×10^5 GBq/mg ^{99m}Tc
2.85×10^5 mCi/mg ^{32}P or
1.05×10^4 GBq/mg ^{32}P
6.0×10^5 mCi/mg ^{67}Ga or
2.22×10^4 GBq/mg ^{67}Ga
10. 74.3 hr

Chapter 5
4. (a) 550.9 mCi (20.4 GBq)
   (b) 477.1 mCi (17.7 GBq)
7. (a) 0.50 ml
   (b) 0.30 ml
   (c) 0.20 ml
10. 351 mCi (13.0 GBq)

Chapter 7
2. 3×10^5 particles

Chapter 8
6. Yield: 91.6%
   Impurity: 8.4%

Chapter 10
2. 269 mrad (2.69×10^{-3} Gy)
3. 25 rad (0.25 Gy)
4. 200 rem (2 Sv)

Chapter 11
5. (a) 89 mR/hr
   (b) 22.2 mR/hr
6. 37.5 mR/hr

Chapter 12
  5. 3852 ml
  6. 12 days

Chapter 13
  5. 34.9%
  15. 117 ml/min

Index